EX LIBRIS

UNIVERSITATIS SANCTI JOANNIS

LIPIDS, LIPOPROTEINS, AND DRUGS

ADVANCES IN EXPERIMENTAL MEDICINE AND BIOLOGY

Recent Volumes in this Series

LIPIDS, LIPOPROTEINS, AND DRUGS

Edited by

David Kritchevsky
The Wistar Institute
Philadelphia, Pennsylvania

Rodolfo Paoletti
Institute of Pharmacology and Pharmacognosy
University of Milan
Milan, Italy

and

William L. Holmes
Division of Research
The Lankenau Hospital
Philadelphia, Pennsylvania

PLENUM PRESS • NEW YORK AND LONDON

Library of Congress Cataloging in Publication Data

International Symposium on Drugs Affecting Lipid Metabolism, 5th, Milan, 1974.
  Lipids, lipoproteins, and drugs.

  (Advances in experimental medicine and biology; v. 63)
  Sponsored by Italian Society of Pharmacology, Fondazione Giovanni Lorenzini,
Milan Italy, International Society for Biochemical Pharmacology.
  Includes bibliographical references and index.
  1. Lipid metabolism–Congresses. 2. Lipid metabolism disorders–Congresses. 3.
Drugs–Physiological effect–Congresses. I. Kritchevsky, David, 1920-   II.
Paoletti, Rodolfo. III. Holmes, William L., 1918-   IV. Societá Italiana di
farmacologia. V. Fondazione Giovanni Lorenzini. VI. International Society of
Biomedical Pharmacology. VII. Title. VIII. Series. [DNLM: 1. Lipids–Metabolism–
Congresses. 2. Lipoproteins–Metabolism–Congresses. 3. Metabolic diseases–Drug
therapy–Congresses. 4. Metabolism–Drug effects–Congresses. W1 AD559 v. 63/
QU85 I596 1974L]
QP751.I64 1974   615'.739   75-31790
ISBN-13: 978-1-4684-3260-2   e-ISBN-13: 978-1-4684-3258-9
DOI: 10.1007/978-1-4684-3258-9

Proceedings of the Fifth International Symposium on Drugs
Affecting Lipid Metabolism held in Milan, Italy, September 9-12, 1974

Symposium sponsored by

Italian Society of Pharmacology
Fondazione Giovanni Lorenzini, Milan, Italy
International Society for Biochemical Pharmacology

© 1975 Plenum Press, New York
Softcover reprint of the hardcover 1st edition 1975

A Division of Plenum Publishing Corporation
227 West 17th Street, New York, N.Y. 10011

United Kingdom edition published by Plenum Press, London
A Division of Plenum Publishing Company, Ltd.
Davis House (4th Floor), 8 Scrubs Lane, Harlesden, London, NW10 6SE, England

INTERNATIONAL ORGANIZING COMMITTEE

S. Bergstrom
L. A. Carlson
S. Garattini
W. L. Holmes
D. Kritchevsky
M. F. Oliver
R. Paoletti
G. Schettler
D. Steinberg

LOCAL ORGANIZING COMMITTEE

R. Paoletti
R. Fumagalli
S. Gorini
C. R. Sirtori

SCIENTIFIC SECRETARIES

W. L. Holmes
R. Paoletti

The Organizing Committee gratefully acknowledges the contributions of the following organizations:

BAYER-ITALIA S. p. A. , Milan, Italy
BOEHRINGER MANNHEIM GmbH, Mannheim, West Germany
BOOTS COMPANY LTD. , Nottingham, England
BYK GULDEN ITALIA S. p. A. , Cormano, Milan, Italy
CARLO ERBA S. p. A. , Milan, Italy
CIBA-GEIGY S. p. A. , Origgio, Varese, Italy
THE DOW CHEMICAL COMPANY, Indianapolis, Indiana, USA
FARMITALIA S. p. A. , Milan, Italy
F. I. R. M. A. S. p. A. , Florence, Italy
HOECHST PHARMACEUTICALS, INC. , Somerville, New Jersey,
                                          USA
HOFFMANN-LA ROCHE, INC. , Nutley, New Jersey, USA
IMPERIAL CHEMICAL INDUSTRIES, LTD. , Macclesfield, England
I. S. F. S. p. A. , Trezzanos/Naviglio, Milan, Italy
ISTITUTO DE ANGELI S. p. A. , Milan, Italy
ISTITUTO FARMACOLOGICO SERONO, Rome, Italy
LILLY RESEARCH LABORATORIES, Indianapolis, Indiana, USA
MEAD JOHNSON LABORATORIES, Evansville, Illinois, USA
E. MERCK, Darmstadt, Germany
MERCK SHARP AND DOHME INTERNATIONAL, Rahway,
                                          New Jersey, USA
MIDY S. p. A. , Milan, Italy
MILAN-FARMA, Milan, Italy
NATTERMANN INTERNATIONAL GmbH, Koln, West Germany
ORTHO PHARMACEUTICALS, Raritan, New Jersey, USA
PFIZER, INC. , Groton, Connecticutt, USA
THE PROCTER AND GAMBLE COMPANY, Cincinnati, Ohio, USA
SANDOZ AG, Basle, Switzerland
ROCHE S. p. A. , Milan, Italy
SANDOZ-WANDER, INC. , East Hanover, New Jersey, USA
SCHERING CORPORATION, Bloomfield, New Jersey, USA
SEARLE LABORATORIES, Chicago, Illinois, USA
SIGMA-TAU S. p. A. , Rome, Italy
SUMITOMO CHEMICAL COMPANY, LTD. , Osaka, Japan
SMITH KLINE AND FRENCH LABORATORIES, Philadelphia,
                                          Pennsylvania, USA
SYNTEX LABORATORIES, INC. , Palo Alto, California, USA
THE UPJOHN COMPANY, Kalamazoo, Michigan, USA
U. S. V. PHARMACEUTICAL CORPORATION, Tuckahoe, New York,
                                          USA
THE WELLCOME RESEARCH LABORATORIES, London, England
BURROUGHS WELLCOME COMPANY, Research Triangle Park,
                                          North Carolina, USA

The generosity of these donors made it possible for us to arrange this Symposium, which was attended by over four hundred scientists from all over the world.

PREFACE

The First International Symposium on Drugs Affecting Lipid Metabolism was held in Milan in 1960. In the succeeding symposia, as in the first, new data and new ideas emerged which stimulated further research in the field. The present volume comprises the proceedings of the Fifth Symposium. In the area of lipoproteins, we have progressed from descriptions of their chemistry to discussion of their physiology and of their control of cholesterol metabolism at the cellular level. Workshop sessions explored thrombosis as affected by drugs, risk factors other than diet, animal models for atherosclerosis research and the organization of lipid clinics and clinical trials. All these topics represent advances in knowledge over the last decade. In the area of drugs a number of new compounds were introduced, many of them offering new structural concepts for hypocholesteremic activity. We expect that the next Symposium will offer as many new hypotheses and avenues of approach as did this one.

We gratefully acknowledge the assistance of Dr. Sergio Gorini and the Lorenzini Foundation and the contributions of Drs. Cesare Sirtori and Remo Fumagalli all of which helped to assure the success of this Symposium. We also wish to thank Miss Jane T. Kolimaga for her assistance in the preparation of this volume.

David Kritchevsky
Rodolfo Paoletti
William L. Holmes

CONTENTS

APPROACHES TO TREATMENT OF HYPERLIPIDEMIAS

DRUGS AND THROMBOSIS

RISK FACTORS OTHER THAN DIET

ANIMAL MODELS FOR ATHEROSCLEROSIS RESEARCH

SCOPE AND ORGANIZATION OF A LIPID CLINIC
AND CLINICAL TRIALS

OPENING REMARKS

W. L. Holmes, Ph. D.

Division of Research, Lankenau Hospital
Philadelphia, Pennsylvania

When the first of these symposia was organized some fourteen
years ago, the subject matter was limited almost exclusively to
drugs affecting lipids. This format was maintained for both the
second and third symposia, however the scope of the program for
the fourth meeting held in Philadelphia in 1971 was broadened
somewhat to include new basic information, providing it was relevant. In organizing this fifth symposium, the program committee
attempted to follow the same guidelines used in Philadelphia, and
we hope that our efforts will meet with your approval.

As one reflects on the developments of the past three years
it is obvious that there have been tremendous advances in atherosclerosis research. We have witnessed a veritable explosion in
the lipoprotein field. For example, methods of phenotyping have
been improved markedly, our knowledge of lipoprotein chemistry
has increased by leaps and bounds, we now recognize seven or
eight apoproteins rather than two as thought only a few years ago,
the amino acid sequence of several of these apoproteins has been
elucidated, and distinct biological functions of some of the apos
are now beginning to emerge. This morning we will hear about
the structural features of lipoproteins required for binding of
various lipids and about the metabolic fate of certain of the lipoproteins. Later in the week, Dr. Steinberg will point out that a
large fraction of hyperlipidemias are due to defects in the rate of
removal of lipoproteins from plasma rather than to increased
rates of production and secretion, and of the impact this new

1

knowledge may have on future approaches to pharmacologic control
of hyperlipoproteinemias.

Another new and exciting area of investigation to be presented
at this meeting for the first time is concerned with the genetics of
hyperlipoproteinemias. Many of us were privileged last Fall in
Austria and Berlin, to hear Drs. Goldstein and Brown present
their work on cultured fibroblasts as a model system for studying
the regulation of cholesterol metabolism in human cells. This
morning they will add another chapter to this fascinating story in
discussing the role of an LDL receptor site on the cell wall in
regulating cholesterol metabolism in man. During the workshop
session on risk factors, Dr. Glueck will review the genetics of
the common familial hyperlipoproteinemias with an emphasis on
their frequency of occurrence and the clinical importance of early
diagnosis through the use of family screening and lipid sampling
methods.

Another approach to lowering serum lipids, especially the
serum cholesterol concentration, will be discussed by Dr.
Buchwald, when he reviews 11 years of clinical experience with
the partial ileal bypass operation. It is of interest to note that
this operation is now being used in a secondary prevention trial
in the USA by a group of four clinics spearheaded by the Minnesota
group. I believe that Dr. Buchwald will make definite recommendations for the greater usage of this procedure in the control of
hyperlipidemias that do not respond to other methods.

It is now many years since Dr. Page pointed out that atherosclerosis is a multifactorial disease, a fact which has become
more and more obvious in the intervening period. It has become
abundantly clear that we must take into consideration the many
so-called risk factors in planning successful approaches to the
prevention of atherosclerotic vascular disease. As a consequence
we have included in this symposium a session on drugs and thrombosis, and another on risk factors other than diet, including diabetes, hypertension, genetics, smoking and neural-psychological
factors. The final morning of the program will be devoted to a
round table discussion of the scope and organization of lipid clinics
and clinical trials in five different countries. This session should
be of enormous interest to all of us.

A cursory inspection of the program would indicate a continuing growing interest in this field of <u>Drugs Affecting Lipids.</u> This
year some 70 papers received from 20 different countries will
present data on 37 drugs of natural products. Some of these represent new drugs being presented for the first time, some we have
heard about before, and this week will receive new data on long-
term clinical trials.

Finally, on behalf of the organizing committee, I want to express my sincere thanks to our many sponsors who have made
this program possible through their generous financial support.
Also, a special note of thanks goes to Professor Paoletti and his
able staff for the magnificent manner in which they have organized
this symposium.

Chemistry and Physiology
of Lipoproteins

THE INTERACTION OF APOLIPOPROTEIN-ALANINE (ApoC-III)

WITH LIPIDS: STUDY OF STRUCTURAL FEATURES REQUIRED

FOR BINDING

Joel D. Morrisett*, Henry J. Pownall, James T. Sparrow, Richard L. Jackson*, and Antonio M. Gotto, Jr.

Baylor College of Medicine and The Methodist Hospital, Houston, Texas

Abbreviations: ApoLp-Ala, apolipoprotein-alanine or apoC-III, the most abundant of the human C-proteins; VLDL, very low density lipoproteins, normally isolated at d < 1.006 g/ml; LDL, low density lipoproteins, normally isolated at d 1.006-1.063 g/ml; PC, phosphatidylcholine.

INTRODUCTION

The plasma very low density lipoproteins (VLDL) are the major vehicle for the transport in human blood of endogenously synthesized triglycerides. VLDL particles contain about 50% triglyceride, 20% cholesterol, 20% phospholipid, and 10% protein, by weight (1). The plasma of subjects with Type IV or V hyperlipoproteinemia (2) is rich in VLDL and is a convenient source of these lipoproteins. After the delipidation of VLDL with mixed organic solvents such as chloroform-methanol (2:1) or diethyl ether-ethanol (3:1), the resulting lipid-free apoproteins can be separated on Sephadex G-150 into two major fractions (3). The protein(s) that elutes at the void volume is identical in many respects to the major

---

* Established Investigators of the American Heart Association.

apoprotein(s) of LDL (4). The other fraction, which is not excluded from the gel, contains a mixture of several apoproteins which can be fractionated on DEAE-cellulose (Figure 1) and have been referred to collectively as the C-proteins (5), the D-peptides (6) or Fraction V (7a). One of these apoproteins, apoLP-Ala (apoC-III), has been studied extensively. It exists as a linear polypeptide containing 79 amino acids (Figure 2) and has a calculated molecular weight of 8751, excluding carbohydrate (8, 9). The amino acid composition of apoLP-Ala is distinguished by absence of isoleucine, cystine, and cystein (Table I). To threonine-74 is attached an oligosaccharide containing one residue each of galactose and galactosamine, and either 0, 1, or 2 residues of N-acetylneuraminic acid which produces three polymorphic forms of this glycoprotein (6, 7b).

This interesting protein has been the subject of intensive study in our laboratory for the past three years. The purpose of the present report is to summarize these studies and the conclusions which have been drawn from them.

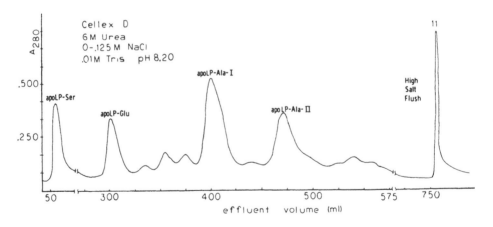

Figure 1: Chromatographic behaviour of the C-proteins on DEAE cellulose (3).

APOLIPOPROTEIN-ALANINE

H₂N-Ser-Glu-Ala-Glu-Asp-Ala-Ser-Leu-Leu-Ser-Phe-Met-Gln-Gly-Tyr-Met-Lys-His-Ala-Thr-Lys-Thr-Ala-Lys-Asp-Ala-Leu-
1   5   10   15   20   25

Ser-Ser-Val-Gln-Ser-Gln-Gln-Val-Ala-Ala-Gln-Gln-Arg- Gly -Trp-Val-Thr-Asp-Gly-Phe- Ser -Ser-Leu-Lys-Asp-Tyr-Trp-
30   35   40   45   50

Ser -Thr-Val-Lys-Asp-Lys- Phe -Ser-Glu-Phe-Trp-Asp-Leu-Asp-Pro-Glu-Val-Arg-Pro-Thr-Ser-Ala-Val-Ala-Ala-COOH
55   60   65   70   75   79

$$\left(Gal, Gal\right)-\left(NAN\right)_{0,1,2}$$
$$\underset{NH_2}{|}$$

Figure 2: Amino acid sequence of apoLP-Ala as determined by Shulman et al (8) and Brewer et al (9).

TABLE I

Amino Acid Composition of apoLP-Ala from Human
Plasma Very Low Density Lipoproteins (9)

Amino Acid	No. of Residues	Amino Acid	No. of Residues
Aspartic Acid	7	Isoleucine	0
Threonine	5	Leucine	5
Serine	11	Tyrosine	2
Glutamic Acid	5	Phenylalanine	4
Glutamine	5	Lysine	6
Proline	2	Histidine	1
Glycine	3	Arginine	2
Alanine	10	Tryptophan	3
Valine	6		
Methionine	2	Total	79
		Mol. Wt.	8751

EFFECT OF PHOSPHATIDYLCHOLINE ON THE PHYSICAL
PROPERTIES OF ApoLP-Ala

The lipid-free form of apoLP-Ala exhibits the spectral characteristics of a disordered peptide containing relatively small per-
centages of β-structure or α-helix. The addition of aliquots of
sonicated egg yolk phosphatidylcholine (PC) to the apoprotein results in a step-wise decrease in the ellipticity at 222 nm as determined by circular dichroism (Fig. 3). A linear plot of the ellipticity at 222 nm vs. the PC:apoprotein molar ratio indicates significant structural changes in the apoprotein until a ratio of approximately 50:1 is reached (Figure 4). At higher ratios, no further
spectral changes are observed. This titration experiment indicates
that PC causes the α-helical structure of apoLP-Ala to increase
from 22 to 54% and suggests that the stoichiometry of a resulting
lipid-protein complex would be about 50:1 (10).

ApoLP-Ala contains three tryptophan residues (sequence positions 42, 54, 65 in Fig. 2), one or more of which are sensitive to
the polarity of the protein's environment. This fortunate circum-
stance permits a fluorescence titration experiment analogues to
that described above employing circular dichroism. Titration of
the apoprotein with aliquots of sonicated egg yolk PC results in a
step-wise blue shift of the tryptophan fluorescence (Figure 5). The
plot of the wavelength shift against the lipid:protein molar ratio
gives a curve (Figure 6) with a plateau effect similar to that observed by circular dichroism (Figure 4). A limiting value of about
11 nm is reached when the ratio is about 90:1 (10).

Fluorescence quenching experiments have been performed to
determine the steric accessibility of the tryptophan residues of
apoLP-Ala alone, and when associated with sonicated egg yolk PC.
Iodide and pyridinium ions produce diffusion controlled fluorescence
quenching of tryptophan according to Stern-Volmer kinetics (17).
In apoLP-Ala the quenching efficiency is also a function of whether
the tryptophans are exposed or buried (11). Comparison of the
quenching efficiency of the apoprotein to that of tryptophan reveals
that 38% of the three tryptophan residues in the apoprotein are exposed to solvent and quencher. The greater steric accessibility
observed with <u>positively</u> charged pyridinium ion (Figure 7B) as
quencher suggests that one or more tryptophan residues are located
in a relatively <u>negatively</u> charged environment. The addition of PC
to apoLP-Ala reduces the steric accessibility of iodide ions to the

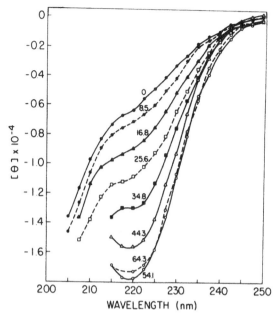

Figure 3: Titration of apoLP-Ala with egg yolk PC monitored by circular dichroism. The number adjacent to each curve represents the lipid:protein molar ratio (10).

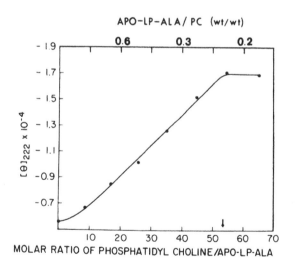

Figure 4: Plot of mean residue ellipticity at 222 nm against the PC:apoLP-Ala molar ratio. Data points were taken from Figure 3 (10).

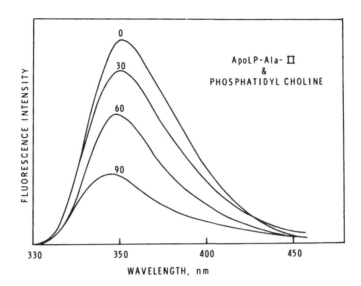

Figure 5: Titration of apoLP-Ala with egg yolk PC monitored by intrinsic tryptophan fluorescence. The decreasing spectral amplitudes are due to dilution effects (10).

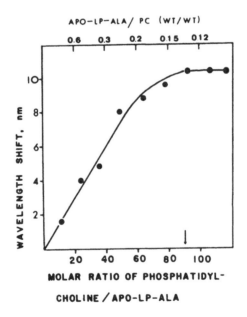

Figure 6: Plot of fluorescence wavelength shift against the PC: apoLP-Ala molar ratio. Data points were taken from experiments similar to that illustrated in Figure 5 (10).

tryptophan residues to about 33% of the value for the apoprotein alone (Figure 7A). With pyridinium ion, this accessibility is reduced to 50% after lipid binding. This difference indicates preferential phospholipid interaction with a positively charged region of the protein which contains tryptophan residues that are accessible to solvent (11).

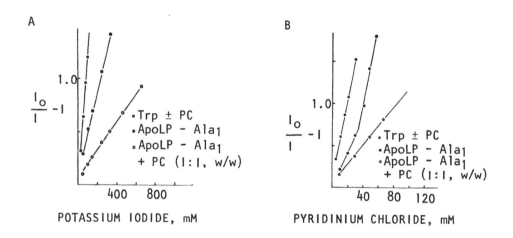

Figure 7: Quenching of intrinsic tryptophan fluorescence of apoLP-Ala by iodide (A) and pyridinium (B) ions. The addition of phosphatidylcholine to the amino acid tryptophan has no effect on its spectral properties, whereas the addition of phosphatidylcholine to the tryptophan containing apoprotein, apoLP-Ala, markedly reduces the accessibility of the quenching ions to the fluorophores (11).

EFFECT OF ApoLP-ALA ON THE PHYSICAL PROPERTIES
OF PHOSPHATIDYLCHOLINE

The observation that egg yolk PC brings about striking changes in the physical structure of the apoprotein raises the question of whether the protein has a concomitant effect on the structure of the phospholipid vesicles. Initial experiments employing electron microscopy suggested that it does (12). The addition of increasing amounts of the apoprotein to a homogeneous population of bilamellar vesicles is accompanied by the formation of linear aggregates of flattened vesicles (Figure 8). At a lipid:protein ratio of about 36:1, these linearly aligned vesicles appear to split open and fuse with adjacent stacks of like structure (Figure 8). Similar morphological changes have also been produced by bile salts (13). However, proteins which do not bind PC do not cause rouleaux formation. These experiments raise the important question of whether these structures actually exist in solution or whether they represent a composite effect of lipid-protein interaction, negative staining and drying (12). This question is considered further under "Structure of a Phosphatidylcholine Vesicle-Apoprotein Complex."

Dimyristoyl PC normally exhibits an abrupt gel → liquid crystalline phas transition at ~23° as determined by colorimetric studies (14) and by paramagnetic resonance (15). When apoLP-Ala is added to visicles of this lipid, a significant alteration in this transition is observed with the spin label, di-tertiarybutylnitroxide (16). This alteration involves both broadening and elevation of the transition (Figure 9). That the transition of the phospholipid is still detectable after apoprotein binding indicates that the bilayer structure of the lipid is retained. The apoprotein also has the effect of decreasing the translational diffusion of pyrene (20-50%) and of lowering the partitioning of the spin label (~50%) into the hydrophobic region of the phospholipid.

The thermotropic transition of dimyristoyl PC is also accompanied by a reversible decrease in the light scattering of vesicles of this phospholipid (20). The addition of apoLP-Ala to these vesicles markedly enhances the magnitude of this effect and also renders it irreversible (Figure 10). Each of the above experiments demonstrates the remarkable ability of apoLP-Ala to induce significant changes in the structure of PC.

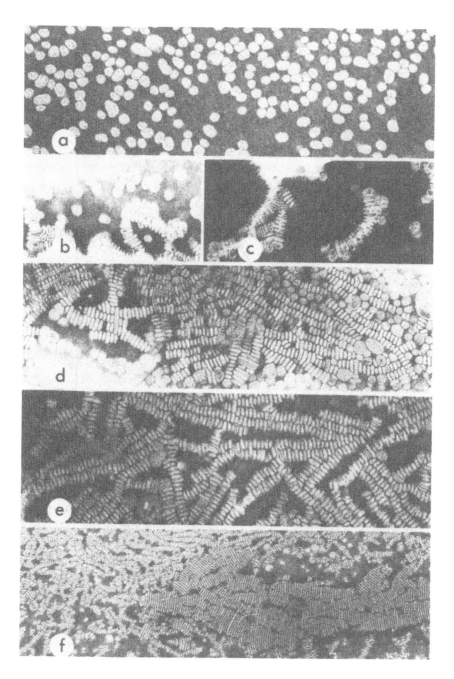

Figure 8: Electron micrographs of phosphotungstate-stained bilamellar vesicles in the absence (a) and presence (b-f) of increasing
amounts of apoLP-Ala. In panels b and c, the PC:apoprotein molar
ratio is 290:1. In panel f, this ratio is 36:1 (12).

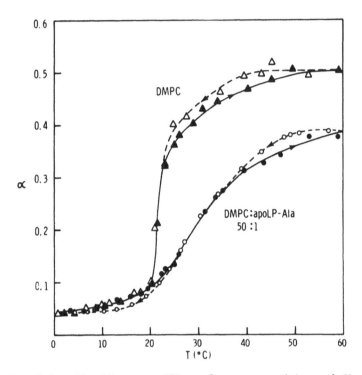

<u>Figure 9</u>: Gel → liquid crystalline phase transition of dimyristoyl
PC alone and complexed to apoLP-Ala (16) as determined by
paramagnetic resonance. The transition was detected by the spin
lable, di-tertiarybutylinitroxide, using a method similar to that
described by Shimshick and McConnell (15). The ratio of label
dissolved in the fluid hydrophobic and aqueous environment is
given by the quantity α.

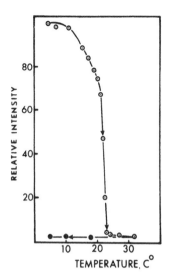

Figure 10: Temperature dependence of the light scattering (400 nm) of dimyristoyl PC liposomes in the presence of apoLP-Ala. In the absence of the apoprotein, this effect is not nearly so large nor is it irreversible. Lipid:protein molar ratio is 50:1.

STRUCTURAL FEATURES OF LIPIDS REQUIRED FOR MAXIMUM BINDING TO ApoLP-ALA

Acyl Chain Structure

Most of the studies described above have employed egg yolk PC which is a heterogeneous mixture of phosphatidylcholine molecules whose acyl chains differ widely in their length and number of double bonds. To determine the effect of chain length and unsaturation on the interaction of PC with apoLP-Ala, a systematic study involving chemically homogeneous lipids was performed. Generally, those PC molecules whose acyl chains are in a liquid crystalline form interact more efficiently than those of the gel state as judged by the shift in tryptophan fluorescence maximum (Figure 11) and ultracentrifugal behavior. The PC molecules which contain acyl chains of 6, 10, 12 or 14 carbon atoms have transition temperatures at or below room temperature, the temperature at which these experiments were conducted. For dipalmitoyl PC (di-$C_{16:0}$), the efficiency of interaction is clearly dependent on whether this lipid exists above or below its transition temperature of 41°. While this particular lipid interacts to a significant extent with apoLP-Ala at or above shorter chain phospholipids. The

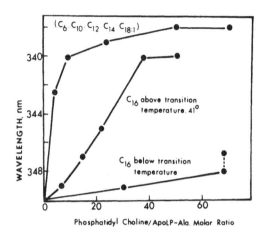

Figure 11: Effect of various diacyl phosphatidylcholines on the intrinsic tryptophan fluorescence maximum of apoLP-Ala (18).

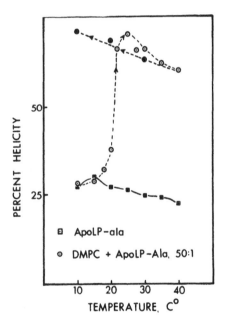

Figure 12: Temperature dependence of the α-helicity of apoLP-Ala in the presence (dotted line) and absence (solid line) of dimyristoyl PC (19).

reason for this difference is probably due to thermal dissociative
effects which tend to diminish the strength of binding at $\gtrsim 35°$.

As mentioned above, dimyristoyl PC (di-$C_{14:0}$) undergoes a
gel → crystalline transition at 23° (14, 15), a temperature which
is experimentally convenient. The striking effect of this transition
on the interaction of apoLP-Ala and dimyristoyl PC is readily
observed by circular dichroism (Figure 12). An abrupt increase
in the percent of α-helicity in the protein occurs near 23° (19).
Once a complex is formed from the interacting species, lowering
the temperature below the transition temperature of the phospholipid does not result in dissociation of the complex. This phenomenon is further illustrated by abrupt and irreversible changes in
the wavelength of maximum tyrptophan fluorescence (Figure 13).

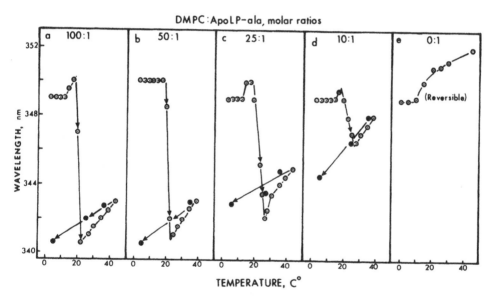

Figure 13: Dependence of the wavelength of intrinsic tryptophan
fluorescence of apoLP-Ala-dimyristoyl PC complexes on temperature and lipid:protein ratio. As this ratio is increased from 0-50,
there is a concomitant increase in the magnitude of the wavelength
shift. No further increase is observed above this level (19, 21).
Open (closed) circles are data points taken during increasing
(decreasing) temperature.

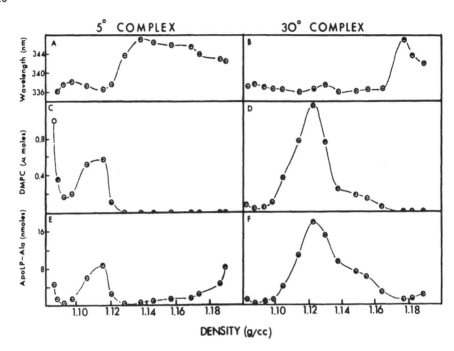

Figure 14: Ultracentrifugal behavior of dimyristoyl PC-apoLP-Ala complexes formed at 5° and 30°. Density gradients were fractionated and analyzed for intrinsic tryptophan fluorescence (upper panels), phospholipid content (central panels), and protein content (bottom panels). Stoichiometry of the complex formed at 5° is exactly the same (66:1) as that formed at 30°. However, the yield of the complex formed at 30° is significantly greater than that obtained at 5° (21).

The extent of the blue shift is dependent on the lipid:apoprotein molar ratio up to a level of about 50:1. At higher ratios, there is no further increase in the magnitude of this change. This stoichiometry compares well with that determined independently by circular dichroism (Figure 4). The ultracentrifugal behavior of dimyristoyl PC-apoLP-Ala complexes formed below (5°) and above (30°) the transition temperature of the phospholipid (23°) is shown in Figure 14. Below the transition temperature, a slow time-dependent formation of the complex occurs but is not complete after the three days required for ultracentrifugation. Both unbound lipid (Figure 14C) and unbound protein (Figure 14E) are present in these gradients. However, the lipid:protein molar ratio of the complex which is formed at 5° is exactly the same (66:1) as that

observed for the complex formed above the transition temperature
at 30°. These experiments provide conclusive evidence that interaction between apoLP-Ala and phosphatidylcholine vesicles is more
efficient when the acyl chains of the phospholipid exist in a liquid
crystalline than a gel state.

Polar Head Group Structure

To determine the effect of polar head group structure of lipids
on their interaction with apoLP-Ala, a number of different amphipathic molecules were studied. For this study, three criteria were
used to evaluate the relative strength of interaction of these lipids
with the apoprotein: a) wavelength shift of maximum tryptophan
fluorescence, b) increase in α-helical content, and c) the amount
of apoprotein which could be ultracentrifugally isolated in a lipid-
bound form. Of the lipids examined, lysolecithin, sphingomyelin,
and phosphatidylcholine exhibited the strongest binding as evaluated
by these three criteria (Figure 15). Significantly, each of these
phospholipids contains a permanent zwitterionic polar head group.
Although in a certain pH range, phosphatidylethanolamine is also
zwitterionic, it does not contain the quaternary ammonium group
which allows extensive polar head group hydration (22) thereby
attenuating head group-head group interaction. The abscence of
this structural feature in phosphatidylethanolamine prevents extensive hydration of the polar head region and thereby maximizes
head group-head group intereation. The apparent requirement
for a permanent zwitterionic polar head group in the phospholipid
suggests that a complementary ion pair on the protein might be
involved in lipid-protein interaction. This possibility is considered
further under "Structural Features of ApoLP-ALA Required for
Binding to Phosphatidylcholine. "

Physical Form of the Lipid

The interaction of apoLP-Ala with PC depends not only upon
the chemical structure of the lipid molecules, but also on the
physical form of the phospholipid particles they comprise. A
sonicated dispersion of PC usually contains a mixture of single-
shelled, bilamellar vesicles and larger multi-lamellar vesicles
of various sizes (23). These two types of liposomes differ sufficiently in size to allow their separation by gel filtration chromatography. The smaller vesicles ($\sim$210 Å diameter) bind efficiently

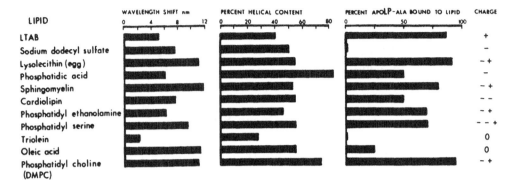

Figure 15: Physical properties of apoLP-Ala in the presence of various polar and nonpolar lipids. The magnitude of the lipid-protein interaction as judged by all three criteria together is greatest for those lipids which are neutrally charged and contain a permanent zwitterionic polar head group.

to apoLP-Ala as evidenced by the large α-helicity and fluorescence maximum changes they induce in the apoprotein (24). In contrast, the larger multi-shelled liposomes expose a much lower outer surface area per unit weight phospholipid and hence do not interact with the apoprotein nearly as efficiently. This difference in binding is further illustrated by comparing the lipid-protein complexes which are formed from these two types of vesicles. The multi-lamellar vesicles form a heterogeneous population of complexes which vary widely in their lipid:protein ratio and hydrated density (Figure 16A). The bilamellar vesicles, however, form a more homogeneous mixture of complexes which exhibit a rather narrow range of lipid:protein ratios and hydrated densities (Figure 16B) (24). The more favorable apoprotein-binding properties of the smaller single-shelled liposomes and the uniformity of the complexes which they form indicate that they are the phospholipid form of choice.

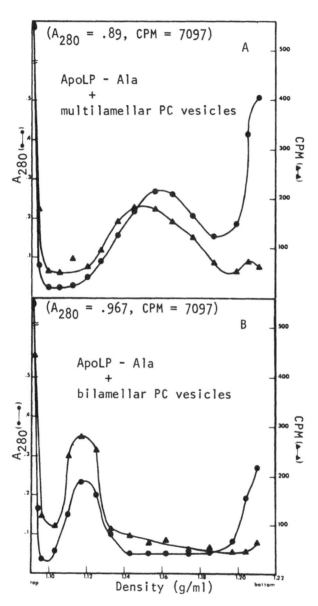

Figure 16: Ultracentrifugal behavior of PC vesicle-apoLP-Ala complexes on KBr density gradients (24).

STRUCTURE OF A PHOSPHATIDYLCHOLINE
VESICLE-APOPROTEIN COMPLEX

Gel filtration, laser light scattering, and analytical ultracentrifugation have been used to determine the structure of a PC
vesicle-apoLP-Ala complex.   Mixing egg yolk PC bilamellar vesicles and apoLP-Ala (without sonication) at a molar ratio of 50:1
results in the formation of a complex which elutes from a Sepharose 6B column at about the same volume as the PC vesicles
alone (Figure 17).   Chemical analysis of this complex indicates
a lipid:protein ratio of 48:1.   Not only does this experiment provide direct evidence for the formation of a stable lipid-protein
complex, but also establishes that the multivesicular aggregates
observed by electron microscopy do not exist in solution as suggested in Figure 8 (12).

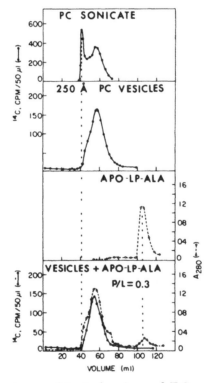

Figure 17: Chromatographic behavior of PC vesicles, apoLP-Ala,
and a mixture of these species on a 0.9 x 100 cm column of
Sepharose 6B (25).

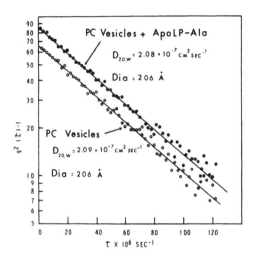

Figure 18: Clipped correlation function for scattered light from a suspension of PC vesicles and vesicles plus apoLP-Ala. A least squares fit of the data points to a straight line indicates the homogeneity of the scattering species (25).

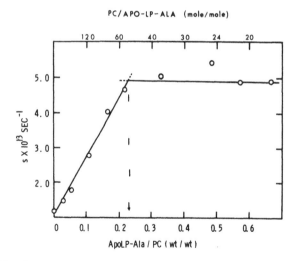

Figure 19: Sedimentation velocity experiments in which the observed sedimentation coefficient of the apoLP-Ala-PC vesicle complex was measured as a function of the apoprotein:PC mass ratio (25).

The diffusion coefficient of the bilamellar vesicles as measured by laser light scattering is $(2.0 \pm 0.03) \times 10^{-7}$ cm^2 sec^{-1} (Figure 18). This value is not detectably changed when sufficient apoLP-Ala is added to give a protein-lipid mixture with a molar ratio of 1:50 or a weight ratio of 0.3:1. While both the gel filtration and light scattering experiments lead to the same conclusion that PC vesicle-apoprotein complexes are not aggregated, they give no information regarding the location of the apoprotein in the complex. To obtain information concerning this point, analytical ultracentrifugation experiments were performed. When the sedimentation coefficient of PC vesicles is measured after sequential additions of apoLP-Ala, the observed sedimentation coefficient increases from 1.19 S to a limiting value of 4.93 S (Figure 19) which is reached when the protein:lipid ratio is 0.23 g/g (25). This weight ratio corresponds to a molar ratio of about 1:53 or about 46 apoLP-Ala molecules per PC vesicle. Sedimentation equilibrium analysis of vesicles saturated with apoprotein (apoprotein:PC = 0.32 g/g) indicates a molecular weight of 1.26×10^6 if it is assumed that the partial specific volumes of the PC vesicle and the apoprotein remain unchanged after their interaction. While this experiment rules out the possibility that PC vesicles undergo apoprotein induced aggregation in solution as suggested by electron microscopy, it requires the resolution of a seemingly inconsistent results, since a molecular weight for the vesicle-apoprotein complex (1.26×10^6) which is lower than that of the vesicle alone (1.86×10^6) is not consistent with complex formation if the original structure of the vesicle is maintained in the complex. This apparent inconsistency is probably related to a change in the partial specific volume of the PC vesicle after binding apoprotein. The hydrodynamic data lead to the conclusion that both the hydration shell around the vesicle as well as the volume occupied by the nonpolar portion of the bilayer are changed upon complex formation with apoLP-Ala (Figure 20). This view is consistent with a model where the apolipoprotein is bound to hydrophobic sites within the vesicle with parts of the protein protruding into the polar head region so that interactions with the hydrophilic sites on the surface of the bilayer can occur (26).

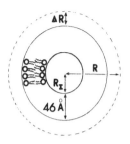

$$R = \Delta R + 46 \overset{\circ}{A} + R_I = 103 \overset{\circ}{A}$$

Figure 20: Spherical model of PC bilamellar vesicle. ΔR indicates the hydration shell displaced by the apoprotein (25).

STRUCTURAL FEATURES OF ApoLP-ALA REQUIRED FOR BINDING TO PHOSPHATIDYLCHOLINE

ApoLP-Ala contains three pairs of amino acids whose side
chains are oppositely charged (Lys-24, Asp-25; Lys-51, Asp-52;
and Lys-58, Asp-59; Fig. 2). To test whether one or more of
these ion pairs might be involved in PC binding, synthetic fragments spanning residues 41-79 (I), 48-79 (II), 55-79 (III) and
61-79 (IV) were synthesized by solid phase techniques (27). These
fragments contain 2, 2, 1, and 0 ion pairs, respectively. After
purification to homogeneity, these peptides were tested for their
ability to interact with phosphatidylcholine. The addition of a 50-
fold molar excess of sonicated egg yolk PC to the synthetic fragments causes a significant increase in the α-helical content of the
two longer fragments (I and II) but not in the two shorter ones
(III and IV) (Figure 21). The effect of PC on the structure of these
peptides was also evaluated by monitoring the fluorescence maxima
of the tryptophan residue(s). The two longest peptides (I and II)
which contain two ion pairs, showed significant blue shifts in the
intrinsic tryptophan fluorescence, while the two shorter peptides
(III and IV) showed only very small spectral shifts (Table II).
Evaluation of the phospholipid-binding ability of these four synthetic
fragments was also tested by a competitive dehydrogenase assay
(Figure 22). Again, the two shorter fragments (III and IV) showed
only nominal inhibition of the reactivation of this enzyme, while
the two larger fragments (I and II) inhibited the reactivation to a
significant extent. ApoLP Ala-(41-79), which corresponds to the
C-terminal half of the naturally-occurring apoprotein, appears

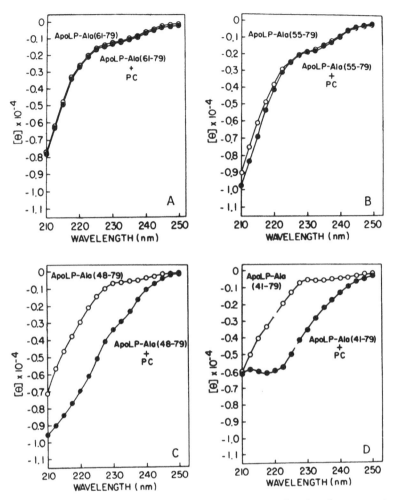

Figure 21: Circular dichroic spectra of synthetic fragments of apoLP-Ala alone (open circles) and in the presence of a 50-fold molar excess of egg yolk PC (closed circles) (28).

to be about 25% as effective as the native material in inhibiting the reactivation of this enzyme. The lipid-binding properties of these synthetic peptides were further tested by examination of their ability to form phospholipid-peptide complexes which could float at density 1.064. Results of these experiments indicated that less than 15% of the two shorter peptide fragments (III and IV) formed stable PC complexes which floated, while the longer fragments (I and II) formed these complexes to the extent, 87 and 51%,

Table II

Intrinsic Tryptophan Fluorescence of apoLP-Ala and Synthetic
Peptide Fragments in the Presence and Absence of
50-fold Molar Excess of Egg Yolk PC

Peptide	max With PC	max Without PC	Δ max
ApoLP-Ala (natural)	345	333	12.0
ApoLP-Ala (41-79)	349	337	12.0
ApoLP-Ala (49-79)	341.4	335.5	5.9
ApoLP-Ala (55-79)	348.3	349.1	0.8
ApoLP-Ala (61-79)	349	346.5	2.5

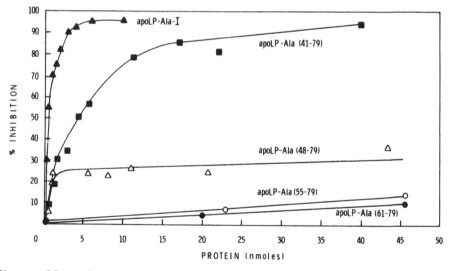

Figure 22: Inhibition by apoLP-Ala and synthetic peptide fragments
of the reactivation of β-hydroxybutyrate apodehydrogenase by sonicated egg yolk PC (28).

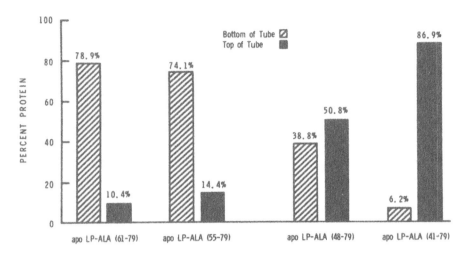

<u>Figure 23:</u> Formation of PC-synthetic peptide complexes. The percent of protein complexed was determined from that amount which could be ultracentrifugally floated at density 1.064 g/ml.

respectively (Figure 23). The results of these studies strongly suggest, but by no means conclusively prove, that ion pairs play an important role in the binding of phosphatidylcholine and related phospholipids to apolipoproteins. Recent experiments involving apoLP-Ala (48-79) in which Asp-52 and/or Asp-59 are substituted by asparagine also suggest the importance of these ion pairs in the phospholipid binding (29).

A MODEL FOR LIPID-APOLIPOPROTEIN INTERACTION

The results of studies on apoLP-Ala and three other apolipo-proteins which have been sequenced [apoLP-Gln-I (30), apoLP-Gln-II (31) and apoLP-Ser (32, 33)] have allowed the development of an hypothesis which describes in considerable detail the inter-action of plasma apolipoproteins and lipids. A full statement of this hypothesis as it relates to the total structure of lipoprotein particles is outside the scope of this paper, but is discussed in detail elsewhere (34, 35). The conclusions of the studies described above form the basis for the development of this hypothesis. These conclusions are: 1) zwitterionic phospholipids undergo the strongest

interaction with apoLP-Ala, 2) apoprotein-phospholipid interaction is maximal when the fatty acyl chains are in a liquid crystalline state, 3) the binding of phosphatidylcholine to apolipoprotein
is accompanied by an increase in the α-helical content of the apoprotein, 4) pairs of amino acids which exist in a 1, 2 sequence
relationship* and have oppositely charged side chains may confer
on an apolipoprotein special phospholipid-binding properties.
Examination of a space-filling model of apoLP-Ala which has
about 50% of the polypeptide chain in the α-helical configuration
(based on the circular dichroism results in Fig. 3 and 4) reveals
that certain helical segments contain oppositely charged side
chains which are oriented in a manner which allows their electro-
static interaction with the complementary polar head groups of
zwitterionic phospholipids. While we do not feel this type of interaction is the major one, it may be important in stabilizing the hydrophobic bonding between the fatty acyl chains of the phospholipids
and the apolar residues of the apoprotein. An important feature
of these helical peptide segments which contain ion pairs is that
one side is polar and the opposite side is hydrophobic. Each of
these sides occupies a full half of the cylindrical surface of the
helix. On the polar side, there is a unique distribution of charged
residues. While the negatively charged acidic amino acids are
clustered in the middle of the surface, positively charged basic
amino acids are oriented toward the outer edges (Figure 2). These
structural features would not only allow close steric contact between the charged amino acid side chains and oppositely charged
groups of the phospholipid, but would also permit the segment containing C_2-C_5 of the fatty acyl chains to interact with the hydrophobic side of the helix and possibly even with the hydrocarbon side
chains of such amino acids as lysine and arginine. Recent studies
on synthetic model peptides (29) indicate that the hydrophobic index
of the nonpolar side of the helix is an important determinant of the
strength of phospholipid binding. This amphipathic model is consistent with experimental data from phospholipid binding studies
on not only apoLP-Ala, but also apoA-I, apoA-II, and apoC-I. Experiments designed to test the validity of different aspects of this
model are currently underway in our laboratory.

---

* Actually, either a 1, 2 or a 1, 4 sequence relationship will allow
these side chains to be spatially close to each other when the peptide backbone is in an α-helix. ApoA-I contains 26 non-degenera-
tive 1, 4 ion pairs and 12 non-overlapping 1, 2 pairs (30).

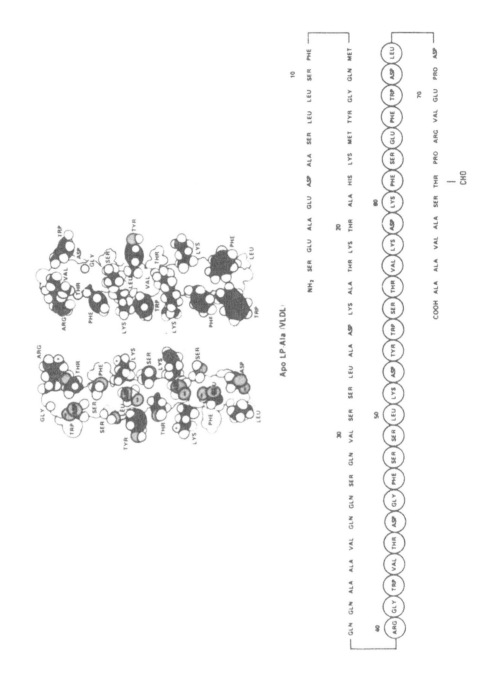

Apo LP-Ala (VLDL)

ACKNOWLEDGEMENTS

The authors are indebted to Drs. David Taunton, Ramon Segura, Henry Hoff, and Nordean Baker for helpful discussions during the course of this work.   They are particularly grateful to Mr. Joe Chen, Miss Irene Cardona, and Mr. Richard Plumlee for technical assistance, and to Ms. Debbie Mason for help in preparation of the manuscript (TBTGA).

This work has been supported in part by a grant from the NHLI for a Specialized Center of Research in Atherosclerosis (HL-14194), by an NIH General Clinical Research Center grant (RR-00350), by a grant from the John A. Hartford Foundation, Inc. and by a Lipid Research Clinic contract (71-2156).

REFERENCES

1. Skipski, J. P. In: Blood Lipids and Lipoproteins: Quantitation, Composition, and Metabolism. G. J. Nelson, editor. Wiley-Interscience, New York, 1972, p. 471.

2. Fredrickson, D. S. and Levy, R. I. In: The Metabolic Basis of Inherited Diseases. Third Edition. J. B. Stanbury, J. B. Wyngaarden, D. S. Fredrickson, editors. McGraw-Hill, New York, 1972, p. 545.

3. Brown, W. V., Levy, R. I. and Fredrickson, D. S. J. Biol. Chem. 244: 5687, 1969.

4. Gotto, A. M., Brown, W. V., Levy, R. I., Birnbaumer, M. E., and Fredrickson, D. S. J. Clin. Invest. 51: 1486, 1972.

5. Alaupovic, P. Atherosclerosis 13:141, 1971.

6. Brown, W. V., Levy, R. I. and Fredrickson, D. S. J. Biol. Chem. 245: 6588, 1970.

7a. Scanu, A., Toth, J., Edelstein, C., Koga, S. and Stiller, E. Biochemistry 8: 3309, 1969.

Figure 24: Molecular model of the amphipathic helical region (residues 40-67) of apoLP-Ala. The model on the left (right) illustrates the hydrophilic (hydrophobic) side of the amphipathic helix. In the middle of the polar face are localized the negatively charged amino acids while the positively charged residues are located mostly on the lateral edges (26).

7b. Albers, J. J. and Scanu, A. M. Biochim. Biophys. Acta 236: 29, 1971.

8. Shulman, R. S. , Herbert, P. N. , Fredrickson, D. S., Wehrly, K. , and Brewer, H. B. J. Biol. Chem. 249: 4969, 1974.

9. Brewer, H. B. , Shulman, R. , Herbert, P. , Ronan, R. and Wehrly, K. J. Biol. Chem. 249: 4975, 1974.

10. Morrisett, J. D. , David, J. S. K. , Pownall, H. J. , and Gotto, A. M. Biochemistry 12: 1290, 1973.

11. Pownall, H. J. and Smith, L. C. Biochemistry 13: 2590, 1974.

12. Hoff, H. F. , Morrisett, J. D. and Gotto, A. M. Biochim. Biophys. Acta 296: 653, 1973.

13. Howell, J. L , Lucy, J. A. , Pirola, R. C. and Bouchier, I. A. D. Biochim. Biophys. Acta 210: 1, 1970.

14. Hinz, H-J and Sturtevant, J. M. J. Biol. Chem. 247: 6071, 1972.

15. Shimshick, E. J. and McConnell, H. M. Biochemistry 12: 2351, 1973.

16. Novosad, Z. F. , Pownall, H. P. , Gotto, A. M. and Morrisett, J. D. In preparation.

17. Birks, J. B. Photophysics of Aromatic Molecules. Wiley-Interscience, London, 1970, Chapter 10.

18. Pownall, H. J. , Morrisett, J. D. , Sparrow, J. T. , and Gotto, A. M. Biochem. Biophys. Res. Commun. 60: 779, 1974.

19. Pownall, H. J. , Morrisett, J. D. , Sparrow, J. T. , and Gotto, A. M. Biochem. Biophys. Res. Commun. 60: 779, 1974.

20. Tsong, T. Y. Proc. Nat. Acad. Sci. (USA) 71: 2684, 1974.

21. Pownall, H. J. , Morrisett, J. D. , Sparrow, J. T. , and Gotto, A. M. Submitted for publication.

22. Phillips, M. C. , Finer, E. G. , and Hauser, H. Biochim. Biophys. Acta 290: 397, 1972.

23. Huang, C. Biochemistry 8: 344, 1969.

24. Morrisett, J. D. and Gotto, A. M. In preparation.

25. Morrisett, J. D. , Gallagher, J. G. , Aune, K.C., and Gotto, A. M. Biochemistry 13: 4765, 1974.

26. Segrest, J. P. , Jackson, R. L. , Morrisett, J. D. and Gotto, A. M. FEBS Letters 38: 247, 1974.

27. Merrifield, R. B. Adv. Enzy. 32: 221, 1969.

28. Sparrow, J. T. , Gotto, A. M. and Morrisett, J. D. Proc. Nat. Acad. Sci. (USA) 70: 2124, 1973.

29. Sparrow, J T. , Gotto, A. M. and Morrisett, J. D. Unpublished results.

30. Baker, H. N. , Delahunty, T. , Gotto, A. M. and Jackson, R. L. Proc. Nat. Acad. Sci. (USA) 71: 3631, 1974.

31. Brewer, H. B., Lux, S. E., Ronan, R., and John, K. M.
    Proc. Nat. Acad. Sci. (USA) 69: 1304, 1972.
32. Shulman, R., Herbert, P., Wehrly, K., Chesebro, B.,
    Levy, R. I., and Fredrickson, D. S.   Circulation 45: II: 246.
33. Jackson, R. L., Sparrow, J. T., Baker, H. N., Morrisett,
    J. D., Taunton, O. D., and Gotto, A. M.   J. Biol. Chem. 249:
    5308, 1974.
34. Morrisett, J. D., Jackson, R. L. and Gotto, A. M.   Ann.
    Rev. Biochem., in press.
35. Jackson, R. L., Morrisett, J. D., Gotto, A. M., and Segrest,
    J. P.   Mol. Cell. Biochem., in press.

LIPOPROTEINS AND LIPID TRANSPORT

Richard J. Havel

Cardiovascular Research Institute and Department of
Medicine, University of California, San Francisco,
California

Abbreviations used in this paper:

VLDL, LDL and HDL are very low density, low density and
high density lipoproteins; LCAT is lecithin-cholesterol acyl
transferase; A-apoproteins refer to the two major apoproteins
of HDL, B-apoprotein to the major apoprotein of LDL and C-apoproteins to the three proteins of low molecular weight that are
shared between VLDL and HDL in humans and rats.

Lipids are transported in blood plasma in association with
proteins. Some polar lipids are transported by albumin (free fatty
acids, bile acids) or by specific binding proteins (retinol-binding
protein). Nonpolar lipids are transported in large complexes
containing polar lipids and specific apoproteins (which serve
functions beyond that of "packaged"). These complexes comprise
the macromolecular particles that we generally think of when we
apply the term "lipoproteins" to blood plasma and other extracellular fluids. These lipoproteins and their role in transport of
nonpolar lipids are the subject of this short and eclectic review.

A striking feature of the plasma lipoproteins is the lability of
their concentration in a given species under differing physiological
and pathological states and also among different animal species.
Among mammals, these differences cannot be explained solely on

the basis of differences in the rate at which the nonpolar lipids
are transported in the blood.   Even within species, rates of
transport vary among particles that differ from each other in
rather subtle ways and evidence for species differences in the
pathways of metabolism of a given lipoprotein class is also
emerging.

This subject was reviewed very briefly at the last of these
Symposia (1).   Here I will develop the subject somewhat more
extensively and will emphasize new developments during the past
three years.   Finally, aspects of human hyperlipoproteinemias
that have been illuminated by these developments will be discussed.

LIPOPROTEIN STRUCTURE

Increasing evidence supports the "pseudomicellar" model for
the structure of the major lipoprotein classes in normal human
blood plasma.   It envisions lipoproteins as spherical particles
composed of a liquid core of nonpolar lipids (chiefly triglycerides
and cholesteryl esters) covered by a monomolecular film of polar
lipids (chiefly phospholipids and cholesterol) and apoproteins that
differ among lipoprotein classes.   Variation in size is related to
the volume of the apolar core, whereas the surface has essentially
a constant mean thickness on the order of 22 Å (i. e. , that of a
monolayer of a phospholipid-cholesterol mixture).   Regions of the
various apoproteins may penetrate the monolayer or intereact with
the polar groups of the lipids in the manner described elsewhere
in this volume by Dr. Gotto.   A spherical shape is indicated from
electron microscopy, using both negative and positive staining
methods (2, 3) and from viscometry (4).   Evidence for the location
of core and surface components includes the precise relationship
between the chemical composition and the size of very low density
lipoprotein particles having a narrow range of diameters (5).   This
relationship also predicts the diameter of human LDL to the 220 Å
and that of HDL to be 120 Å.   The value for LDL corresponds
closely with the observed diameter by electron microscopy of
216 Å (2, 4), whereas the value for HDL (d 1.063-1.21) exceeds
those obtained from electron microscopy of 100 Å for HDL_2 and
75 Å for HDL_3 (6).   Low angle x-ray diffraction patterns of HDL
(7-9) also support this model but the pattern of LDL is more complex and difficult to interpret (10, 11).   The observation of tem-
perature-dependent changes in the structure of LDL (12) may

provide a clue to this complexity. Subunit structures proposed for
both HDL (2, 6) and LDL (13) may reflect artifacts of negative
staining procedures and it may be concluded that there is presently
no compelling reason to discard the pseudomicellar model for any
of these lipoprotein classes.

As will be discussed later, the pseudomicellar model has
been very useful in the interpretation of changes in composition
that occur during the metabolism of triglyceride-rich lipoproteins,
as first proposed by Schumaker and Adams (14). They pointed out
that removal of nonpolar lipid from the core must be accompanied
by removal of surface components if a basic pseudomicellar structure is to be maintained. This deduction has received strong support from studies of lipoprotein catabolism. These studies indicate
that the surface components of lipoproteins not only determine the
size of lipoproteins but that they also critically influence their
metabolism. In fact, all of the major groups of apolipoproteins
have now been shown to influence the binding of lipoproteins to
surface receptors on cells or the activity of key enzymes of lipid
transport (15-17).

TRIGLYCERIDE-RICH LIPOPROTEINS

Synthesis and Secretion

Triglyceride-rich lipoproteins are synthesized in the endoplasmic reticulum of parenchymal cells of liver and intestinal
mucosa. Particles resembling VLDL can be visualized at the
smooth-surfaced ends of cisternae of the rough endoplasmic reticulum in liver and the B apoprotein, which is considered to be
essential for secretion of triglyceride-rich lipoproteins, has been
found by an immunocytochemical technique in association with
these particles and in the rough endoplasmic reticulum (18). Although similar particles are also evident in cisternae of the smooth
endoplasmic reticulum, they cannot be shown to contain the B
apoprotein. This has led to the suggestion that triglyceride-rich
particles synthesized there receive the protein when they move to
the region of the rough reticulum (18). The lipoprotein particles
are concentrated in secretory vesicles of the Golgi apparatus.
These migrate, under the influence of the microtubular system
(19, 20), to the cell surface and discharge their contents into the
space of Disse. Presumably, an analogous situation obtains in

the synthesis of chylomicrons from exogenous lipids in the small
intestinal mucosa.

The composition of the core of nascent VLDL in the hepatic
Golgi apparatus closely resembles, whereas the surface monolayer differs from, that of plasma VLDL (21). Nascent VLDL
contain more phospholipids and less of the soluble proteins of
low molecular weight ("C" apoproteins) and cholesterol than do
plasma VLDL. VLDL secreted from rat livers perfused with
lysine-^{3}H contain radioactivity in all component proteins (B and
C apoproteins as well as proteins of intermediate molecular
weight), but most is in the B apoprotein (22). By contrast, lipoproteins secreted from similarly perfused small intestine contain most of the radioactivity in a major protein of intermediate
molecular weight that is virtually absent in VLDL and no radioactivity is found in the C apoproteins that migrate rapidly in polyacrylamide gels (22). Presumably, the protein that contains most
of the radioactivity is the major "A" apoprotein of HDL. Thus,
the soluble surface protein components of triglyceride-rich lipoproteins secreted from liver and gut differ substantially although
both contain the B apoprotein.

Catabolism - The First Step

Evidence from several sources indicates that the surface of
triglyceride-rich lipoproteins is modified once they enter the
extracellular environment. This modification depends upon exposure to a large amount of HDL. [1] Both chylomicrons (23) and
hepatogenous VLDL (21) acquire C apoproteins from HDL. For
chylomicrons in both rats and humans, this evidently represents
a "total" acquisition (22, 23), whereas for rat VLDL it represents
a substantial increment, accompanied by increased electrophoretic
mobility (21). The content of cholesterol in the surface also increases while that of phospholipid falls (21). These reciprocal
transfers of surface components seem to preserve the original
surface area and hence the original size of each particle. One of
the C apoproteins increases the affinity of the particles for lipoprotein lipase and increases the catalytic rate of the enzyme on
component triglycerides (24). This protein has no effect on the
apparent Km at physiological pH. Hydrolysis normally occurs

---

[1]Triglyceride-rich lipoproteins may be exposed to some HDL in
secretory vesicles of the Golgi apparatus.

rapidly at the surface of blood capillaries in several tissues (most notably adipose tissue and heart). Normally, the partially degraded particles ("remnants") are rapidly metabolized by the liver. They accumulate, however, in hepatectomized animals from which they can be isolated and characterized.

Remnants produced from lymph chylomicrons and plasma VLDL have been obtained from a functionally eviscerated ("supradiaphragmatic") rat preparation (25). Collection of remnants from plasma VLDL was accomplished simply by harvesting lipoproteins from the supradiaphragmatic (living) part of the animal one hour after tying off the portal vein and the vena cava and aorta just below the diaphragm. Preliminary studies on the formation of remnants from chylomicrons indicated that they overlapped VLDL remnants in size and density. Therefore, to study chylomicron remnants, animals were rendered free of d < 1.006 lipoproteins by injecting them with 4-aminopyrazolopyrimidine (26) 18 hours before injecting chylomicrons into supradiaphragmatic preparations. The density of some remnants was in the range of normal LDL (1.006 - 1.063) but most remained in the range of VLDL (< 1.006). Remnants of d < 1.006 that were derived from large chylomicrons (mean diameter about 1500 Å), small chylomicrons (mean diameter about 700 Å) and plasma VLDL (mean diameter about 570 Å) differed little in size (mean diameters 400-600 Å). Studies with remnants formed from precursors labeled with cholesterol-^{3}H and palmitate-^{14}C showed that in all cases 70-90 per cent of the triglyceride in the original particles had been removed while the other core component, cholesteryl esters, was retained. Although lipoprotein lipase does not hydrolyze the 2-acyl linkage, monoglycerides did not accumulate in the particle, presumably because of rapid acyl migration or because the polar monoglycerides left the particle surface and were rapidly removed from the blood. A normal relationship (5) between the size of the remnants and the fraction of particle volume occupied by polar lipids and proteins was preserved and they generally retained a round shape when examined by electron microscopy. Calculations showed that the remnants retained their original complement of B apoprotein and cholesterol[2]

---

[2]Content of B-apoprotein was higher in chylomicrons and their remnants (ca 1.2x10^{6} daltons per particle) than it was in VLDL and VLDL-remnants (ca 0.6x10^{6} daltons per particle). Content of cholesteryl esters in remnants actually increased, suggesting that preformed cholesteryl esters had been transferred from lipoproteins of higher density.

but had lost most of their phospholipids and a considerable fraction of the other proteins. In particular, those C-apoproteins that migrate rapidly in polyacrylamide gels were substantially depleted and the proteins of intermediate weight became predominant. Loss of soluble proteins from plasma VLDL was smaller in animals that had received 4-aminopyrazolopyrimidine. Since the amount of HDL was substantially reduced in these animals, it seems likely that removal of some surface components may have been impaired. This interpretation was supported by the presence of particles appearing to have a "membranous" structure in those drug-treated animals injected with large chylomicrons. Removal of phospholipids, however, was greater in remnants from drug-treated than from untreated supradiaphragmatic rats. Both the phospholipids and the C-apoproteins are evidently transferred to HDL (23) and this process seems to occur spontaneously when sufficient triglycerides have been removed by action of lipoprotein lipase. Some C-apoproteins are retained but the remnant particles become a progressively poorer substrate for lipoprotein lipase as triglyceride is lost; the catalytic rate falls abruptly after 50% has been removed (27). Just why this is so is not certain, but other soluble apoproteins (15, 28) and cholesterol (29) inhibit the co-factor property of the active protein for lipoprotein lipase in in vitro systems. The C-apoproteins are utilized repeatedly by newly secreted triglyceride-rich lipoproteins, whereas the phospholipids presumably are metabolized by action of LCAT on HDL as described below.

Catabolism - The Second Step

Remnant particles, whether derived from chylomicrons or VLDL, contain only a fraction of the triglycerides, phospholipids and C proteins originally present, but they retain all of the cholesteryl esters and B-apoprotein and the bulk of the cholesterol. In addition, at least in the case of VLDL, they retain the major protein of intermediate molecular weight, which is unusually rich in arginine.

Earlier studies in rats, dogs and sheep (30-32) showed that chylomicron cholesteryl esters and cholesterol are rapidly and almost completely taken up by the liver. The efficiency of this process is such that these remnants must have a life span in blood of about 2 minutes. More recent work has shown that VLDL remnants are rapidly metabolized in the rat and indicate that the liver also accounts for removal of almost all of their component cholesteryl esters and cholesterol (33). Rapid uptake of both core and surface components of these particles by the liver suggests that the entire particle may be removed as a unit. This possibility is supported by the demonstration that hepatic removal of the B-apoprotein of VLDL is similarly rapid and complete in the rat (34). In these experiments, VLDL-proteins were labeled by injecting donor animals with lysine-^{3}H and the bulk of the radioactivity in apoproteins other than the B-apoprotein was removed by molecular exchange during incubation with unlabeled HDL. When the product, which contained about 90% of the ^{3}H in the B-apoprotein, was injected into recipient rats, most of the radioactivity was rapidly taken up by the liver. Similar results have been obtained using VLDL in which all the proteins were labeled with ^{125}I (35).

Since the liver rapidly takes up remnants from the blood, but not their precursors, the hepatic parenchymal cell must recognize a unique difference in the surface of the remnant particle. It has been suggested than an hepatic lipase, which, like lipoprotein lipase, is rapidly released into the blood by heparin (indicating a location close to the bloodstream), may be involved in uptake of the triglycerides remaining in remnants in the dog (32). During constant intravenous infusion of chylomicrons into unanesthetized dogs bearing indwelling vascular catheters, about 20% of the component triglycerides was taken up by the liver; of this, about 40% was released as free fatty acids. Studies with the purified hepatic lipase have failed to provide evidence that lipoproteins contain a co-factor for this enzyme, analogous to that for lipoprotein lipase (36, 37). If the entire particle is taken up as the studies summarized above suggest, the surface of liver cells may contain a receptor for the particle which is not an enzyme and uptake may be by adsorptive endocytosis.

In humans, LDL are thought to be a major catabolic product of the metabolism of VLDL (38). The studies cited above have shown that this is not so for the rat. However, a small amount (ca 3%) of labeled B-apoprotein, the major apoprotein of LDL, did appear in the appropriate density fraction (1.019-1.063) when B-apoprotein labeled VLDL were injected into intact rats. Furthermore, when lysine-^{3}H was injected into rats, the specific activities of the B-apoprotein in VLDL and LDL showed a precursor-product relationship (34). This suggests that remnants may follow two pathways: first, incorporation as a unit into the liver; second, conversion, presumably also involving the liver, to LDL. In the latter case, most of the remaining triglyceride as well as proteins other than the B-apoprotein are removed from the particle to form the smaller LDL, whose core is composed almost entirely of cholesteryl esters[3]. This particle is no longer recognized by the same hepatic receptor or enzyme involved in the metabolism of remnants. Since the extent to which these two pathways of remnant metabolism are used in the rat and humans correlates with the grossly different concentrations of LDL in these two species, the relative use of these two pathways may be an important determinant of the prevailing level of LDL. The fate of remnant components removed during the formation of LDL is unknown, but recycling of the arginine-rich protein seems likely because it is also present in HDL and in proteins of $d > 1.21$ in humans (39). The various steps in the metabolism of VLDL are shown schematically in Figure 1.

LIPOPROTEINS AND CHOLESTEROL TRANSPORT

The liver seems to be the primary site of removal of HDL from the blood (40). Therefore, cholesteryl esters carried by HDL or in remnants of triglyceride-rich lipoproteins are transported to the organ in which cholesterol is excreted from the body. Those cholesteryl esters that enter LDL, either from catabolism of triglyceride-rich lipoproteins or by transfer from HDL, may have a different fate. Recent studies suggest that removal of LDL from the blood is not impaired by hepatectomy (41) and a high affinity receptor for LDL is present on the surface of fibroblasts (17). As discussed elsewhere in this volume by Dr. Goldstein, binding to this receptor is rapidly followed by hydrolysis of the esters and the B-apoprotein. Although the physiological significance of the LDL-receptor is uncertain, different lipoproteins may therefore have quite different functions in transport of cholesterol - VLDL and HDL serving to remove cholesterol derived from the

---

[3]Only a fraction of the cholesteryl esters of rat LDL originates in cholesteryl esters of VLDL; the remainder is derived from LCAT and presumably is transferred to LDL from HDL (33).

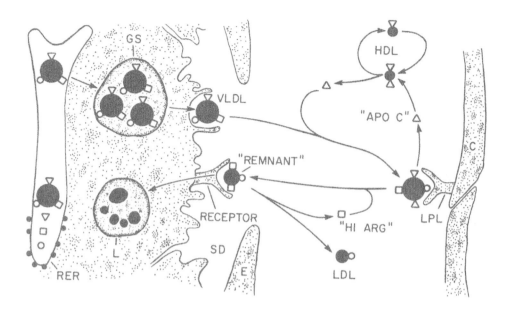

Figure 1: This diagram indicates some of the steps in the synthesis, secretion and catabolism of VLDL. It emphasizes the participation of HDL in the provision of certain proteins to the newly secreted particle and the role of the liver in the second step of VLDL catabolism. The existence of an hepatic "receptor" is based upon indirect evidence (see text).

Abbreviations: RER - rough endoplasmic reticulum; GS - Golgi saccule; L - lysosome; SD - space of Disse; E - endothelial cell; LPL - lipoprotein lipase.

diet or various tissues from the body by transport to the liver and LDL serving to supply cholesterol (mainly as esters) needed for membrane synthesis. However, LDL-cholesterol is ultimately derived from dietary cholesterol transported in chylomicrons or from cholesterol secreted from the liver in VLDL (plus a small amount secreted in HDL). Key roles for LCAT and for HDL in the transport of cholesterol to the liver are also suggested by the genetic disorders of LCAT deficiency and Tangier disease, whereas that of LDL may find negative expression in abetalipoproteinemia.

HIGH DENSITY LIPOPROTEINS

Synthesis and Secretion

Like the triglyceride-rich lipoproteins, HDL are synthesized
in parenchymal cells of the liver and intestinal mucosa. Recent
studies with perfused liver indicate that newly secreted HDL have
considerably less cholesteryl esters than do plasma HDL. The
liver also secretes LCAT, which acts upon HDL-lipids in the
presence of the major A protein to yield cholesteryl esters and
lysolecithin. Demonstration of the low content of cholesteryl
esters has therefore required addition of an inhibitor of the enzyme to the perfusion medium (42) or use of a non-recirculating
perfusion system (43). Because newly secreted HDL are composed
almost entirely of polar lipids together with a substantial amount
of protein, it is not surprising that their structure differs from
that of plasma HDL. By negative staining electron microscopy,
they appear as circular discs, about 44 x 190 Å (42). In thin
sections, they show trilaminar structure. These images are best
interpreted as a bilayer, the edges of which are covered by protein. The component proteins of the newly secreted HDL seem to
be similar to those of plasma - both slowly migrating bands and
the typical rapidly migrating C proteins are present (42). HDL obtained from livers perfused with lysine-^{3}H contain appreciable
radioactivity in both regions, but primarily in the slowly migrating
bands (22). HDL obtained similarly from perfused small intestine
contain radioactivity only in the slowly migrating bands, as is the
case of triglyceride-rich lipoproteins (22). Their detailed composition and structure have not been determined.

Metabolism

The action of LCAT upon newly secreted HDL evidently converts the disc-shaped particle into a sphere in which cholesteryl
esters comprise about 20% of the particle volume. The newly
formed bilayer particle is thereby converted to a typical pseudomicellar lipoprotein. In the rat, virtually all component cholesteryl
esters of HDL appear to be derived from the action of LCAT (33).
Labeled cholesteryl esters of VLDL do not appear in HDL and the
HDL esters are primarily cholesteryl arachidonate, whereas those
of VLDL are mainly oleate esters with very little arachidonate.
The composition of cholesteryl esters of rat LDL is intermediate

between that of HDL and VLDL but resembles the former more closely, suggesting that they are also mainly derived from the action of LCAT. Since LDL do not contain the co-factor protein for LCAT (16), these esters presumably are transferred to LDL from HDL by a nonenzymatic mechanism, involving exchange of core components (44).

About 85% of HDL phospholipid is lecithin, one of the substrates for LCAT. The lysolecithin formed by this enzyme leaves the surface of HDL and is bound to albumin (45). It is then rapidly removed from the blood and re-acylated. Both of the lipids of the HDL surface are therefore removed by action of the enzyme. Replacement of surface components presumably occurs by transfer from the plasma membrane of various cells, such as the erythrocyte, and from triglyceride-rich lipoproteins as remnants are formed. During alimentary lipemia in humans, the content of phospholipids in HDL increases substantially (23, 46). This is not surprising because phospholipids comprise most of the surface of chylomicrons and they comprise the bulk of the surface that is lost during formation of remnants (25). Most of the increase in HDL-phospholipid occurs in the density fraction 1.063-1.125 (23). These HDL are larger than those of higher density (1.125-1.21) and their surface contains a higher proportion of phospholipids. The composition of HDL evidently is not fixed, but depends upon the availability of component lipids. Since lymph chylomicrons (47) unlike plasma chylomicrons and VLDL (48) contain a substantial complement of A-apoproteins, the possibility that HDL are also formed directly during their metabolism needs to be considered. When mixed with lecithin, these proteins form disc-shaped particles closely resembling HDL secreted from rat liver (49).

The increased availability of substrates of the LCAT reaction during alimentary lipemia in humans is accompanied by increased enzyme activity (50). This increased activity may not be dependent upon an increase in the enzyme protein because addition of chylomicrons to serum itself increases the enzymatic rate. Cholesteryl esters inhibit LCAT (51) so that it is likely that the enzyme acts more rapidly on HDL newly secreted from the liver or produced during formation of remnants which are poor in cholesteryl esters. Methods commonly used to assay LCAT do not take the quality of the substrate lipoprotein into account and may therefore not reflect the catalytic rate in vivo. The key role of HDL in cholesterol transport and the fate of LCAT-derived cholesteryl esters are indicated in Figure 2.

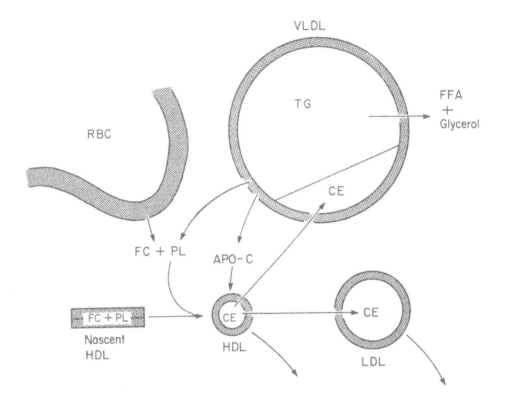

<u>Figure 2</u>: This diagram depicts the action of LCAT upon nascent discoid HDL to form the pseudomicellar HDL of plasma. It also indicates some of the sources of the surface lipid substrates of the enzyme and the transfer of some of the product cholesteryl esters to other lipoproteins.

    <u>Abbreviations:</u> RBC - red blood cell; TG - triglycerides; CE - cholesteryl esters; FC - (free) cholesterol; PL - phospholipids; FFA - free fatty acids.

    Although lipoprotein metabolism is commonly considered in terms of the discrete classes that are separated by flotation or by other methods, such as electrophoresis and gel chromatography, the metabolic events described above may occur in part when the surfaces of the particles interact and exchange component lipids and proteins. Such interactions would of course be interrupted when the particles are separated physically.

LIPID TRANSPORT IN LIPOPROTEINS AND
HUMAN HYPERLIPOPROTEINEMIAS

Primary Dysbetalipoproteinemia

Both structural and dynamic studies strongly suggest that remnants of triglyceride-rich lipoproteins accumulate in this disorder. Two populations of abnormal particles exist in the post-absorptive state (52-55). One, comprising the bulk of them, is a cholesteryl ester-rich, β-migrating VLDL of about 300 Å diameter; the other, averaging about 800 Å diameter, is unusually rich in cholesteryl esters and the B-apoprotein for its size. Since VLDL and, during alimentary lipemia, chylomicrons of normal composition are also present (48, 52, 54), the two groups of abnormal particles could represent remnants rather than an abnormal secretory product. Detailed analysis supports this view. As shown in Table 1, the smaller of the two abnormal particles contains, per particle, more cholesteryl esters and less triglyceride than do normal VLDL, consistent with the VLDL remnants isolated from functionally hepatectomized rats. In addition, the putative human VLDL remnants also contain a complement of cholesterol and of the B and arginine-rich apoproteins similar to their presumed precursors, whereas phospholipids and the C-apoproteins are substantially reduced.

Comparable differences are observed between plasma chylomicrons and the larger of the two abnormal populations. As in the rat, each of these particles contains more B-apoprotein than do VLDL or their remnants. Content of the arginine-rich protein is several fold higher. The putative chylomicron remnants have lost most of their original complement of triglycerides and phospholipids and, again like the rat, phospholipids account for most of the loss of surface components. They differ from chylomicron remnants of the rat by their larger size. This may be related to the substantially larger amount of cholesteryl esters in the core of human chylomicrons. Evidently, cholesteryl esters produced by LCAT are transferred to both of the remnants populations in exchange for triglycerides during their prolonged life-span in the blood. As in other human hyperlipemias, LDL and HDL in dysbetalipoproteinemia contain more triglycerides and less cholesteryl esters than normal (56).

The composition of individual human LDL, also shown in Table 1, indicates preservation only of the B-apoprotein, whereas

Table 1

PROPERTIES OF INDIVIDUAL HUMAN SERUM
LIPOPROTEIN PARTICLES

	Chylomicrons		VLDL		LDL
	Normal	Dysbetalipo-proteinemia	Normal	Dysbetalipo-proteinemia	Normal
Diameter (Å)	1200	825	400	330	216
Density (g/cm^3)	0.931	0.951	0.970	1.000	1.035
Molecular Weight (daltons x 10^{-6})	504	153	19.2	11.3	3.06
Chemical Composition (daltons x 10^{-6})					
Cholesteryl esters	18	54	1.8	3.3	1.33
Triglycerides	431	74	11.7	3.9	0.10
Total Core	449	128	13.5	7.2	1.43
Cholesterol	10	9	1.0	0.9	0.31
Phospholipids	35	13	3.1	2.0	0.63
Proteins					
Apo-B	1.2	1.3	0.74	0.68	0.67
Arginine-rich	2.4	1.6	0.19	0.25	
R-ser	0.8	0.4	0.04	0.02	
R-glu	1.5	0.2	0.19	0.04	0.02
R-ala's	4.3	0.6	0.70	0.15	
Total Surface	55	26	5.9	4.0	1.63

Values for chylomicrons and VLDL are calculated from data in references 5 and 48 with corrections for chromogenicity of the individual proteins in Amidoschwarz-stained polyacrylamide gels (Kane, J.P. and Havel, R.J., unpublished data).

Values for LDL (d 1.025-1.045) are from reference 4.

content of all other components is substantially lower than that of either "remnant" population. Conversion of remnants to LDL evidently is accompanied by loss of most of the core cholesteryl esters and triglycerides as well as the surface cholesterol and phospholipids together with virtually all of the arginine-rich protein and the remaining C-apoproteins. The conversion may occur in the liver, but this remains to be shown.

Kinetic studies with protein-labeled (^{125}I) and triglyceride-labeled VLDL (57, 58) also indicate that pre-beta VLDL are the precursor of beta-VLDL in dysbetalipoproteinemia. The apparent accumulation of remnants of chylomicrons and VLDL as well as delayed conversion of protein in β-VLDL to LDL (57) is consistent with the suggestion that hepatic catabolism of remnants is specifically deficient in this disorder. It is also possible that the pathway is simply overloaded (59). In cholesterol-fed rabbits and in other mammals fed cholesterol-rich diets (60, 61), the VLDL are cholesterol-rich and contain a large amount of the arginine-rich protein. These could represent remnants that accumulate because hepatic uptake has become saturated. This possibility, however, remains to be tested.

Lecithin-Cholesterol Acyl Transferase Deficiency

The variety of abnormal lipoproteins that accumulate in this disorder and their possible relationship to the enzymatic defect have been reviewed recently in detail (62). The largest particles (> 1000 Å diameter) are found in both VLDL and LDL. They are composed largely of unesterified cholesterol and phospholipids (mainly lecithin) and appear in negative stains by electron microscopy as flattened rounded structures which resemble the "membranous" particles formed in supradiaphragmatic rats treated with 4-aminopyrazolopyrimidine after they receive chylomicrons intravenously. The "membranous" quality of these particles in human LCAT-deficiency is supported by the occasional occurrence of myelin figures in the large particle fractions separated from VLDL and LDL by gel filtration. That they are indeed abnormal chylomicron remnants is suggested by the fact that their concentration increases substantially (62) when affected individuals are fed fat-rich diets, with or without added cholesterol. Their low content of cholesteryl esters is to be expected because virtually none is available for transfer from the HDL and smaller LDL. It

seems likely that they consist of a film of phospholipids and
cholesterol together with a small amount of protein enclosing a
small but variable amount of nonpolar lipid and cholesterol[4].
Possibly, the "core" of these particles also contains a separate
aqueous phase as described below for another abnormal particle
in LCAT-deficiency and in cholestasis. The occurrence of such
remnants in LCAT-deficiency is strong evidence that LCAT
normally participates in the metabolism of surface lipids of chylomicrons. Presumably, excessive surface lipids are also produced
during the metabolism of VLDL, but the total amount may be substantially reduced when diets poor in fat are fed.

The HDL in LCAT-deficiency comprise small amounts of two
abnormal populations of particles, neither of which resembles
normal HDL (63-66). The larger closely resembles in chemical
composition as well as in appearance the bilayer discs secreted
from rat liver and may therefore represent the product of normal
hepatic (and possibly also intestinal) secretion, unmodified by
action of the enzyme. The other particle is round but smaller than
normal HDL, about 50 Å in diameter. It contains primarily the
major A-apoprotein (R-gin$_1$) together with cholesterol and phospholipids (67). Its concentration, but not that of the larger HDL, increases when affected individuals are fed fat-rich diets (62). It
has already been pointed out that lymph chylomicrons are rich in
A-apoproteins, whereas plasma chylomicrons are not, and it
seems likely that exchange of these apoproteins for other surface
components of HDL occurs normally after chylomicrons enter the
blood. This interchange would be expected to be blunted in individuals with LCAT-deficiency because of the paucity of HDL; the
small HDL might then be produced directly when lipoprotein lipase
acts upon chylomicrons. It has been suggested that the larger HDL
also are formed during this process (62); however, since they are
not affected by fat-feeding, it seems more likely that they are formed
by the normal secretory pathway as described above.

The LDL in LCAT deficiency contain, in addition to the large
membranous structures already described, two other populations
(65, 66, 68-70). One consists of particles resembling normal LDL

---

[4] Stable monolayers of lecithin can contain up to an equimolar a-
mount of cholesterol. The molar content of cholesterol considerably exceeds that of phospholipids in the large particles so the remainder may be dissolved in their nonpolar core.

and containing primarily the B-apoprotein. These particles differ
from normal LDL in that their core consists mainly of triglycerides
rather than cholesteryl esters (70).   They thus resemble LDL from
severely hyperlipemic subjects without LCAT-deficiency in whom
exchange of lipids has modified the composition of the core.   The
last population consists of particles of intermediate size, about
500 Å in diameter.   It is composed of an approximately 1:1 molar
mixture of cholesterol and phospholipids together with a small
amount of protein and very little nonpolar lipid.   The protein includes a substantial amount of albumin together with C-apoproteins
(68, 69, 71).   The chemical composition and electron microscopic
appearance of these particles, as well as their immunological
properties (68, 69, 71), closely resemble those of the abnormal
lipoprotein of cholestasis described in the next section and it therefore seems likely that they are spherical vesicles enclosing an
aqueous compartment.   The amount present is much smaller than
that found in many patients with cholestasis.   Possibly, they represent another form of remnant, but their concentration is only
slightly affected by dietary fat (62).   Other mechanisms for their
formation will be discussed in the next section.

Cholestasis

The characteristic abnormal LDL that accumulates in cholestasis has an invariant composition and structure.   It is composed
almost entirely of polar lipids (cholesterol and phospholipids,
mainly choline phosphatides, in a 1:1 molar ratio) together with
about 3% by weight of protein, including albumin and all of the apoproteins of normal VLDL except for the B-apoprotein (72, 73).   Its
structure as a vesicle with a lipid bilayer wall is established (73).
Its flattened appearance by electron microscopy in negative stains
(73, 74) results from drying since, when fixed material is observed
in thin sections, the vesicle is spherical (75).   Its stained wall has
the characteristic trilaminar appearance of cell membranes, con-
firming the bilayer structure deduced from x-ray diffraction.
Vesicles with identical appearance can be formed from 1:1 molar
mixtures of lecithin and cholesterol.   Measurement of the trapped
volume of such vesicles, formed in the presence of inulin-^{3}H,
also indicates a spherical shape (75).   Since the albumin associated
with the particle is not accessible to its antibody (72, 74), it may
be dissolved in the inner aqueous compartment, whereas the specific apoproteins are associated in the usual manner with the wall.

The HDL in patients with cholestasis usually are composed primarily of bilayer discs with the same dimensions as those normally secreted from perfused rat liver (68, 75, 76). Their composition is also closely similar to those from rat liver and they contain the usual complement of HDL-apoproteins (77). The concentration of normal pseudomicellar HDL is usually very low but not invariably so (77) and many patients with cholestasis evidently have abundant activity of LCAT in their plasma (78, 79). The consistent presence of a substantial amount of cholesteryl esters in plasma, of which about one-half is cholesteryl linoleate (77), provides additional evidence that this enzyme continues to catalyze transfer of acyl chains from lecithin to cholesterol. Most of these cholesteryl esters are in beta-migrating, pseudomicellar LDL of the usual dimensions. Their core, however, contains about one-half triglycerides by weight (77), a replacement of triglycerides for cholesteryl esters resembling, albeit less pronounced than, that of primary LCAT deficiency.

The mechanisms for the accumulation of the abnormal vesicular lipoprotein and the HDL discs has not been established. Perhaps the most parsimonius explanation is that the vesicles arise from the discs, which constitute a normal product of secretion (75). This could occur if the normal action of LCAT were impaired, for example by association of conjugated bile salts with the discs, or if bile salts "destabilize" the discs so they are unable to accumulate cholesteryl esters and gradually fuse to form stable vesicles (80). In either case, the presumed normal conversion of bilayer discs to pseudomicellar HDL would be impaired as suggested by the usually low concentration of normal HDL. The cholesteryl esters that are synthesized would presumably accumulate in other pseudomicellar lipoproteins (VLDL and LDL), as is in fact observed. It is also possible that the liver "regurgitates" micelles, normally secreted into the bile, into the blood and that these micelles are destabilized by loss of the bile salts to albumin with resultant formation of vesicles, discs, or both. Except for a small amount of multilamellar structures in LDL, evidence for accumulation of abnormal remnants of triglyceride-rich lipoproteins in cholestasis has not been obtained and VLDL in these subjects have a normal composition (77). Ample amounts of C-apoproteins are present, although transfer to newly secreted triglyceride-rich lipoproteins presumably occurs mainly from the vesicle rather than from HDL. The paucity of abnormal remnants suggests that LCAT is active in metabolizing surface components of triglyceride-rich lipoproteins, however chylomicron formation may be impaired because of lack of bile salts in the intestine. Therefore, although the lipoprotein abnormalities in cholestasis differ from those of primary LCAT deficiency, the extent to which defective function of LCAT contributes to the extraordinary accumulation of the vesicular lipoprotein in cholestasis remains uncertain.

CONCLUSION

Continued advances in the delineation of pathways of lipid transport in lipoproteins now provide substantial information on all phases of plasma triglyceride transport. Analysis of certain genetic human disorders, together with studies in experimental animals, has begun to show how lipoproteins transport cholesterol as esters of long chain fatty acids. Both triglycerides and cholesterol are esters of long chain fatty acids. Both triglycerides and cholesteryl esters are transported in the "core" of lipoproteins, but the polar lipids and the apoproteins at the aqueous interface critically determine the interactions with enzymes and cellular receptors that control this complex transport system. Differences in pathways as well as in rates of lipid transport appear to underlie the large interspecies variations in lipoprotein concentrations.

ACKNOWLEDGEMENT

The research cited by the author and his colleagues (C. J. Fielding, R. L. Hamilton, J. P. Kane and T. Sata) was supported by grants (HL-14237 and HL-06285) from the U. S. Public Health Service.

REFERENCES

1. Havel, R. J. Adv. Exp. Med. Biol. 26:57, 1972.
2. Forte, G. M. , Nichols, A. V. and Glaeser, R. M. Chem. Phys. Lipids 2: 396, 1958.
3. Hamilton, R. L. In: Proc. 1958 Deuel Conference on Lipids. G. Cowgill, D. L. Estrich, P. D. S. Woods, eds., U. S. Government Printing Office, Washington, D. C. , p. 1.
4. Kane, J. P. Dissertation, University of California, San Francisco, 1971.
5. Sata, T. , Havel, R. J. and Jones, A. L. J. Lipid Res. 13: 757, 1972.
6. Forte, T. and Nichols, A. V. Adv. Lipid Res. 10:1, 1972.
7. Laggner, P. , Muller, K. and Kratky, O. FEBS Letters 33: 77, 1973.
8. Muller, K. , Laggner, P. , Kratky, O. , Kostner, G. , Holasek, A. , and Glatter, O. FEBS Letters 40: 213, 1974.
9. Shipley, G. G. , Atkinson, D. and Scanu, A. M. J. Supramolecular Structure 1: 98, 1972.
10. Mateu, L. , Tardiu, A. , Luzatti, V. , Aggerback, L. and Scanu, A. M. J. Mol. Biol. 70: 105, 1972.
11. Laggner, P. , Muller, K. , Kratky, O. , Kostner, G. and Holasek, A. Conference on Serum Lipoproteins, Graz. , 1973, p. 47.
12. Chen, G. C. and Kane, J. P. Biochemistry 13: 3330, 1974.
13. Pollard, H. , Scanu, A. M. and Taylor, E. W. Proc. Nat. Acad. Sci. (U. S. A.) 64: 304, 1969.
14. Schumaker, V. N. and Adams, G. H. J. Theoret. Biol. 26: 89, 1970.
15. Havel, R. J. , Fielding, C. J. , Olivecrona, T. , Shore, V. G. , Fielding, P. E. and Eglrud, T. Biochemistry 12: 1828, 1973.
16. Fielding, C. J. , Shore, V. G. and Fielding, P. E. Biochem. Biophys. Res. Comm. 46: 1493, 1972.
17. Brown, M. S. and Goldstein, J. L. Proc. Nat. Acad. Sci. (U. S. A.) 71: 788, 1974.
18. Alexander, C. A. , Hamilton, R. L. and Havel, R. J. Proc. 32nd Ann. Electron Microscopy Soc. Amer. , 1974, p. 238.
19. Le Marchand, J. , Singh, A. , Assimacopoulos-Jeannet, F. , Orci, L. , Rouiller, C. and Jeanrenaud, B. J. Biol. Chem. 248: 6862, 1973.
20. Stein, O. and Stein, Y. Biochim. Biophys. Acta 306: 142, 1973.
21. Hamilton, R. L. Adv. Exp. Med. Biol. 26: 7, 1973.

22. Windmueller, H. G. , Herbert, P. N. and Levy, R. I.
    J. Lipid Res. 14: 215, 1973.
23. Havel, R. J. , Kane, J. P. and Kashyap, M. L.   J. Clin.
    Invest. 52: 32, 1973.
24. Fielding, C. J.   Biochim. Biophys. Acta 316: 66, 1973.
25. Mjøs, O. D. , Faergeman, O. , Hamilton, R. L. and Havel,
    R. J.   Europ. J. Clin. Invest. 4: 382, 1974.
26. Shiff, T. S. , Roheim, P. S. and Eder, H. A.   J. Lipid Res.
    12: 596, 1971.
27. Fielding, C. J. and Higgins, J. M.   Fed. Proc. 33: 351, 1974.
28. Brown, W. V. and Baginsky, M. L.   Biochem. Biophys. Res.
    Res. Comm. 46: 375, 1972.
29. Fielding, C. J.   Biochim. Biophys. Acta 218: 221, 1970.
30. Goodman, D. S.   J. Clin. Invest. 41: 1886, 1962.
31. Nestel, P. J. , Havel, R. J. and Bezman, A.   J. Clin. Invest.
    42: 1313, 1963.
32. Bergman, E. N. , Havel, R. J.   Wolfe, B. M. and Bøhmer, T.
    J. Clin. Invest. 50: 1831, 1971.
33. Faergeman, O. and Havel, R. J.   J. Clin. Invest. , in press.
34. Faergeman, O. , Sata, T. , Kane, J. P. and Havel, R. J.
    Circulation 50 Suppl. III : 114, 1974.
35. Eisenberg, S. and Rachmilewitz, D.   Biochim. Biophys.
    Acta 326: 378, 1973.
36. Greten, H. , Walter, B. and Brown, W. V.   FEBS Letters
    27: 306, 1972.
37. Frost, P. and Havel, R. J.   Unpublished data
38. Bilheimer, D. W. , Eisenberg, S. and Levy, R. I.   Biochim.
    Biophys. Acta 260: 212, 1972.
39. Sata, T. and Havel, R. J.   Unpublished data
40. Rachmilewitz, D. , Stein, O. , Roheim, P. S. and Stein, Y.
    Biochim. Biophys. Acta 270: 414, 1972.
41. Sniderman, A. L. , Carew, T. E. , Chandler, J. G. and
    Steinberg, D.   Science 183: 526, 1974.
42. Hamilton, R. L. , Williams, M. C. , Havel, R. J. and Fielding,
    C. J.   Proc. 3rd Intl. Symp. on Atherosclerosis, abstr. 50,
    1973.
43. Marsh, J. B.   J. Lipid Res. 15: 544, 1974.
44. Nichols, A .V. and Smith, L.   J. Lipid Res. 6: 206, 1965.
45. Glomset, J. A.   J. Lipid Res. 9: 155, 1968.
46. Havel, R. J.   J. Clin. Invest. 36: 848, 1957.
47. Kostner, G. and Holasek, A.   Biochemistry 11: 1217, 1972.
48. Havel, R. J. and Kane, J. P.   Proc. Nat. Acad. Sci. U. S. A.
    70: 2015, 1973.

49. Forte, T. , Nichols, A. V. , Gong, E. L. , Lux, S. and Levy, R. I. Biochim. Biophys. Acta 248: 381, 1974.

50. Marcel, Y. L. and Vezina, C. J. Biol. Chem. 248: 8254, 1973.

51. Fielding, C. J. , Shore, V. G. and Fielding, P. E. Biochim. Biophys. Acta 270: 513, 1972.

52. Hazzard, W. R. , Porte, D. , Jr. , and Bierman, E. L. J. Clin. Invest. 49: 1853, 1970.

53. Hazzard, W. R. , Lindgren, F. L. and Bierman, E. L. Biochim. Biophys. Acta 202: 517, 1970.

54. Quarfordt, S. , Levy, R. I. and Fredrickson, D. S. J. Clin. Invest. 50: 75, 1971.

55. Sata, T. , Havel, R. J. and Jones, A. L. J. Lipid Res. 13: 757, 1972.

56. Havel, R. J. and Kane, J. P. Unpublished data

57. Bilheimer, D. W. , Eisenberg, S. and Levy, R. I. Circulation 44 Suppl. 2: 56, 1971.

58. Quarfordt, S. H. , Levy, R. I. and Fredrickson, D. S. Biochim. Biophys. Acta 296: 572, 1973.

59. Hall, M., III, Bilheimer, D. W. , Phair, R. D. , Levy, R. I. and Berman, M. Circulation 50 Suppl. III: 114, 1974.

60. Shore, V. G. , Shore, B. and Hart, R. G. Biochemistry 13: 1579, 1974.

61. Mahley, R. W. , Weisgraber, K. H. and Innearity, T. Circulation Res. , in press.

62. Glomset, J. A. and Norum, K. R. Adv. Lipid Res. 11: 1, 1973.

63. Torsvik, H. , Solaas, M. H. and Gjone, E. Clin. Genetics 1: 139, 1970.

64. Torsvik, H. Clin. Genetics 1: 310, 1970.

65. Norum, K. R. , Glomset, J. A. , Nichols, A. V. and Forte, T. J. Clin. Invest. 50: 1131, 1971.

66. Forte, T. , Norum, K. R. , Glomset, J. A. and Nichols, A. V. J. Clin. Invest. 50: 1141, 1971.

67. Torsvik, H. Clin. Genetics 3: 188, 1972.

68. Untermann, G. , Schoenbrun, W. , Langer, K. H. and Dieker, P. Humangenetik 16: 245, 1972.

69. Torsvik, H. , Berg, K. , Magnani, H. N. , McConathy, W. J. , Alaupovic, P. , and Gjone, E. FEBS Letters 24: 165, 1972.

70. Glomset, J. A. , Nichols, A. V. , Norum, K. R. , King, W. and Forte, T. J. Clin. Invest. 52: 1078, 1973.

71. McConathy, W. J. , Alaupovic, P. , Curry, M. D. , Magnani, H. N. , Torsvik, H. , Berg, K. and Gjone, E. Biochim. Biophys. Acta 326: 406, 1973.

72. Siedel, D. , Alaupovic, P. , Furman, R. H. and McConathy, W. J. J. Clin. Invest. 49: 2396, 1970.

73. Hamilton, R. L. , Havel, R. J. , Kane, J. P. , Blaurock, A. E. and Sata, T. Science 172: 475, 1971.

74. Seidel, D. , Agostini, B. and Muller, P. Biochim. Biophys. Acta 160: 146, 1972.

75. Hamilton, R. L. , Havel, R. J. and Williams, M. C. Fed. Proc. 33: 351, 1974.

76. Forte, T. , Nichols, A. , Glomset, J. and Norum, K. Biochim. Biophys. Acta 33 Suppl. 137: 121, 1974.

77. Havel, R. J. , Hamilton, R. L. , Kane, J. P. and Shore, V. G. Unpublished data

78. Kepkay, D. L. , Poon, R. and Simon, J. S. J. Lab. Clin. Med. 81: 172, 1973.

79. Ritland, S. , Blomhoff, J. P. and Gjone, E. Clin. Chim. Acta 49: 251, 1973.

80. Hamilton, R. L. and Kayden, H. J. In: Biochemical Pathology. A Molecular Approach to Disease, Vol. V, Liver: Pathobiology. E. Farber, ed. , in press.

PATHWAYS OF LIPOPROTEIN METABOLISM: INTEGRATION OF STRUCTURE, FUNCTION AND METABOLISM

S. Eisenberg[1], D. Rachmilewitz[1], R. I. Levy[2], D. W. Bilheimer[3], and F. T. Lindgren[4]

[1] - Lipid Research Laboratory, Department of Medicine B, Hadassah University Hospital, Jerusalem, Israel; [2] - Division of Heart and Vaschular Diseases, National Heart and Lung Institute, Bethesda, Maryland; [3] - University of Texas, Southwestern Medical School, Dallas, Texas; [4] - University of California, Donner Laboratories, Berkeley, California

The plasma lipoproteins are complex structures composed of proteins and lipids and involved with the transport of lipids in the circulation. The various lipoproteins are customarily separated into several groups following their flotation properties in salt solutions. Lipoproteins thus obtained differ in size, particle weight, lipid and protein composition, electrophoretic mobility and other physical and chemical properties. Yet, the lipoprotein system resembles more a continuous spectrum of particles of changing composition than families of distinct and discernible character. This is especially true for the lower density lipoproteins - chylomicrons, VLDL and LDL. Clearly, the classification of lipoproteins is somewhat arbitrary and a functional approach towards the lipoproteins is needed.

The studies on the protein moiety of lipoproteins, initiated by Drs. B. and V. Shore in the late 1960's, are an example of the complexity of the lipoprotein system (1-4). In the human, several different apoproteins have been isolated and characterized. They are easily separated on polyacrylamide gels (Figure 1A). Apoprotein

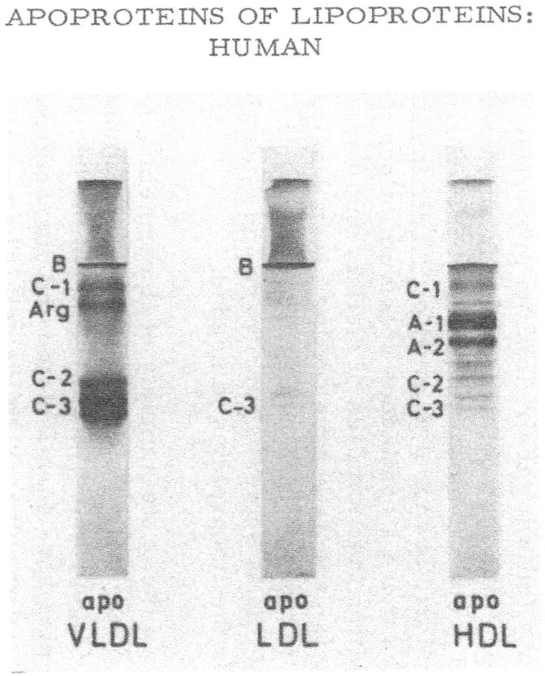

1A

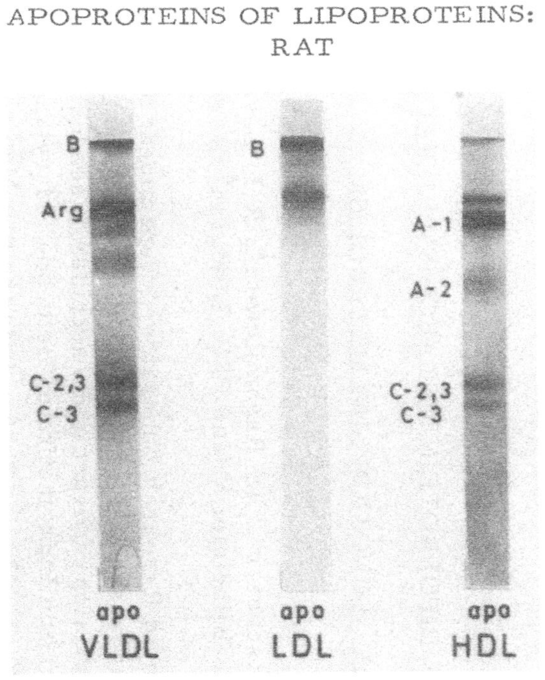

1B

<u>Figure 1:</u> Polyacrylamide gel electrophoresis of apolipoproteins. A. Human B. Rat

B is the major protein of plasma LDL, and is present in VLDL
(20-60% of total protein) (5, 6). Apoprotein C is a mixture of
three different and discernible proteins - C-I, C-II and two forms
of C-III (7-10). The C proteins constitute 40-80% of the VLDL
proteins, are regularly found in HDL and are present in minute
amounts in LDL. It has now been established that apoprotein C-II
is a specific protein cofactor, obligatory for triglyceride hydrolysis
by lipoprotein lipase (11). The other C proteins may also play
important roles in regulating the activity of this enzyme (12). Apoproteins A-I and A-II are the major proteins of HDL (1-5, 13, 14).
Their presence in small amounts in chylomicrons and VLDL has
been reported by several investigators (15, 16). The arginine-rich
protein is an apoprotein found in VLDL and constitutes 5-15% of
its total protein (4, 17, 18). It may also be present in HDL and LDL.
Each lipoprotein is thus characterized by a specific apoprotein
composition; each apoprotein however, is present in more than one
lipoprotein family. Analogous apoproteins of rat plasma lipoproteins are very similar to those of the human in their physical and
chemical properties, and distribution among lipoproteins (19, 20)
(Figure 1B).

The studies reported here were designed to define the metabolic relationship among lipoproteins and to elucidate the role of
lipolytic enzymes, in particular the lipoprotein lipase system, in
the process of interconversion of human and rat plasma lipoproteins.

METABOLISM OF VLDL IN HUMANS (21-23)

VLDL was isolated from normal humans and patients with
hyperlipoproteinemia at a density of less than 1.006 g/ml. The
VLDL was labeled with 125-iodine by a modification of MacFarlane's
iodine monochloride method and reinjected into the donor subject.
Plasma, isolated at time intervals after the injection, was separated
into 4 lipoproteins: VLDL (d < 1.006), Intermediate Density Lipoproteins (IDL) (d = 1.006-1.019), LDL (d = 1.019-1.063) and HDL
(d = 1.063-1.21).

Radioactivity associated with different apoproteins was determined after delipidation and polyacrylamide gel electrophoresis.
Individual apoproteins were sliced off the gel and counted. In the
original ^{125}I-VLDL, 50% of the radioactivity was associated with
apoprotein B and 40% with apoproteins C-II and C-III. Preliminary

in vitro experiments have demonstrated that apoprotein C was
readily transferred from VLDL to HDL and vice versa, whereas
apoprotein B was always recovered with the density range of VLDL.
During the first 24 hours after the injection of ^{125}I-VLDL to normal
humans, however, radioactivity disappeared rapidly from VLDL
and appeared in all other lipoprotein fractions. At the end of this
period, only about 10% of the injected radioactivity was associated
with VLDL. As expected, radioactivity was transferred to HDL
already 10 minutes after the injection. It was due predominantly
to ^{125}I-apoprotein C. Labeled proteins were also transferred with
time to IDL and LDL. Radioactivity in IDL peaked 6-12 hours after
the injection and that of LDL 24 hours after the injection. At that
time, about 50% of the plasma radioactivity was associated with
LDL and 25% each with VLDL and HDL. When the radioactivity
associated with apoprotein B and apoprotein C in VLDL was determined, we found that labeled apoprotein B was the major apoprotein
transferred to IDL and LDL. It was also the major labeled protein
of these lipoproteins, accounting for more than 80% of their radioactivity. The $t_{1/2}$ of labelled apoprotein B in VLDL ranged between 2-4 hours. The activity of apoprotein B in VLDL, IDL and
LDL suggested a precursor-product relationship between these
lipoproteins. These experiments have clearly demonstrated that
apoprotein B and apoprotein C in VLDL are metabolized by different
routes. Apoprotein C is distributed between VLDL and HDL; apoprotein B constitutes the precursor of the protein moiety of plasma
LDL, and is transferred unidirectionally from VLDL to LDL
through the formation in plasma of a short-lived lipoprotein form
of intermediate density (Figure 2). Plasma LDL therefore may be
regarded as a final breakdown product of VLDL.

The role of activation of lipoprotein lipase in the metabolic
process of conversion of lipoproteins was studied in humans injected with ^{125}I-VLDL and heparin (24). The activation of the lipoprotein-lipase system resulted in a rapid hydrolysis of triglycerides;
transfer of ^{125}I-apoprotein C to HDL; and accumulation of apoprotein
B-rich lipoproteins in the density range of the small VLDL particles
of Sf rate 20-60 and intermediate lipoprotein. The subsequent
transfer of apoprotein B to LDL occurred long after the cessation
of accelerated triglyceride hydrolysis. It was similar to that observed in humans not injected with heparin. We have concluded
from the study that lipoprotein lipases play a major role in the first
stage of VLDL metabolism - the formation of the intermediate
lipoprotein. It may have no role in the conversion of IDL to LDL.

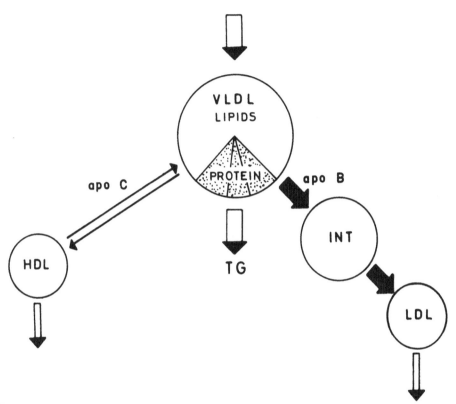

Figure 2: Schematic representation of the pathways of metabolism of human plasma VLDL apoproteins.

METABOLISM OF VLDL IN RATS

The fate of VLDL apoproteins in rats was similar to that observed in humans (25, 26). In this species, a dichotomy of VLDL apoproteins metabolism was also observed: apoprotein C was distributed between VLDL and HDL, and apoprotein B was transferred unidirectionally to LDL. The time course of the transfer reactions was, however, much more rapid than that found in humans, and the $t_{1/2}$ of apoprotein B in VLDL was less than 10 minutes. Of interest was the comparison of the behaviour of four different preparations of labeled apoprotein C: of VLDL origin, HDL origin and purified apoproteins isolated by gel chromatography on Sephadex G-150 from either lipoprotein. The half life time in circulation (8-10 hours) and the distribution of labeled apoprotein C among lipoproteins was similar in all preparations and was independent of the origin or type (purified and part of a lipoprotein) of apoprotein C studied. The experiment thus strengthened the hypothesis that apoprotein C in plasma represents an apoprotein pool discernible from all other apoproteins and lipoproteins. Its presence in any lipoprotein family therefore reflects functional-structural features independent of density, size or other properties as used operationally to define lipoproteins.

When the metabolic fate of apoprotein B in VLDL and LDL was determined in detail, we found unexpectedly that during the first 2 hours of the study, more than 80% of the labeled apoprotein B injected as part of the ^{125}I-VLDL has disappeared from the circulation. Labeled apoprotein B constituted about 17% of the injected radioactivity. The peak of radioactivity in LDL did not exceed 2.5% of the injected dose, and 2 hours after the injection, ^{125}I-apoprotein B in VLDL and LDL amounted to only 1.7% of the injected dose. Since several additional experiments have demonstrated that apoprotein B is not cleared from circulation when the metabolism of VLDL is delayed, and since labeled LDL decays from rat plasma at a relatively slow rate ($t_{1/2}$ 4-6 hours [25-28]), we have concluded that the clearance of apoprotein B from circulation in normal rats occurred at the stage of formation of the intermediate lipoprotein. Similar observations were reported by Faergeman et al., using VLDL labeled in its protein moiety with ^{14}C-lysine (29). Thus, in rats, an additional pathway of lipoprotein metabolism could be delineated: an extremely rapid clearance from circulation of a partially degraded VLDL or intermediate lipoprotein (Figure 3). This pathway doubtlessly explains the low

levels of rat plasma LDL in the face of a high rate of apoprotein B
synthesis and secretion as an integral part of VLDL.   Together
with Drs. O. and Y. Stein, we were able to demonstrate that the
major site of catabolism of VLDL apoproteins is the liver (30).
The study has also indicated that VLDL particles become attached
to the sinusoidal liver cell boundary prior to being catabolized.   At
this site, the following lipolytic enzymes were demonstrated: triglyceride hydrolase, phospholipase and cholesterol hydrolase.
The binding of VLDL to cell boundaries may therefore represent
an initial phase of hydrolysis of esterified lipids, proceeding the
interionization of the lipoprotein.

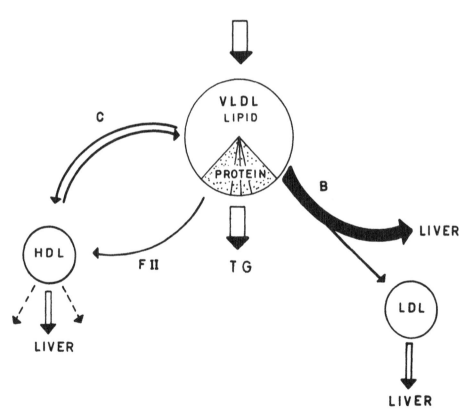

Figure 3: Schematic representation of the pathways of metabolism
of rat plasma VLDL apoproteins.

CHARACTERIZATION OF THE INTERMEDIATE LIPOPROTEINS: STUDIES IN RATS

Partially degraded VLDL particles were prepared by incubation of radio-iodinated VLDL with lipoprotein lipase rich (post heparin) plasma (31, 32). Similar to the previous experiments, we have analyzed the radioactivity associated with the various lipoproteins isolated by flotation and have determined the content of labeled lipids and labeled apoproteins in each lipoprotein. A schematic representation of a typical experiment is shown in Figure 4. We have chosen to carry the incubations on with whole plasma rather than any of the partially purified lipoprotein lipases since we aimed at mimicking the in vivo situation as much as possible. Indeed, as far as the ^{125}I-apoprotein composition of the various lipoproteins is concerned, the in vitro produced intermediate lipoprotein was indistinguishable from that isolated from rats injected with ^{125}I-VLDL and heparin.

After the interaction of ^{125}I-VLDL with post-heparin plasma, about one-third to one-half of the radioactivity in lipids and apoproteins disappeared from the density range of the VLDL (d < 1.019 g/ml) and was recovered with higher density lipoproteins, predominantly HDL. Labeled apoproteins of lipoproteins were analyzed after delipidation and polyacrylamide gel electrophoresis. The main difference between VLDL incubated with normal (control) plasma and VLDL incubated with lipoprotein lipase rich (post heparin) plasma, was the almost complete disappearance of labeled apoprotein C from the latter lipoprotein (Figure 5). In sharp contrast, more than 80% of the labeled apoprotein B was associated with the partially degraded VLDL. About one-third of labeled apoproteins at the upper half of the gels (predominantly the arginine-rich protein) have also disappeared from the density range of the partially degraded VLDL (intermediate lipoprotein). The small increase in LDL radioactivity was due primarily to labeled apoprotein B. However, it did not exceed 10-15% of the labeled apoprotein B introduced into the incubation mixture.

The pattern of labeled apoproteins in the two forms of HDL (d = 1.04-1.085 and 1.085-1.21 g/ml) was similar after the incubation of ^{125}I-VLDL with either normal or post-heparin plasma, and HDL contained most of the ^{125}I-apoprotein C which disappeared from the density range of VLDL. In several additional experiments we were able to demonstrate that the disappearance of apoprotein C

EFFECT OF HEPARIN ON VLDL IN VITRO

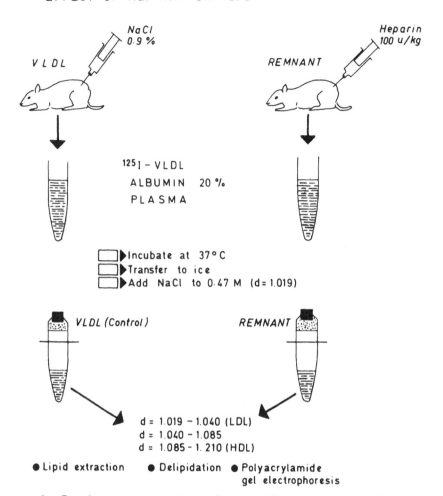

Figure 4: In vitro preparation of partially degraded VLDL (IDL, Remnant).

from VLDL was graded and related, at least in part, to the degree of lipolysis. Thus, ^{125}I-apoprotein C content in VLDL was inversely proportional to the time of incubation and proportional to the amount of VLDL added to the incubation mixture.

VLDL and the intermediate lipoprotein were isolated in large amounts and further characterized. The contribution of protein to the mass of the particles was 14% and 19%, respectively. The two lipoproteins differed in lipid composition. Triglycerides,

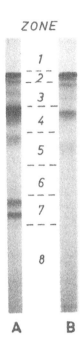

Figure 5: Polyacrylamide gel electrophoresis of apoproteins isolated after incubation of VLDL with plasma obtained from normal
rats (A) and rats injected with heparin (B).

phospholipids and cholesterol constituted 62%, 14% and 9% of the
VLDL mass, and 46%, 20% and 15% of the mass of the intermediate
lipoprotein. Individual apoproteins were separated by gel chromatography on Sephadex G-150. Three apoprotein fractions were
isolated: apoprotein B; an apoprotein fraction designated VS-2 and
containing predominantly the arginine-rich protein; and apoprotein
C. The percent distribution of protein among the three fractions
was identical in original VLDL, and in VLDL incubated with normal
plasma, and was 21%, 22% and 57%, respectively. In contrast,
the intermediate lipoprotein isolated after incubation of VLDL with
post-heparin plasma was composed of 57% apoprotein B, 34% apoprotein VS-2 and only 9% apoprotein C. A major difference between
VLDL and its degraded form - the intermediate lipoprotein - therefore was their apoprotein composition.

We next measured the mean flotation rate (Sf) of the two lipoproteins and determined their mean diameter using analytical

ultracentrifugation and electron microscopy. The mean Sf rate of
VLDL was 115 and that of the intermediate lipoprotein 30.5. The
diameter of VLDL particles varied between 300-600 Å, with a
mean of 427 Å. Intermediate lipoprotein particles were more
homogeneous with regard to their diameter with a mean diameter
of 269 Å.

The composition of lipoproteins is customarily presented as
percent contribution of lipid and protein constituents to the total
mass. Since lipoproteins are discrete and definite entities, an
attempt to determine the properties of a <u>single particle</u> should be
made. We have estimated the weight of a single particle from the
mean of Sf rate of VLDL and intermediate lipoprotein. The values
obtained were 23×10^6 and 7.0×10^6 daltons. The ratio of these
values was very similar to that of their calculated volumes. Since
the relative contribution of individual components to the mass of
the particles was determined, we were able to calculate the
absolute content of each constituent in <u>one particle</u> (Table 1). Apoprotein B content in one VLDL particle and one intermediate lipoprotein particle was virtually identical - 0.7 million daltons. Such
a result is possible only when <u>one and only one intermediate lipoprotein particle is produced from each VLDL particle.</u> In contrast,
the content of all other constituents in VLDL particles is reduced
after their interaction with lipoprotein-lipase rich plasma. The
intermediate lipoprotein contained about 20% of the VLDL triglycerides, 41% phospholipids, 37% unesterified cholesterol, 68%
cholesteryl esters, 60% apoprotein VS-2 and only 7% of the original
apoprotein C.

THE INTERMEDIATE LIPOPROTEIN OF HUMAN ORIGIN

In the human, data on the content of lipids and proteins in
VLDL and LDL subfractions of different Sf rates was published by
Eisenberg, Bilheimer, Levy and Lindgren (24, 33); Lindgren and
coworkers (34); and Hammond and Fisher (35). When all these
results are plotted to express the absolute amount of each constituent in a single particle, the pattern obtained is similar to that
described in rats. Again, the amount of triglycerides, phospholipids, unesterified cholesterol and cholesteryl esters in one particle diminished as the particle became smaller. The content of
apoprotein C in LDL particles decreased to an almost undetectable
level. In sharp contrast, apoprotein B content was similar in all

Table 1

LIPID AND APOPROTEIN CONTENT OF SINGLE VLDL AND
INTERMEDIATE LIPOPROTEIN (IDL) PARTICLES

Constituent	VLDL	IDL
	daltons x 10^{-6}/particle	
Particle weight	23.1	7.0
Lipids	19.9	5.7
Triglyceride	14.1	3.1
Phospholipid	3.3	1.4
Cholesterol, Free	1.5	0.5
Cholesterol, Esterified	1.0	0.7
Apoproteins	3.2	1.3
Apoprotein B	0.70	0.73
Apoprotein VS-2	0.73	0.44
Apoprotein C	1.80	0.12

particles which vary in weight between 30 x 10^6 to 2.2 x 10^6 daltons. Thus, one to one relationship between VLDL and LDL particles must exist also in the humans. These results indicate that a "fundamental substructure" containing a constant amount of apoprotein B exists in each particle regardless of its size, weight, origin or content of other lipid and protein constituents. The amount of apoprotein B in the fundamental substructure is about 0.4 million daltons. During the metabolism of these lipoproteins, they lose not only triglycerides, but also some of each of their other constituents, except for the apoprotein B fundamental substructure.

METABOLIC RELATIONSHIPS AMONG LIPOPROTEINS

Functionally, five lipoproteins are defined: Chylomicrons, VLDL, IDL, LDL and HDL. They are defined by their function and metabolism rather than composition, size, flotation properties, apoprotein content, etc. All lipoproteins participate in the exceedingly important process of triglyceride transport. Chylomicrons and VLDL are the primary triglyceride carrying lipoproteins. They are regarded as bistructural lipoproteins containing apoprotein B and apoprotein C subunits. They are susceptible to the activity of extrahepatic lipoprotein lipase which results in the disintegration of the complex lipoproteins and dissociation of the two subunits. Apoprotein C subunits are transferred to HDL; apoprotein B subunits are converted to IDL and LDL.

The normal metabolism of VLDL and chylomicrons is initiated by triglyceride hydrolysis; the pathway, however, involves many phases of delipidation and deproteination of the particle. It is taking place at close proximity to the capillary endothelial cells, a site of activity of extrahepatic lipoprotein lipases. The triglyceride-rich lipoproteins become attached to the enzyme sites by a mechanism yet unknown. The overall process of lipoprotein degradation involves hydrolysis of triglycerides and removal of phospholipids (predominantly lecithin), cholesterol (predominantly unesterified) and apoprotein C. Some or most of the lecithin molecules are also hydrolized to form lysolecithin which is removed rapidly from the circulation (36). Apoprotein C, possibly complemented with phospholipids and cholesterol, is transferred to HDL. Partially degraded particles are then released from the enzyme site into the circulation. They have lost some of their apoprotein C subunits. They contain the full complement of apoprotein B present in the original particle. These particles are found in plasma sub-fraction of Sf rates lower than the original particles and are capable of interacting again with the endothelial lipoprotein lipase. The degradation of any one particle thus occurs in multiple similar steps and during interaction of the particle with many endothelial lipase sites. After multiple interactions, the particle loses most of its triglycerides as well as phospholipids, free cholesterol and apoprotein C. Its further interaction with endothelial lipoprotein lipase sites of extrahepatic tissues becomes limited or is even completely inhibited. From a metabolic point of view, this particle represents the true intermediate lipoprotein.

The intermediate lipoprotein is thus defined by its mode of formation. It is even more importantly defined by its unique meta-bolic fate. In rats, most of the intermediate lipoprotein is re-moved from the circulation. In humans, it is metabolized to form "a final breakdown lipoprotein" - the LDL - by a mechanism yet unknown. We suggest that this pathway involves primarily the hepatic lipoprotein lipase, and occurs in the liver. LDL, HDL and possibly also IDL are therefore the lipoprotein forms which are cleared from circulation by tissue cells. Aberrations of one or more of the multiple pathways of the integrated scheme of lipoprotein metabolism may result in formation of excessive plasma lipoprotein levels. Understanding of these pathways, however, may provide a rational basis for the treatment of the lipid trans-port disorders.

REFERENCES

1. Shore, B. and V. Shore. Biochemistry 7: 2773, 1968.
2. Shore, B. and V. Shore. Biochemistry 7: 3996, 1968.
3. Shore, B. and V. Shore. Biochemistry 8: 4510, 1969.
4. Shore, B. and V. Shore. In: Blood Lipids and Lipoproteins, G. Nelson, editor. Interscience, New York, 1972.
5. Fredrickson, D. S., S. Lux and P. Herbert. Adv. Exptl. Med. and Biol. 26: 25, 1972.
6. Gotto, A. M., W. V. Brown, R. I. Levy, M. E. Birnbaumer, and D. S. Fredrickson. J. Clin. Invest. 51: 1486, 1972.
7. W. V. Brown, R. I. Levy and D. S. Fredrickson. J. Biol. Chem. 244: 5687, 1969.

8. Brown, W. V., R. I. Levy and D. S. Fredrickson. Biochim. Biophys. Acta 200: 573, 1970.

9. Brown, W. V., R. I. Levy and D. S. Fredrickson. J. Biol. Chem. 245: 6588, 1970.

10. Albers, J. J. and A. M. Scanu. Biochim. Biophys. Acta 236: 97, 1971.

11. LaRosa, J. C., R. I. Levy, P. Herbert, S. E. Lux, and D. S. Fredrickson. Biochem. Biophys. Res. Commun. 41: 57, 1970.

12. Brown, W. V. and M. L. Baginsky. Biochem. Biophys. Res. Commun. 46: 375, 1972.

13. Scanu, A. M., J. Toth, C. Edelstein, S. Koga, and E. Stiller. Biochemistry 8: 3309, 1969.

14. Kostner, G. and P. Alaupovic. FEBS Letters 15: 320, 1971.

15. Kostner, G. and A. Holasek. Biochemistry 11: 1217, 1972.

16. Pearlstein, E., P. Eggena and F. Aladjem. Immunochemistry 8: 865, 1971.

17. Shore, B. and V. Shore. Biochem. Biophys. Res. Commun. 58: 1, 1974.

18. Shelburne, F. A. and S. H. Quarfordt. J. Biol. Chem. 249: 1428, 1974.

19. Bersot, T. P., W. V. Brown, R. I. Levy, H. G. Windmueller, and D. S. Fredrickson. Biochemistry 9: 3427, 1970.

20. Koga, S., L. Bolis, and A. M. Scanu. Biochim. Biophys. Acta 236: 416, 1971.

21. Bilheimer, D. W., S. Eisenberg, and R. I. Levy. J. Clin. Invest. 40: 480, 1971.

22. Bilheimer, D. W., S. Eisenberg, and R. I. Levy. Biochim. Biophys. Acta 260: 212, 1972.

23. Eisenberg, S., D. W. Bilheimer, and R. I. Levy. Biochim. Biophys. Acta 280: 94, 1972.

24. Eisenberg, S., D. W. Bilheimer, R. I. Levy and F. T. Lindgren. Biochim. Biophys. Acta 326: 361, 1973.

25. Eisenberg, S. and D. Rachmilewitz. Biochim. Biophys. Acta 326: 378, 1973.

26. Eisenberg, S. and D. Rachmilewitz. Biochim. Biophys. Acta 326: 391, 1973.

27. Hay, R. V., L. A. Pottenger, A. L. Reingold, G. S. Getz, and R. W. Wissler. Biochem. Biophys. Res. Commun. 44: 1471, 1971.

28. Roheim, P. S., H. Hirsch, D. Edelstein and D. Rachmilewitz. Biochim. Biophys. Acta 278: 517, 1972.

29. Faergeman, O., T. Sata, J. P. Kane, and R. J. Havel. Circulation (Suppl. III): 114, 1974.

30. Stein, O. , D. Rachmilewitz, L. Sanger, S. Eisenberg, and
    Y. Stein. Biochim. Biophys. Acta 360: 205, 1974.
31. Eisenberg, S. and D. Rachmilewitz. Circulation (Suppl. IV):
    111, 1973.
32. Eisenberg, S. and D. Rachmilewitz. In preparation.
33. Eisenberg, S. , D. W. Bilheimer, R. I. Levy and F. T. Lindgren.
    Biochim. Biophys. Acta 260: 329, 1972.
34. Lindgren, F. T. , L. C. Jensen and F. T. Hatch. In: Blood
    Lipids and Lipoproteins. G. Nelson, editor. Interscience,
    New York, 1972.
35. Hammond, M. G. and W. Fisher. J. Biol. Chem. 246: 5454,
    1971.
36. Eisenberg, S. Unpublished observations.

STEROID REQUIREMENTS FOR SUPPRESSION OF HMG CoA

REDUCTASE ACTIVITY IN CULTURED HUMAN FIBROBLASTS

Joseph L. Goldstein, Jerry R. Faust,
Gloria Y. Brunschede and Michael S. Brown

Department of Internal Medicine, University of Texas
Southwestern Medical School, Dallas, Texas

The rate of cholesterol synthesis in cultured human fibro-blasts is determined by the activity of 3-hydroxy-3-methylglutaryl coenzyme A reductase (HMG CoA reductase) (1-3). The activity of this enzyme in normal fibroblasts becomes suppressed when low density lipoproteins (LDL) bind to specific receptors on the cell surface (4, 5) and deliver cholesterol and cholesteryl esters to the cell (6). High density lipoproteins (HDL), which do not bind to the LDL receptor (4, 5), do not increase the cellular con-tent of cholesterol and cholesteryl esters (6) nor do they suppress HMG CoA reductase activity and cholesterol synthesis (1, 3). Cultured fibroblasts from subjects with the autosomal dominant disorder familial hypercholesterolemia are deficient in the LDL receptor (4, 5, 7). As a result, LDL does not bind to the cells (4, 5, 7), cholesterol is not transferred intracellularly (6), HMG CoA reductase activity is not suppressed, and cholesterol is over-produced (2, 3).

Considered together, the evidence to date suggests that it is the accumulation of cholesterol delivered to the cell by LDL that results in suppression of HMG CoA reductase activity. The de-tailed intermediate biochemical events by which the sterol acts inside the cell are not known.

Although the fibroblasts from homozygotes with familial

hypercholesterolemia do not respond to LDL, these mutant cells show a normal suppression of HMG CoA reductase activity when incubated with cholesterol added in a nonlipoprotein form (3, 8). Such nonlipoprotein cholesterol can enter the cell in the absence of the LDL receptor and thus suppress enzyme activity.

STEROID STRUCTURAL REQUIREMENTS FOR SUPPRESSION

In view of the potential theoretical and practical implications of sterol-mediated suppression of HMG CoA reductase activity, we have recently tested the effect of 47 steroid compounds on the activity of this enzyme in human fibroblasts. In these studies, the test steroid was dissolved in ethanol and the ethanolic steroid solution was then added to the medium surrounding the monolayers of fibroblasts (8). After an appropriate period of incubation, the cells were then harvested and a cell-free extract was prepared for measurement of HMG CoA reductase activity (8).

As a group, the C-17, C-18 and C-19 steroids had little to no effect on HMG CoA reductase (8). However, many of the C-27 sterols that were tested proved to be significantly more potent than cholesterol in their ability to suppress the activity of this enzyme. In particular, the addition of a second hydroxyl or keto group to the cholesterol molecule increased the effectiveness of the sterol by appoximately 100-fold when expressed on a weight bases. The additional oxy function was effective when placed at any of a variety of positions on the sterol nucleus or side chain, provided that the 3-position was always occupied with either a hydroxyl or keto group (Fig. 1). The lack of specificity for the location of the additional oxy group suggested that its effect was to increase the polarity of the sterol molecule rather than to enhance its interaction with a specific intracellular receptor.

7-OXY CHOLESTEROL ANALOGUES

To study further the action of these potent sterol analogues, 7-ketocholesterol was selected as a model compound. When incubated with fibroblasts from either normal subjects or patients with familial hypercholesterolemia, 7-ketocholesterol not only was 100 times more potent than cholesterol on a molar basis, but it also acted much more quickly, suppressing HMG CoA reductase

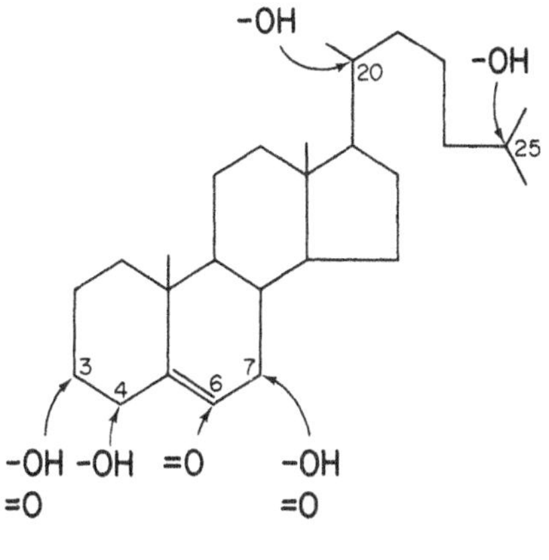

Figure 1: Structural modifications of cholesterol that enhance its ability to suppress HMG CoA reductase activity in human fibro-blasts from both normal subjects and patients with familial hyper-cholesterolemia. In the presence of either a hydroxyl or a keto group at position 3, the addition of a single oxy function (either as a hydroxyl or keto group) to positions 4, 6, 7, 20, or 25 resulted in a marked increase in the potency of suppression of HMG CoA re-ductase activity as compared to that of cholesterol. These high potency sterol analogues included: 5-cholesten-3β, 4β-diol, 6-ketocholestanol, 7α-hydroxycholesterol, 7β-hydroxycholesterol, 7-ketocholesterol, 20α hydroxycholesterol, and 25α-hydroxycho-lesterol.

activity by more than 90 per cent in 2 hours (8). The effect of 7-ketocholesterol on this enzyme was highly specific. Whereas the incorporation of $[^{14}C]$acetate into sterols was reduced by more than 90 per cent in 2 hours, the incorporation of $[^{14}C]$mevalonate into sterols was not significantly affected. Moreover, the in-corporation of $[^{14}C]$acetate into saponifiable lipids and the incor-poration of $[^{3}H]$leucine into protein were similarly unaffected (8).

Reduction of the 7-keto group to give either 7α-hydroxy or 7β-hydroxycholesterol did not affect the ability of the sterol to suppress HMG CoA reductase activity (Figure 2). On the other hand, when the 7-hydroxyl group was esterified with benzoic acid (5-cholesten-3β, 7β-diol-7-benzoate), all inhibitory activity was lost. Inhibitory activity was also reduced when the 3-hydroxyl

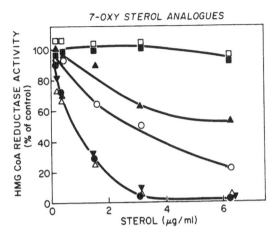

Figure 2: Effect of varying concentrations of 7-oxy cholesterol
analogues on HMG CoA reductase activity of normal human fibroblasts. Cells were grown to near confluence in 60 x 15 mm petri
dishes as previously described (8). After 24 hours of growth in
medium containing lipoprotein-deficient human serum (5 mg pro-
tein/ml), the culture medium was replaced with 2 ml of fresh
growth medium containing lipoprotein deficient serum (5 mg pro-
tein/ml) and the indicated amount of sterol added in 20 μl of ethanol.
After incubation at 37° for 4 hours, cell-free extracts were prepared and assayed for HMG CoA reductase activity (8). The sterols
tested were: □, 5-cholesten-3β, 7β-diol-7-benzoate; ■, 5α-
cholestan-7-one; ▲, 5β-cholestan-3α, 7α, 12α-triol; 0, 3, 5-chole-
stadien-7-one; Δ, 7α-hydroxy-cholesterol; ▽, 7β-hydroxychole-
sterol; and ●, 7-ketocholesterol.

group was absent and the B ring saturated (5α-cholestan-7-one).
Two other 7-oxy sterols, 5β-cholesten-3α, 7α, 12α-triol and 3, 5-
cholestadien-7-one, were significantly more effective than cholesterol, but were less potent than 7-ketocholesterol (Figure 2).
using cultured mouse L cells and liver cells, Kandutsch and Chen
have also found that 7-oxy derivatives of cholesterol are much
more potent than the parent compound in suppression of HMG CoA
reductase activity and cholesterol synthesis (9).

UPTAKE OF 7-KETOCHOLESTEROL BY FIBROBLASTS

One reason for the enhanced potency of 7-ketocholesterol

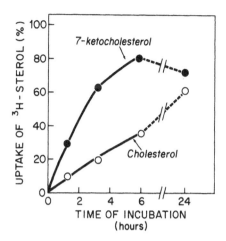

Figure 3: Time course of uptake of 7-ketocholesterol[1, 2-^{3}H] and cholesterol[1, 2-^{3}H] by normal human fibroblasts. Cells were grown to near confluence in 60 x 15 mm petri dishes as previously described (4, 5). After 24 hours of growth in medium containing human lipoprotein-deficient serum (2. 5 mg protein/ml), 2 μCi of either cholesterol[1, 2-^{3}H] (New England Nuclear Corp. , 52. 6 Ci/mmole) or 7-ketocholesterol[1, 2-^{3}H] (52. 6 Ci/mmole, synthesized as previously described [10]) were dissolved in 20 μl of ethanol and added to the lipoprotein-deficient medium surrounding the cell monolayers. After incubation at 37° for the indicated time, each cell monolayer was washed extensively at 4° in a buffer containing 50 mM Tris-Dl, pH 7. 4; 0. 15 M NaCl, and 2 mg/ml of bovine serum albumin (4). The cellular content of ^{3}H-sterol was then determined by counting an aliquot of a chloroform:methanol (2:1) extract. To confirm the identity of the ^{3}H-radioactivity, aliquots of the chloroform:methanol extract at each time point were sub-jected to thin layer chromatography on silica gel using benzene: ethyl acetate (1:1). In each case, more than 95% of the radio-activity was located in the appropriate sterol. Each point repre-sents the mean of values obtained from duplicate dishes.

relative to cholesterol may be that the more polar analogue is taken up more rapidly by the cells. When an equimolar concentration of tracer amounts of cholesterol[1, 2-^{3}H] and 7-ketocholesterol [1, 2-^{3}H] were incubated with monolayers of normal fibroblasts, the initial rate of cellular uptake was approximately 3-fold greater for the 7-keto derivative (Figure 3). Thin-layer chromatography

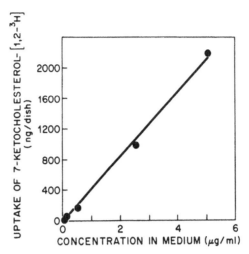

Figure 4: Relation of the rate of cellular uptake of 7-ketocholesterol to its concentration in the medium. Normal human fibroblasts were grown to confluence in 60 x 15 mm petri dishes as previously described (4, 5). After 24 hours of growth in medium containing human lipoprotein-deficient serum (2. 5 mg protein/ml), the cells were incugated with the indicated final concentration of 7-keto-cholesterol[1, 2-^{3}H] added to the 2 ml of medium in 20 μl of ethanol. After incubation at 37° for 6 hours, each cell monolayer was washed extensively at 4° as described in the legend to Figure 3, after which the washed cells were scraped into and dissolved in 1 ml of 0. 1 N NaOH. The cellular content of 7-ketocholesterol was then determined by counting a 0. 7 ml aliquot of this solution in 15 ml of Aquasol (New England Nuclear Corp.). Each point represents the mean of values obtained from duplicate dishes. The average content of total cell protein in each dish was 0. 3 mg.

of extracts from the cells indicated that at each time point the bulk of the radioactivity taken up by the cells (e. g. , 97% for 7-ketocholesterol and 95% for cholesterol) had not been converted to other metabolites.

At concentrations of 7-ketocholesterol up to 5 μg/ml, the initial rate of uptake was linearly proportional to the initial concentration in the medium (Figure 4), suggesting that in the concentration range that suppresses HMG CoA reductase activity no saturable uptake process for 7-ketocholesterol appears to be involved.

IMPLICATIONS

The observation that derivatives of cholesterol can be used to suppress the synthesis of this sterol in human cells raises several timely questions. First, Is the true physiologic intracellular regulator of HMG CoA reductase activity cholesterol itself or one of its polar metabolites, such as 7α-hydroxycholesterol, the first committed intermediate in bile acid synthesis? Two findings in the present study mitigate against the likelihood that 7α-hydroxycholesterol is the physiologic regulator: 1) other cholesterol analogues with oxy functions located at widely varying sites on the sterol molecule were equally as potent as 7α-hydroxycholesterol, and 2) we have been unable to demonstrate significant conversion of cholesterol$[1, 2-^3H]$ to any more polar metabolite in cultured human fibroblasts. Second, Do these potent sterol compounds suppress HMG CoA reductase activity by altering the catalytic capacity of the enzyme or do they act by reducing the number of enzyme molecules through an alteration in the rate of synthesis and/or degradation of the enzyme? Thus far, we (8) and others (9) have not been able to demonstrate in vitro that 7-ketocholesterol has a direct inhibitory effect on cell-free preparations of HMG CoA reductase. Finally, Will these potent compounds prove useful in vivo in suppressing cholesterol synthesis in patients with hypercholesterolemia?

ACKNOWLEDGEMENTS

This work was supported by grants from the American Heart Association (72629 and 74983) and the National Institutes of Health (GM 19258 and HL 16024). Joseph L. Goldstein is a recipient of a Research Career Development Award 1-Kr-GM-70, 277 from the United States Public Health Service. Michael S. Brown is an Established Investigator of the American Heart Association.

REFERENCES

1. Brown, M. S., Dana, S. E., and Goldstein, J. L. Proc. Nat. Acad. Sci. USA 70: 2162-2166, 1973.
2. Goldstein, J. L. and Brown, M. S. Proc. Nat. Acad. Sci. USA 70: 2804-2808, 1973.

3. Brown, M. S., Dana, S. E., and Goldstein, J. L. J. Biol. Chem. 249: 789-796, 1974.

4. Brown, M. S. and Goldstein, J. L. Proc. Nat. Acad. Sci. USA 71: 788-792, 1974.

5. Goldstein, J. L. and Brown, M. S. J. Biol. Chem., in press.

6. Brown, M. S., Dana, S. E., and Goldstein, J. L. Proc. Nat. Acad. Sci. USA, in press, 1974.

7. Brown, M. S. and Goldstein, J. L. Science 185: 61-63, 1974.

8. Brown, M. S. and Goldstein, J. L. J. Biol. Chem., in press, 1974.

9. Kandutsch, A. A. and Chen, H. W. J. Biol. Chem. 248: 8408-8417, 1973.

10. Chicoye, E., Powrie, W. D., and Fennema, O. Lipids 3: 551-556, 1968.

THE IMMUNOLOGY OF SERUM LIPOPROTEINS

Kenneth W. Walton

Department of Experimental Pathology, University of
Birmingham, England

Human serum lipoproteins are effective antigens when
used to immunize other species. Some human serum lipoproteins,
in certain circumstances (see below) even give rise to isologous
antisera. The immunological specificity of antisera to lipoproteins varies with the circumstances of immunization and the nature
and mode of presentation of the lipoprotein antigen, but reactivity
is invariably directed predominantly, if not exclusively, against
the protein part of the molecule (apolipoprotein). Antisera may
be directed against major or minor antigens.

MAJOR ANTIGENS

If animals are immunized with whole human serum, amongst
the many antibodies obtained there are two defining lipid-contain-
in proteins, with α_1-globulin and α_2- or β_1-globulin mobilities
respectively. These are known as the alpha- and beta-lipoproteins
(Figure 1) which correspond broadly to the total high-density
(THDL) and the total low-density lipoproteins (TLDL), as characterized ultracentrifugally. When suitably isolated and purified such
antisera give a "reaction of non-identity" (Figure 2) in gel-diffusion
reactions suggesting that these two broad classes of lipoproteins
do not have antigenic components in common but are distinct and
different.

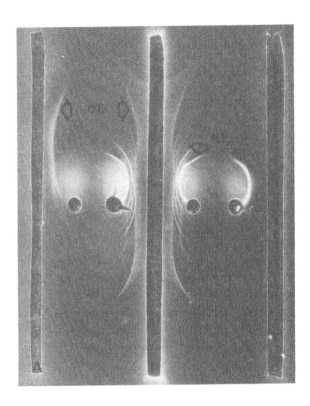

Figure 1: Immunoelectrophoresis of normal serum (in all four wells) against antiserum to whole serum (central trough, P); antiserum to alpha-lipoprotein (THDL) in left-hand trough, marked A; and antiserum to beta-lipoprotein (TLDL) in right-hand trough, marked B. Plate washed, dried and stained with azocarmine for protein with Sudan Black for lipid. Note arcs characteristic for alpha lipoprotein (αL) and beta lipoprotein (βL) marked with arrows. (Reprinted from Walton, 1973b, with permission).

Within each broad class of lipoproteins there is physico-chemical heterogeneity, especially with regard to lipid composition and therefore in relation to density and sedimentation-flotation characteristics. For example, conventionally the THDL are divided into HDL_2 and HDL_3 sub-classes; while TLDL are divided into LDL_2, LDL_1 and VLDL (Table 1). Antisera raised to the lipoproteins from a pool of the sub-classes, or to individual sub-classes (Figure 3). This is because such antisera are directed

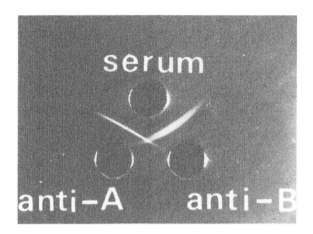

Figure 2: Gel-diffusion reaction of normal serum with antisera raised against intact native alpha lipoprotein (anti-A) and against beta lipoprotein (anti-B). Note crossing of precipitation arcs in "reaction of non-identity." (Reprinted from Walton, 1973b, with permission).

TABLE 1

Molecular and immunological characteristics of lipoproteins

Lipoprotein		Serum Concentration (mg%)	Molecular Weight*	Antigens[†] (apolipoproteins)
TLDL	VLDL	80–150	$6\text{-}50 \times 10^6$	B+C
	LDL_1	25–50	3.4×10^6	B(+C)
	LDL_2	290–340	2.3×10^6	B
Lp(a)		$2\text{--}80^\phi$	$4.8 \times 10^{6\phi}$	$B+Lp(a)^\phi$
THDL	HDL_2	230	4.0×10^5	A(+C)
	HDL_3	70–200	1.75×10^5	A

* From data of Oncley (1963)   [†] Terminology of Alaupovic (1972)

ϕ From data of Ehnholm et al (1971; 1972)

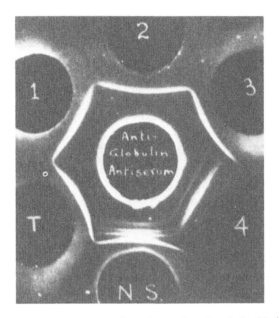

Figure 3: Reaction between polyvalent (anti-globulin) antiserum and lipoprotein fractions. Central well: anti-globulin antiserum; peripheral wells: 1, LDL_2; 2, LDL_1; 3, VLDL; 4, serum freed from TLDL; N. S. , whole serum; T, TLDL (mixture of 1, 2, and 3). Note "reaction of identity" of curved arcs given by T, 1, 2, and 3 with each other and with curved arc nearest to antigen well marked NS showing shared antigen (apolipoprotein B) present in all these specimens (see also Figure 4). (Reprinted from Walton and Darke, 1964, with permission).

predominantly or exclusively against the major antigens <u>common</u> to the sub-class (i. e. , to the antigenic determinants of apolipoprotein B which are common to LDL_2, LDL_1 and VLDL, in the terminology of Alaupovic (1972) or to those apolipoprotein A which is common to HDL_2 and HDL_3).

Apolipoprotein C

On the other hand, in the case of VLDL, it can be verified (as first shown by Gustafson et al, 1964) that, following delipidation of this sub-class, an additional antigen (apolipoprotein C) can be demonstrated. When serum fractions separated by zonal

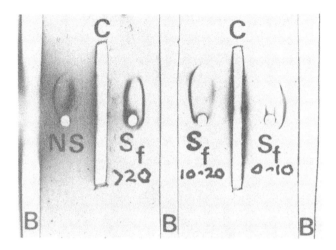

Figure 4: Immunoelectrophoresis of whole serum (well marked NS) and ultracentrifuge fractions against antiserum to apolipoprotein B (troughs marked B) and antiserum to apolipoprotein C (troughs marked C). Note precipitation arcs against whole serum and all fractions with anti-apolipoprotein B; whereas arcs formed strongly against whole serum and VLDL (marked S_f >20), weakly against LDL_1 (marked S_f 10-20) but no reaction with LDL_2 (marked S_f 0-10) with anti-apolipoprotein C. (Reprinted from Walton 1973b, with permission).

ultracentrifugation in a saline density-gradient are examined by immunoelectrophoresis, it is found that anti-apolipoprotein C reacts strongly with whole serum and VLDL, weakly with LDL_1 but not at all with LDL_2 (Figure 4). It has been shown by Kostner and Alaupovic (1972) that apolipoprotein C is also present in HDL.

Apolipoprotein Lp(a)

It was reported by Berg (1963) that some rabbit antisera raised to preparations of human TLDL, isolated from individual donors and cross-absorbed with the TLDL from other donors, contained residual antibodies reacting with the sera of some individuals and not others. The minor antigen thus detected was called the Lp(a) lipoprotein. Population and family studies carried out by a gel-diffusion method suggested that Lp(a) reactivity was a qualitative autosomal dominant genetic marker with a

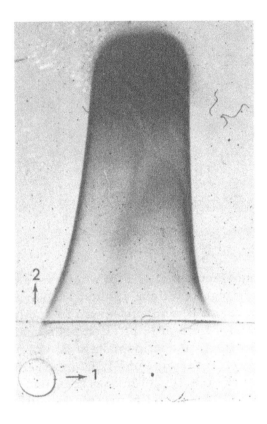

Figure 5: Serum from strongly Lp(a) positive subject subjected to two-dimensional electrophoresis, the second (vertical) dimension being against duospecific antiserum reacting with both apolipoprotein B, apo B, and Lp(a) lipoprotein, apo Lp(a). Note mobility of inner component, Lp(a), corresponding to that of leading (anodal) portion of peak delineating outer component (TLDL). (Reprinted from Walton, 1973b, with permission).

frequency in random Caucasian populations of about 0. 35 (35%).

On the other hand, other investigators (e. g. Rittner and Wichmann, 1967; Ehnholm et al, 1971; Albers and Hazzard, 1974; Walton et al, 1974) using more sensitive and quantitative methods have reported a much higher frequency of Lp(a) reactivity and quantitative variation in concentration of the Lp(a) antigen between individuals.

Table II

Frequency of Lp(a)[+] reactors in unselected population of blood
donors as assessed by dgel-diffusion and by 'rocket' electrophoresis
using sheep anti Lp(a) antiserum.

	Gel-diffusion	'Rocket' technique
No. tested	300	300
No. Lp(a)[+]	133	225
Frequency (%)	44.3	75.0

The work of Simons et al (1970) and of Ehnholm et al (1972)
suggests that immunologically, the Lp(a) lipoprotein consists
essentially of the apolipoprotein B of LDL to which is attached an
additional peptide (the Lpa apolipoprotein) rich in neuraminic acid.
This peptide probably accounts for the somewhat greater density
and faster electrophoretic mobility of the Lp(a) lipoprotein as
compared with LDL (see Figures 5 and 8).

It has been reported from this laboratory (Walton et al, 1974)
that: (a) using one-dimensional 'rocket' electrophoresis (Laurell,
1966) instead of simple gel-diffusion, Lp(a) lipoprotein is detectable in a much higher proportion of a random population (75% - see
Table II); (b) amongst reactors in the random population there is
considerable variation in serum concentration of Lp(a) lipoprotein;
and (c) in hyperlipidemic subjects, still further increase of Lp(a)
reactivity is encountered (Figure 6) but this occurs independent
of the biochemical pattern (Fredrickson Type) of the hyperlipidemia (Table III).

These results suggest that Lp(a) reactivity is not simply
present or absent but shows a variation with concentration which
is to some extent influenced by a general stimulus to overproduc-
tion of lipoproteins (hyperlipidemia). Nevertheless no direct relation was demonstrable between serum lipid and LDL/VLDL
levels on the one hand of of Lp(a) lipoprotein on the other in the
random population. This could be conveniently displayed visually
over a limited range of TLDL concentrations by the 'rocket'

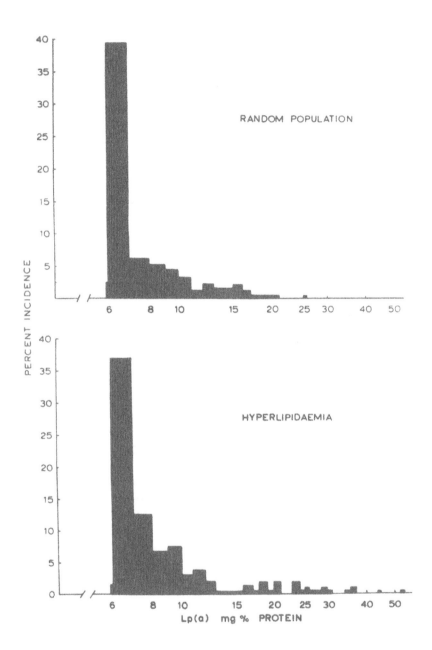

<u>Figure 6:</u>   Comparison of log frequency distribution curves, for
random and hyperlipidemic populations, of Lp(a) lipoprotein
serum levels.   (Reprinted from Walton et al, 1974, with permission).

Table III

Distribution of Lp(a) reactors and non-reactors among
hyperlipidemic subjects typed as recommended by the W. H. O.
(Beaumont et al, 1970)

Type	No. tested	Lp(a)$^+$	Lp(a)$^-$
I	1	1	–
IIA	51	43	8
IIB	97	93	4
III	7	4	3
IV	21	17	4
V	5	0*	5*
Raised pre-β L	60	55	5
Total	242	213	29
Percentage	100	88.0(91.1)[†]	12.0 (8.9)[†]

*Assessment of Lp(a) reactivity in whole serum of
cases of Type V hyperlipidaemia inaccurate for
technical reasons (see Walton et al., 1974).

[†]Figures in parentheses = percentage excluding Type V.

technique by using a duospecific antiserum reacting with both
apolipoprotein B and Lp(a) lipoprotein (Figure 7).

Ag Reactivity

It was first shown by Allison and Blumberg (1961) that the
sera of some patients given many blood transfusions contain iso-
precipitin reactivity against something in the serum of some

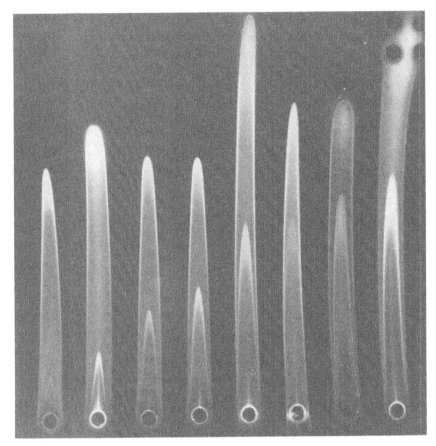

Figure 7: One-dimensional 'rocket' electrophoresis of whole sera against duospecific antiserum reacting with apolipoprotein B (outer 'rocket') and apolipoprotein Lp(a) (inner 'rocket'). Note variation in height of Lp(a) 'rocket' independent of height of apolipoprotein B 'rocket'. (Reprinted from Walton et al, 1974, with permission).

individuals but not others. This was initially designated as the Ag (antigen) factor but was later shown to be TLDL. The reactivity was shown to be inherited as an autosomal dominant trait. Later work (Hirschfeld, 1968; Morganti et al, 1970; Butler et al, 1972) identified four serological factor pairs (Figure 8) which population and family studies showed can be accounted for by assuming

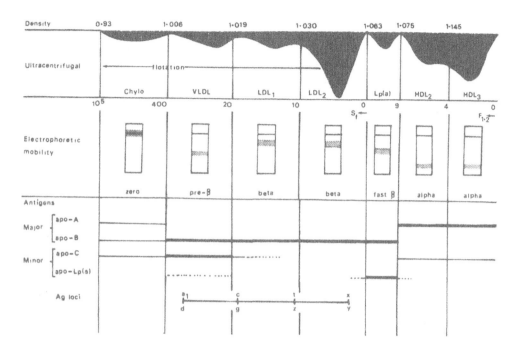

Figure 8: Diagrammatic representation of distribution of major and minor antigens found in serum lipoproteins as characterized in the ultracentrifuge or by electrophoresis on paper or cellulose acetate.

the existence of four closely linked loci, each with co-dominant alleles (Hirschfeld, 1972).

The Ag factors have been found to be distributed throughout the TLDL (i. e. in VLDL, LDL_1 and LDL_2) and to be identifiable only by isologous (human) sera. By analogy with other known human allotypic systems detectable only with isologous sera (e. g. , the Gm and Inv systems on immunoglobulins) and from the distribution of the factors throughout the TLDL, it seems probable that the Ag antigenic determinants may reflect fine differences in the primary structure (amino-acid sequence) of apolipoprotein B, but this has not yet been established.

Table IV

Distribution of commoner Ag phenotypes in hyperlipidemic subjects and their normolipidemic relatives as compared with blood donors, for 7 Ag factors

Reactions with anti-Ag							Normo-lipidaemic	Hyper-lipidaemic	Total (n)	%	Blood donors* %
x	y	a_1	c	g	t	z					
−	+	−	+	+	+	−	10	6	16	13.9	13.5
−	+	+	+	+	+	+	4	10	14	12.2	12.6
−	+	+	+	+	+	−	5	6	11	9.6	4.6
−	+	+	−	+	+	+	2	9	11	9.6	5.5
+	+	+	+	+	+	−	3	7	10	8.7	13.5
+	+	+	+	+	+	+	4	6	10	8.7	0.4
−	+	−	+	−	+	−	2	8	10	8.7	6.7
−	+	−	−	+	+	−	5	3	8	7.0	4.2
+	+	+	−	+	+	+	4	4	8	7.0	7.6
−	+	+	−	+	+	−	3	5	8	7.0	5.0
−	+	−	−	−	+	−	1	2	3	2.6	−
−	+	+	+	−	+	−	1	2	3	2.6	−
Totals							46[†]	69[†]	115[†]		

*Data from sample of 233 blood donors of Berne from Bütler, Morganti and Vierucci (1972).

[†]Phenotypes with frequencies below 1% omitted from this table (3 subjects).

The distribution of the major and minor antigens described above in the lipoproteins as characterized by ultracentrifugation or by simple electrophoresis on solid media is summarized diagrammatically in Figure 8.

APPLICATIONS OF IMMUNOLOGY OF LIPOPROTEINS

Use of Antilipoprotein Antisera in Investigation of Genetics of Hyperlipidemia

The familial incidence of the primary hyperlipidemias is

well-recognized. But epidemiological and family studies have
hitherto been conducted on the basis of comparing cholesterol
values alone or serum lipid patterns (Fredrickson et al, 1967)
between index cases and their relatives, sometimes with confusing
or conflicting results (Hazzard et al, 1974). In our laboratory we
have recently been concerned to see whether the Ag allotypes
(referred to above) might serve as genetic markers more directly
relevant to the study of inheritance patterns in the hyperlipidemias.
So far, 35 families comprising 240 individuals have been identified,
in 116 of whom Ag phenotypes have been determined on the basis

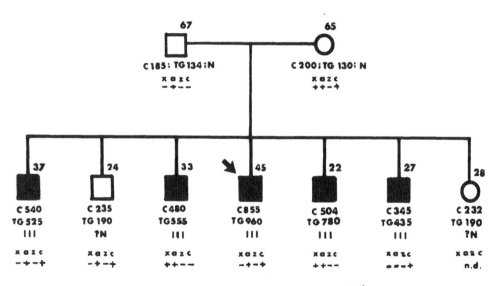

Family A/2 : All y⁺t⁺g⁺.

Figure 9: Distribution of serum lipids (C cholesterol; TG triglycerides in mg/dl), biochemical pattern of alteration of lipoproteins
as determined by cellulose acetate electrophoresis, and Ag phenotypes in a family containing several kindred showing Type II hyperlipidemia. Note that 3 Ag factors in common to all members of
family shown separately from 4 Ag factors differing between individuals. No simple relationship demonstrable between a given
Ag phenotype and expression of hyperlipidemia.

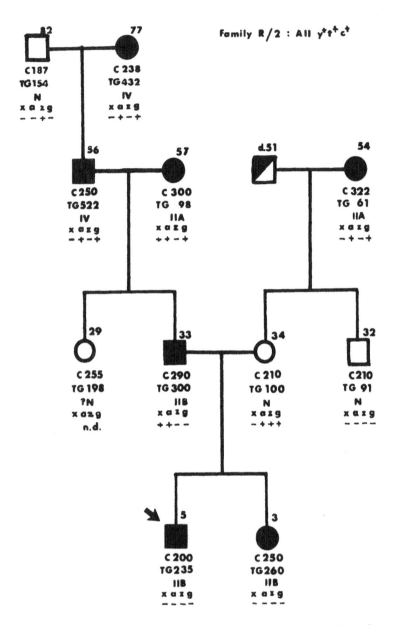

Figure 10: As for Figure 9 in 4 generations of family showing occurrence of Types IV, IIA and IIB hyperlipidemias.

of 7 Ag factors. Some of the results obtained are shown in Table
IV and Figures 9 and 10 from which it can be seen that there is
no simple and direct relationship between a given Ag phenotype
and either expression of a tendancy to hyperlipidemia in general
or of a given biochemical pattern of alteration of lipoproteins
(Fredrickson Type).

Anti-lipoprotein Antisera as Immunohistological Reagents

The association of elevated serum lipids with atherosclerosis
has also been long known. Recent evidence of many kinds, reviewed elsewhere (see Walton, 1969; 1973a; 1974a) suggests that,
among the carriers of serum lipids the TLDL (as opposed to
chylomicra and THDL) are principally implicated, not only in the
formation of arterial lesions, but also in the pathogenesis of the
extravascular lipid deposits (corneal arcus, xanthoma formation)
which frequently accompany atherosclerosis.

For example, using the technique of immunofluorescence,
arterial lesions at all stages of their development (Walton and
Williamson, 1968); lipid deposits in heart valves (Walton,
Williamson and Johnson, 1970); xanthomata (Walton, Thomas and
Dunkerley, 1973); and the corneal arcus (Walton, 1973c) have
been examined. In all these situations it has been shown that at
sites of subendothelial lipid deposition, as revealed by conventional lipid 'stains', it is also possible to demonstrate material
reacting antigenically with antisera detecting apolipoprotein B
but not with antisera detecting apolipoprotein A.

The significance of this observation is, first, that since the
lipid 'stains' are simply pigments with preferential solubility in
fats, they react with lipids but not proteins. On the other hand,
as previously mentioned, anti-lipoprotein antisera react with the
protein part of the molecule (apolipoprotein) and not with the
lipid. Where precise correspondence is demonstrable therefore
between the two techniques it can be inferred that the intact lipoprotein molecule must be present in the lesion.

Second, the reactivity with antisera reacting with apolipoprotein B but not with apolipoprotein A suggests that some component
or components of TLDL but not of THDL is or are concerned in
transporting lipid to the affected sites in lesions. Since TLDL and

THDL contain the same lipids (cholesterol, phospholipids and tri-glycerides) this suggests that it is the nature of the carrier protein for lipids and not that of the lipids which determines the apparently selective <u>retention</u> of TLDL in the atherosclerotic lesion.

The earlier work carried out with this technique (referred to above) used antisera reactive only with apolipoprotein B. Through the kindness of Prof. P. Alaupovic in supplying an antiserum reactive with apolipoprotein C, it was subsequently established that this component is also identifiable in atherosclerotic plaques in both hyperlipidemic and normolipidemic individuals (Walton, 1974b). The topographic distribution of apolipoprotein C was closely similar to that of apolipoprotein B suggesting that both lipoproteins were closely associated spatially, as one would expect them to be if intact VLDL or LDL_1 (carrying both antigens) was present in the lesion along with LDL_2. However the presence of apolipoprotein C in both VLDL and LDL_1 (see Figure 4) means that, from this immunohistological evidence, it is not possible to define precisely the upper limit of molecular size of the components of the TLDL exhibiting atherogenic potential.

Similarly, using fluorescein-labelled anti-Lp(a) lipoprotein antiserum, this antigen has been demonstrated in the arterial lesions of strongly Lp(a) positive individuals, whether hyperlipidemic or normolipidemic (Walton, 1973b; Walton et al, 1974). Once again a close similarity of distribution with that of apolipoprotein B was found consistent with the presence of the intact Lp(a) lipoprotein in the lesion. In the earlier communications (Walton, 1973b; Walton et al, 1974) it was suggested that this finding signified that a lipoprotein with a genetic marker peculiar to a given individual could be demonstrated in that individual's lesions. However, in view of the greater frequency of Lp(a) reactivity subsequently found (Walton et al, 1974) a more factual conclusion might be that minor, as well as major, antigens associated with LDL and/or VLDL can be demonstrated in atherosclerotic lesions.

On the other hand, the molecular size of Lp(a) lipoprotein has been reported to be about 4.8×10^6 by Ehnholm et al (1971). This is larger than LDL_2 (2.3×10^6) or LDL_1 (3.4×10^6) according to the data of Oncley (1963). This is therefore consistent with the finding relating to the distribution of apolipoprotein C in suggesting that lipoproteins of even larger molecular size than LDL_2 are involved in atherogenesis.

ACKNOWLEDGEMENTS

This work was supported by the Medical Research Council and the British Heart Foundation. Figures 1, 2, 4 and 5 are reproduced from Wiss. Veroff. dt. Ges. Ernahrung; Fig. 3 from Immunochemistry; and Figures 6 and 7 from Atherosclerosis with the kind permission of the respective Editors and publishers.

REFERENCES

1. Alaupovic, P.: In Peeters, H. (ed.) Protides of the Biological Fluids, Vol. 19, p. 9, Oxford, Pergamon, 1972.
2. Albers, J. and Hazzard, W.: In Schettler, G. (ed) Atherosclerosis: Proceedings of the 3rd International Symposium, Berlin, Springer Verlag (in press)
3. Allison, A. C. and Blumberg, B. S.: Lancet i, 634, 1961.
4. Beaumont, J. L., Carlson, L. A., Cooper, G. R., Fejfar, Z., Fredrickson, D. S. and Strasser, T.: Bull. Wld. Hlth. Org. 43: 891, 1970.
5. Butler, R., Morganti, G. and Vierucci, A.: In Peeters, H. (ed.) Protides of the Biological Fluids, Vol. 19, p. 161, Oxford, Pergamon, 1972.
6. Berg, K.: Acta Path. Micribiol. Scand. 59: 369, 1963.
7. Ehnholm, C., Garoff, H., Simons, K. and Aro, H.: Biochim. Biophys. Acta 236: 421, 1971.
8. Ehnholm, C., Garoff, H., Renkonen, O. and Simons, K.: Biochemistry 11: 3229, 1972.
9. Fredrickson, D. S., Levy, R. I. and Lees, R. S.: New Engl. J. Med. 267: 32, 94, 148, 215, 273, 1967.
10. Gustafsson, A., Alaupovic, P. and Furman, R. H.: Biochim. Biophys. Acta 84: 767, 1964.
11. Hazzard, W., Goldstein, J., Schrott, H., Motulsky, A. and Bierman, E.: In Schettler, G. (ed.) Atherosclerosis: Proceedings of the 3rd International Symposium, Berlin, Springer Verlag, (in press)
12. Hirschfeld, J.: Ser. Haematol. 1: 38, 1968.
13. Hirschfeld, J.: In Peeters, H. (ed.) Protides of the Biolological Fluids, Vol. 19, p. 157, Oxford, Pergamon, 1972.

14. Kostner, G. and Alaupovic, P. : In Peeters, H. (ed.) Pro-
    tides of the Biological Fluids, Vol. 19, p. 59, Oxford,
    Pergamon, 1972.

15. Laurell, C. B. : Analyt. Biochem. 15: 45, 1966.

16. Morganti, G. , Beolchini, P. E. , Butler, R. , Brunner, E.
    and Vierucci, A. : Humangenetik 10: 244, 1970.

17. Oncley, J. L. : In Folch-Pi, J. L. and Bauer, H. (eds.)
    Brain Lipids and Lipoproteins and the Leucodystrophies,
    p. 1, Amsterdam, Elsevier, 1963.

18. Rittner, C. and Wichmann, D. : Humangenetik 5: 42, 1967.

19. Simons, K. , Ehnholm, C. , Renkonen, O. and Bloth, B. :
    Acta Path. Microbiol. Scand. 78: 459, 1970.

20. Walton, K. W. : In Bittar, E. E. and Bittar, N. (eds.) The
    Biological Basis of Medicine, Vol. 6, pp. 193-223, New
    York, Academic Press, 1969.

21. Walton, K. W. : In Brocklehurst, J. C. (ed.) Textbook of
    Geriatric Medicine and Gerontology, pp. 770112, Edinburgh,
    Churchill Livingstone, 1973a.

22. Walton, K. W. : Wiss. Veroff. dt. Ges. Ernahrung 23: 47,
    1973b.

23. Walton, K. W. : J. Path. 111: 263, 1973c.

24. Walton, K. W. : Amer. J. Cardiol. , in press

25. Walton, K. W. : In Schettler, G. (ed.) Atherosclerosis:
    Proceedings of the 3rd International Symposium, Berlin,
    Springer Verlag, in press

26. Walton, K. W. and Darke, S. J. : Immunochemistry 1: 267,
    1964.

27. Walton, K. W. , Hitchens, J. , Magnani, H. N. and Khan, M. :
    Atherosclerosis, in press

28. Walton, K. W. , Thomas, C. and Dunkerley, D. J. : J. Path.
    109, 271, 1973.

29. Walton, K. W. and Williamson, N. : J. Atheroscler. Res. 8:
    599, 1968.

30. Walton, K. W. , Williamson, N. and Johnson, A. G. : J. Path.
    101: 205, 1970.

Biochemical Pharmacology
of Hypolipidemic Drugs

HORMONE-INDUCED LIPOLYSIS AND THE METABOLIC

PATHWAYS PROVIDING ENERGY TO THE CELL: A POSSIBLE

ROLE OF ATP AS A RATE-LIMITING FACTOR

G. Fassina, P. Dorigo and R. M. Gaion

Institute of Pharmacology, University of Padua, Largo E. Meneghetti 2, 35100 Padua (Italy)

The primary purpose of free fatty acid mobilization from adipose tissue stores, is in the provision of caloric substrate to peripheral tissues. Under this light, hormone-sensitive lipolysis represents a fine regulatory mechanism, rapidly responsive to the most variable conditions and necessities, in accordance with the function of this highly specialized tissue ("Adipose Tissue", 1970; Bjorntorp and Ostman, 1971).

However, apart from the provision of caloric substrate, many other consequences of this phenomenon have been proposed, such as an effect on the coagulation system, on myocardial contractility, and so on. In this context, an excessively rapid free fatty acid mobilization carries many pathophysiologic implications. First of all, there is an increased rate of production of lipoproteins by the liver, which may be a factor in certain types of hyperlipoproteinemia (Havel, 1972; Shafrir and Steinberg, 1960; Windmueller and Spaeth, 1967).

The pharmacological control of lipomobilization (Paoletti and Sirtori, 1973) from adipose tissue is therefore of obvious practical interest. But it is, today, a difficult task to face, because of the fact that the mechanisms responsible for disorders of lipomobilization are still obscure. This is probably due to the

105

discrepancy which exists between our knowledge <u>in vivo</u> and <u>in vitro,</u> on the regulation of the lipolytic process. In other words, while at cellular level the mechanism responsible for the hormone-sensitive lipase activation is sufficiently known in its molecular and biochemical aspects (Butcher, 1970; Steinberg, 1972; Fain, 1973; Khoo et al., 1973), the basic elements involved in the regulation of free fatty acid mobilization <u>in vivo</u>, are, in contrast, much more complex and not yet clarified ("Adipose Tissue," 1970; Bjorntorp and Ostman, 1971; Paoletti and Sirtori, 1973).

All this is shown in Figure 1, where the hormone-sensitive lipolytic process is represented, together with many factors able to stimulate it. The first step is the activation of adenylate cyclase, an enzyme system located in the cell membrane structure. The stimulation of adenylate cyclase induces a very rapid increase in the level of 3', 5'-adenosine monophosphate (cyclic AMP), which in turn activates a protein kinase. This cyclic AMP-dependent protein kinase directly phosphorylates the lipase system, converting it from a less active form to a more active one. Finally, the activated lipase utilizes triglycerides as substrate, whose hydrolysis gives free fatty acid and glycerol as final product.

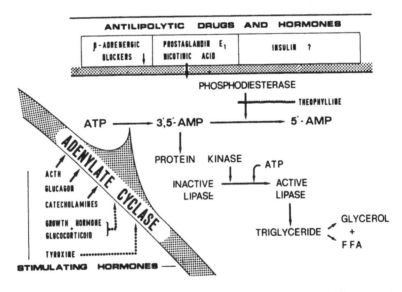

<u>Figure 1:</u> Hormone-sensitive lipolytic process and the most important factors, hormones and drugs, able to influence it <u>in vitro.</u>

Another step has to be noted: the presence of a phosphodiesterase system, which catalizes the cyclic AMP inactivation. There are drugs, such as theophylline and caffeine, that are able to inhibit phosphodiesterase, thus increasing the mean life of cyclic AMP and preserving it in the process. The activity of phosphodiesterase is an important modulating factor, because of the function of cyclic AMP in transmitting the hormone message into the cell, through its level variations (Butcher, 1970). This message is then highly amplified, before its realization in the final response, represented by free fatty acid and glycerol release. The intimate mechanism of this quantitative regulation is still unknown.

Here, the fact has to be stressed that a wide number of nervous and humoral factors, are potentially able to influence this process in vitro, by activating or depressing lipolysis. The more important of them are indicated in Figure 1. The interplay between these factors is extremely complex and, today, it is difficult to establish which of them is the prominent factor, or factors, regulating the fine equilibrium of lipomobilization in vivo. Consequently, the mechanisms responsible for lipid metabolic disorders are still unknown, and the pharmacological control of lipolysis presents serious potential pitfalls.

The problem was considered in a particular light by us, namely, that adipose tissue is an extremely specialized target organ: the fat cell is unique in its capability to respond to such a wide number of hormones of disparate structure with a specific response, lipolysis. Furthermore, the lipolytic activity of a single hormone may vary greatly from one species to another (Braun and Hechter, 1970; Bjorntorp and Ostman, 1971; Burns et al., 1972; Carlson and Butcher, 1972). All this could reflect the high degree of differentiation of adipose cell, in view of its final function, that is, to give a prompt and sensitive response to the organic demand for caloric substrate, a need that differs as regards entity, frequency and periodicity, in various animal species. At cellular level, all this could be supported by a special metabolic feature (reflecting phylogenesis), by a peculiar highly differentiated physiologic mechanism, the most adapted to be subject to a stringent reciprocal control between lipolysis and the energy equilibrium in adipocyte. Differences in this enzyme coordination, and alterations in homeostasis of energy balance, might be responsible for species differences in the sensitivity to hormones, and for disorders in lipomobilization.

This is the focal point of our research: to investigate the relationship between hormone-induced lipolysis and the metabolic
pathways providing energy to the cell. The hypothesis was that
the energy balance, and some alteration in the enzyme systems
regulating it, might be related to disorders of lipomobilization
and, obviously, could offer a new opening in the research of drugs
useful in the pharmacological control of adipose tissue function.

ENERGY CELL PRODUCTION AND THE CONTROL OF
HORMONE-STIMULATED LIPOLYSIS

The first step was to study the effect on adipose tissue of
drugs and of anomalous experimental conditions, such as metabolic
inhibitors and anaerobiosis, all suitable for inducing an altered
equilibrium on energy cell production. The effect of all these factors was parallel tested at three different levels of the process
studied: on the rate of triglyceride hydrolysis (the final step) on
the level of cyclic AMP (the first intracellular transducer of the
hormone message) and, finally, on the level of ATP indicating
the energy production by the adipocyte. All was carried out in
rat adipose tissue incubated in vitro, in the presence of drugs
stimulating lipolysis, such as noradrenaline and theophylline.

Three classes of drugs (Figure 2) were used. (a) Inhibitors
of glycolysis: sodium fluoride and monoiodoacetate. (b) Some
highly specific inhibitors of oxidative phosphorylation (Wainio,
1970): rotenone, piericidin A, antimycin A, 2,4-dinitrophenol,
dicyclohexylcarbodiimide, and oligomycin. They are acting at
various different levels, and by different mechanisms, on the
electron transport chain and energy transfer processes. (c) The
third class of inhibitors is that of ionophorous antibiotics, nigeri-
cin, gramicidin and valinomycin, representative of three groups of
transport-inducing agents (Harris, 1968; Pressman, 1969; Kinsky,
1970; Rottenberg et al., 1970) differing in their cation and proton
specificity, but having as a final common effect the discharge or
reduction of mitochondrial energy.

All the drugs tested were shown to inhibit hormone-induced
lipolysis in adipose tissue (Fassina, 1966; Fassina, 1967;
Fassina et al., 1967; Fassina and Dorigo, 1969; Fassina et al.,
1969; Fassina et al., 1970; Maragno et al., 1971; Dorigo et al.,
1973a; Dorigo et al., 1973b). In particular, the effect of

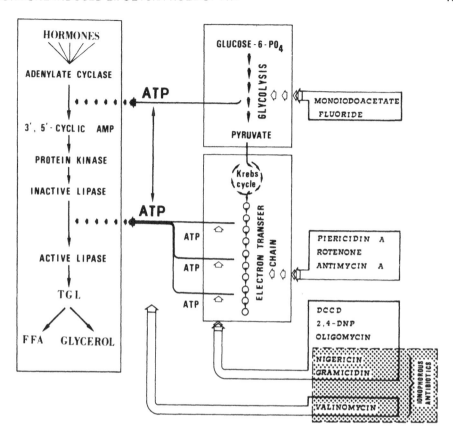

Figure 2: Different groups of metabolic inhibitors, (a) of glycolysis, (b) of oxidative phosphorylation, and (c) ionophorous antibiotics, tested on the hormone-sensitive lipolysis, on cyclic AMP
accumulation and on ATP level in rat adipose tissue in vitro. On
the left, the mechanism of hormone activation of lipolysis. As
indicated, ATP is required at two levels, both before and after
cyclic AMP synthesis. On the right, the two main cellular sources
of ATP, glycolysis and oxidative phosphorylation.

inhibitors and uncouplers of oxidative metabolism indicated that
the oxidative processes have an important role in hormonal action.
Further, the different sige and action mechanism of all these
drugs (Wainio, 1970), indicated that the lipolytic process needs,
not only, an optimal functioning of oxidative processes, but also
respiration coupled with phosphorylation, evidently requiring a
continuous supply of energy.

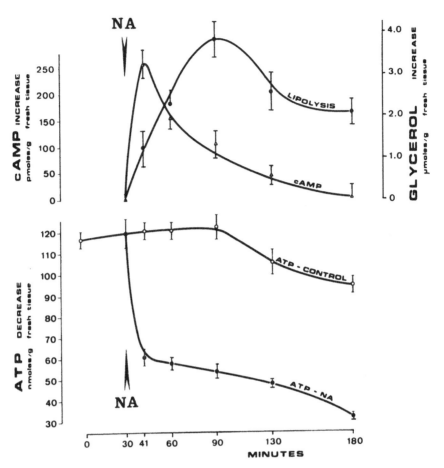

Figure 3: Time-course of ATP level, in parallel with cyclic AMP and lipolysis variations, in rat adipose tissue incubated <u>in vitro.</u>

    On the lower curves, ATP is reported as absolute values; while, on the upper part of the Figure, cyclic AMP increases (tissue + medium) are expressed as differences over the control level (in the assays incubated without noradrenaline) determined at each single time, and integrated. Finally, the stimulation of lipolysis is expressed as glycerol released in the incubation medium at each single time. All the parameters are reported (ordinates) respectively as micro-, nano- or picomoles/g fresh tissue. Epididymal fat samples (200 ± 10 mg) from albino Wistar rats were introduced in 2 ml of Krebs-Ringer bicarbonate containing 3.5% bovine albumin.

    The assays were incubated at 37° in a metabolic shaker. Noradrenaline 10^{-5}M (NA) was added after the first 30 min. After

This is a summary of a great deal of previous work. More recently, a careful study was carried out (Dorigo et al., 1974) by determining the time-course of ATP level variations, in parallel with cyclic AMP, and with lipolysis (Figure 3). The results gave direct evidence that the lipolytic process requires a continuous vast supply of energy.

The concentration of ATP (110-100 nmoles/g of fresh tissue) in adipose tissue incubated for 180 min in the absence of drugs, remains quite constant in time. Only after 90 min the nucleotide level begins to go down. After addition of noradrenaline 10^{-5} M into the incubation medium, the ATP concentration rapidly decreased in the first 10 to 20 min, reaching 50 per cent of the initial level. From then on, we can see a less rapid declining of ATP, reaching a plateau after 60 min; after that, the ATP level began again to decline, in correspondence with the spontaneous decrease of its concentration in the control tissue.

The cyclic AMP increase (Figure 3), though showing a peak 10 min after addition of noradrenaline, and then rapidly decreasing,

---

that, the incubation was continued for the time indicated on the axis of abscissas. ATP extraction and determination by the bioluminescence method of Strehler and Totter (1954) as adapted by Bihler and Jeanrenaud (1970). Cyclic AMP isolation, purification and assay method by the use of protein kinase prepared from bovine heart, according to Kuo and Greengard (1972). Glycerol according to Korn (1955). Other experimental conditions were reported in detail in a previous paper (Fassina et al., 1972b).

Data are the means of 12-32 determinations from 4 experiments, in the case of ATP; of 4 4 determinations from 2 experiments, in the case of cyclic AMP; of 6 determinations from 3 experiments, in the case of lipolysis.

There is an excellent correlation between the progressive stimulation of lipolysis and the decrease of ATP level.

reaches the original value only after more than one hour. It is interesting to observe that cyclic AMP variations just precedes that of lipolysis stimulation. The last one reaches a maximum 60 min after addition of noradrenaline, but it is still present after 2 hours. Parallely, the ATP decrease, even if much more rapid in the first 10 min, reaches a plateau at 60 min after addition of noradrenaline. Thus, on the whole, there is excellent correlation between the progressive stimulation of lipolysis and the decrease of ATP level. That is, the time-course of the two phenomena are closely corresponding.

In greater detail, one can also remark that the curve representing the ATP level seems to reflect, mostly in the first 60 min after addition of noradrenaline, the specular geometric sum of the two other curves representing cyclic AMP increase and lipolysis stimulation (Figure 3).

In summing up, the study using metabolic inhibitors on the relationship between hormone-induced lipolysis and the main cellular sources of ATP (reviewed in: Fassina et al., 1974a), but, mostly, the determination of ATP level in adipose tissue after addition of noradrenaline (Dorigo et al., 1974), strongly supports that the lipolytic process requires a continuous supply of energy, furnished by ATP.

ACTUAL SIGNIFICANCE OF THE LARGE ATP NECESSITY IN THE LIPOLYTIC PROCESS

The next question to be explored was the significance of the large ATP necessity in the process. That is, as ATP is known to be necessary (Fig. 1 and 2) at two different levels in the process, for cyclic AMP formation and to phosphorylate the lipase protein, it was obvious to ask at which level the bulk of ATP consumption was needed. In other words, if the various steps of hormone-stimulated lipolysis are differently dependent, from the quantitative point of view, on the provision of ATP. This problem led to investigation of the action of the different classes of metabolic inhibitors (previously tested on lipolysis) on cyclic AMP accumulation too (Fassina et al., 1972a; Fassina et al., 1972b; Dorigo et al., 1973a; Dorigo et al., 1973b). The comparison between the effect of all these drugs on cyclic AMP accumulation induced by noradrenaline and theophylline and the results previously obtained

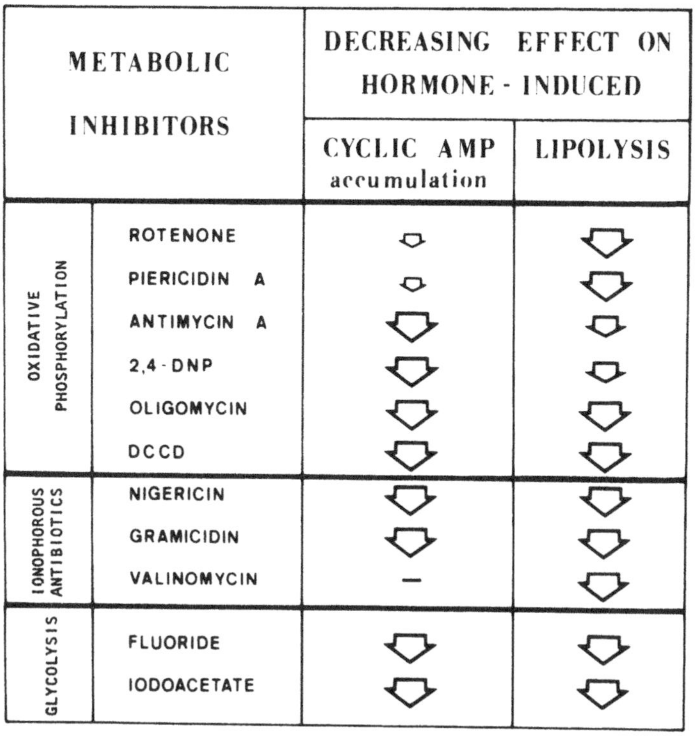

METABOLIC INHIBITORS		DECREASING EFFECT ON HORMONE - INDUCED	
		CYCLIC AMP accumulation	LIPOLYSIS
OXIDATIVE PHOSPHORYLATION	ROTENONE	⇩	⇩
	PIERICIDIN A	⇩	⇩
	ANTIMYCIN A	⇩	⇩
	2,4-DNP	⇩	⇩
	OLIGOMYCIN	⇩	⇩
	DCCD	⇩	⇩
IONOPHOROUS ANTIBIOTICS	NIGERICIN	⇩	⇩
	GRAMICIDIN	⇩	⇩
	VALINOMYCIN	—	⇩
GLYCOLYSIS	FLUORIDE	⇩	⇩
	IODOACETATE	⇩	⇩

Figure 4: Comparison between the effect of oxidative phosphorylation inhibitors, of ionophorous antibiotics, and of glycolysis inhibitors, on hormone-induced cyclic AMP accumulation and lipolysis.

Experimental conditions as indicated in Fig. 3. The absolute values are reported in the original papers (Fassina and Dorigo, 1969; Fassina et al., 1972a and b; Dorigo et al., 1973a and b). The different sizes of the arrows indicate the degree of inhibition exerted by the same concentration of a single drug on each one of the two parameters studied.

Discrepancies between the effects on cyclic AMP level and of lipolysis, are evident mostly in the case of rotenone, piericidin and valinomycin.

on lipolysis (Figure 4), gave stimulating data, with some indications on the relative significance of the two energy producing pathways on the process studied. In fact, some of these drugs did not inhibit cyclic AMP accumulation and lipolysis to the same extent. Rotenone and piericidin were less effective on the cyclic

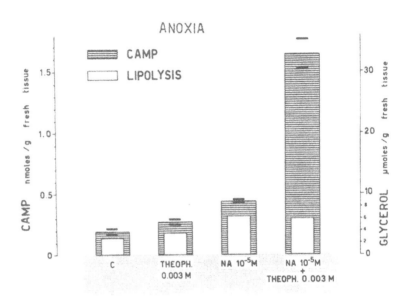

Figure 5: Cyclic AMP accumulation (filled-in columns) and lipolysis (blank columns) induced by noradrenaline, theophylline, and
noradrenaline plus theophylline, in rat adipose tissue under
anaerobic conditions.

C = control values (tissue incubated without drugs). NA =
noradrenaline 10^{-5}M. THEOPH. = theophylline 3 mM. Data are
the means of 12 determinations from three experiments. Cyclic
AMP (picomoles/g fresh tissue) is the sum of tissue plus medium
content, measured after 11 min of incubation. Glycerol (micro-
moles/g fresh tissue) is that released into the incubation medium
after 120 min of incubation. Anaerobiosis was performed by incubating adipose tissue under vacuum, in Thunberg measuring
tubes. All the other experimental conditions were as in Figure
3.

Cyclic AMP in increased (x9) by noradrenaline plus theophylline, whilst lipolysis is only slightly stimulated (x2).

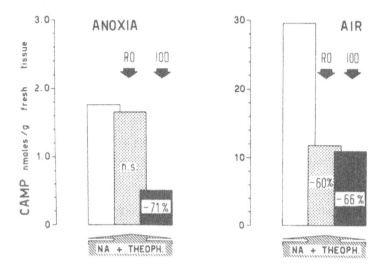

Figure 6: Effect of rotenone and of monoiodoacetate on cyclic AMP accumulation in rat adipose tissue under anaerobic and aerobic conditions.

White columns represent the control value, that is, the cyclic AMP level (tissue + medium) after addition of noradrenaline 10^{-5} M (NA) plus theophylline 3 mM (THEOPH.) RO = rotenone 10^{-5} M. IOD = monoiodoacetate 3 mM. Data are the means of 16 determinations from 4 experiments.

The assays were incubated under vacuum in Thunberg measuring tubes. All the other experimental conditions as in Figure 3.

In anoxia (left) rotenone was ineffective. In air (right), both metabolic inhibitors were active.

AMP level than on lipolysis. Moreover, the increase of cyclic AMP was not modified by valinomycin, quite in contrast with the inhibitory effect of this drug on lipolysis. Glycolysis inhibitors were, instead, equally active on the two steps of the process.

These results seem to indicate that the synthesis of cyclic AMP is related to oxidative phosphorylation in a somewhat

different way than the final lipolytic effect. In order to test this
hypothesis, we studied the effect of drugs inducing lipolysis, on
adipose tissue incubated under anaerobic conditions (Fassina et al. ,
1973; Fassina et al. , 1974a; Dorigo et al. , 1974; Fassina et al. ,
1974b). In anaerobiosis, the supply of energy is quite restricted
and chiefly sustained by glycolysis. In this way, we hoped to
disassociate the two phases of the lipolytic process, that is, to
abolish any correlation between increases in cyclic AMP and activation of lipolysis. And this was so (Fig. 5): in anoxia, cyclic
AMP accumulation is still evident, whilst lipolysis is only slightly
stimulated. More precisely, cyclic AMP was increased, mostly
in the presence of noradrenaline plus theophylline, to levels (about
8-fold the basal value) that would be, in normal conditions, in
oxygen atmosphere, quite sufficient for a maximum stimulation of
lipolysis. But, instead, lipolysis was stimulated very slightly,
that is, only doubled. In air (Fassina et al. , 1973, 1974a and b),
noradrenaline or theophylline, by increasing cyclic AMP 3 to 4-
fold over the control, induces a maximum stimulation of lipolysis
(6 to 7-fold).

This indicates that in anoxic adipose tissue the cyclic AMP
synthesis is still possible (though to a reduced extent) and presumably depends on anaerobic glycolysis. The last suggestion
seems to be confirmed by the findings, always under anaerobic
conditions (Fig. 6), that rotenone (an oxidative phosphorylation
inhibitor) did not impair cyclic AMP accumulation, whilst an
inhibitor of glycolysis, iodoacetate, strongly inhibited it. In air,
as previously mentioned (Fassina et al. , 1967; Fassina et al. ,
1970; Fassina et al. , 1972a) and shown in Figure 6, both metabolic inhibitors were active. Moreover, exogenous glucose
potentiated the increasing effect of noradrenaline and theophylline
on cyclic AMP level in anoxia (Dorigo et al. , 1974; Fassina et al. ,
1974b).

A careful time-course study of the three parameters, cyclic
AMP, lipolysis and ATP, was carried out also in anaerobic conditions (Figure 7). In such a case, the ATP level in adipose tissue

---

The ATP control level rapidly, spontaneously declines (to 50
per cent) inside the first 30 min of incubation. A slight stimulation of lipolysis is evident only during the first 30 min after addition of noradrenaline, when a certain level of ATP is still present.

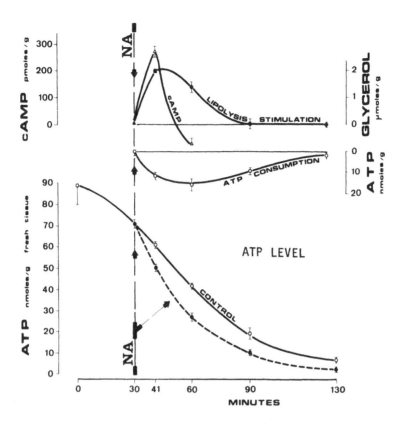

Figure 7: Time-course in anaerobic conditions of ATP level, in parallel with cyclic AMP and lipolysis variations in rat adipose tissue in vitro.

NA = noradrenaline 10^{-5} M, added to the incubation medium after the first 30 min of incubation.

In the lower curves, ATP is reported as absolute values at each time of incubation (abscissas). ATP consumption and cyclic AMP increase (tissue + medium) are expressed as differences from the control, determined at each single time, and integrated. The stimulation of lipolysis is expressed as glycerol released in the incubation medium at each single time. All the parameters are reported (ordinates) respectively as micro-, nano- or pico-molès/g fresh tissue. Each value represents the mean ± s. e. of 8 determinations from 2 experiments.

Anaerobiosis was performed by incubating adipose tissue under vacuum, in Thunberg measuring tubes. All the other experimental conditions were as indicated in Figure 3.

incubated without drugs, rapidly declined, attaining the 50% of
the initial value inside the first 60 min of incubation, while, in
air, the ATP level reminaed constant for one and a half hours at
least, as previously shown (Figure 3). When noradrenaline was
added (Figure 7), a still more rapid fall of ATP was evident. The
ATP consumption showed a parallel time-course behaviour to the
increase of cyclic AMP. Finally, the slight stimulation of lipolysis is evident only at the first stage, that is, during the first 30
min after addition of noradrenaline, when a certain level of ATP is
still present in anoxic adipose tissue. After that, the process
rapidly stops, because of the lack of ATP, which is by then
exhausted.

These results give further evidence that, though cyclic AMP
increase is still present in anaerobiosis, in contrast, lipolysis
as well as ATP consumption are rapidly arresting. A key feature
in this phenomenon is undoubtedly the lack of ATP, consequent to
anoxia.

On the whole, these data indicate that, in anoxia, ATP furnished by glycolysis is sufficient to support cyclic AMP synthesis.
But anaerobic glycolysis is not able to support the final accomplishment of the process. Thus, in anoxia, the message from hormones
can be transmitted, but not amplified or accomplished by the stimulation of lipolysis, because of the lack of ATP from aerobic sources.

CONCLUSIONS

And so, on the basis of the studies summarized here, it appears that cyclic AMP is not the sole modulator of lipolysis. It
is the mediator, the intracellular messenger of hormone stimulus
(Butcher, 1970). But, even though cyclic AMP being the key
intermediate between hormones and their final effect, ATP level
is the rate-limiting factor as regards the intensity and duration of
the stimulated lipolysis. In this way, ATP consumption and provision could represent an important site of regulation, beyond
cyclic AMP formation.

When the optimal physiological conditions are modified, then
ATP could become a causative factor for the accomplishment and
normal running of hormone-induced lipolysis. In extreme situations, like in anoxia, the lack of ATP drastically hinders the

final stimulation of lipolysis. This could be significant regarding the problems encountered in correlating lipolysis with changes in cyclic AMP level, so largely discussed (Fain, 1973, page 79). For instance, as in the case when noradrenaline is present together with theophylline: an enormous accumulation of cyclic AMP is then present (300-fold the control value) while lipolysis is stimulated only 6 to 7-fold, just like in the presence of noradrenaline alone, when the cyclic nucleotide is increased to about 3 to 4-fold. This supramaximal accumulation of cyclic AMP is therefore not related to activation of lipolysis. In our view, this lack of parallelism reflects the rate-limiting function of ATP level, or of some factor strictly related to it.

All this is, firstly, in agreement with the initial hypothesis, of a fine equilibrium necessary between the metabolic sources of energy for a suitable control of lipomobilization. Oxygen consumption, and glucose provision and entrance into the adipocyte, are very important in view of the regulation of the ATP level necessary for the lipolytic process. Secondly, this could be significant in view of the relationship between glucose and lipid metabolism suggested in some metabolic disorders. Finally, it puts forth the possibility that drugs able to influence contemporaneously glucose and lipid metabolism in adipose tissue, may be of interest in the pharmacological control of lipomobilization.

SUMMARY

The relationship between hormone-induced lipolysis and the metabolic pathways providing energy to the adipocyte, was investigated by using different classes of metabolic inhibitors and anomalous experimental conditions (anoxia, fasting, etc.) suitable for inducing an altered equilibrium on energy cell production. The effect of these factors was parallely tested on the levels of cyclic AMP (cAMP), of ATP, and on the rate of triglyceride hydrolysis in the presence of catecholamines, theophylline, and dibutyryl cyclic AMP.

All the inhibitors tested were shown to depress hormone-induced lipolysis, thus, indicating that the process requires a continuous vast supply of energy. ATP consumption in adipose tissue was strictly parallel to the increase of stimulated lipolysis. The time-course of the two phenomena was also closely corres-

ponding. The comparison between the effect of metabolic inhibitors on lipolysis and on cyclic AMP accumulation, suggested that
cAMP synthesis and the final lipolytic process are related to oxidative phorphorylation in a somewhat different way. In view of
this, the response of adipose tissue was tested under anaerobic
conditions, when the supply of energy is more restricted and
chiefly sustained by glycolysis. Cyclic AMP was still increased
to levels quite sufficient for a maximum stimulation of lipolysis,
while instead, the triglyceride hydrolysis, after a brief initial
stimulation, was rapidly stopped. Likewise there was a strong
spontaneous decrease of ATP level. Therefore, when equilibrium
between the metabolic sources of energy is altered, the initial
step (cAMP synthesis) and the final step of induced lipolysis (no
longer present) could be dissociated because of a deficiency of
ATP.

These results indicate that cyclic AMP is not the sole modulator of lipolysis: it is the messenger, but the ATP level is the
rate-limiting factor as regards the intensity and duration of the
process studied. When the optimal physiological conditions are
modified (as in anoxia), then ATP becomes an evident causative
factor for the accomplishment and the normal running of hormone-
induced lipolysis. This could be significant in view of the relationship between glucose and lipid metabolism suggested in some
metabolic disorders.

REFERENCES

1. Jeanrenaud, B. and D. Hepp, eds., Adipose Tissue, Regula-
    tion and Metabolic Functions. Hormone and Metabolic Re-
    search, Suppl. 2, Georg Thieme Verlag and Academic Press,
    1970.
2. Bihler, J. and B. Jeanrenaud. Biochim. Biophys. Acta 202:
    496, 1970.
3. Bjorntorp, P. and J. Ostman. In: Advances in Metabolic
    Disorders, Volume 5, Academic Press, New York, 1971,
    p. 277.
4. Braun, T. and O. Hechter. In: Adipose Tissue, Regulation
    and Metabolic Functions. B. Jeanrenaud and D. Hepp, eds.
    Georg Thiem Verlag and Academic Press, 1970, p. 11.

5. Burns, T. W. , Langley, P. E. and Robison, G. A. In:
    Advances in Cyclic Nucleotide Research, Volume 1,
    P. Greengard, G. A. Robison, eds. , Raven Press, New York.
    1972, p. 63.
6. Butcher, R. W. In: Adipose Tissue, Regulation and Metabolic
    Functions. B. Jeanrenaud and D. Hepp, eds. Georg Thieme
    Verlag and Academic Press, 1970, p. 5.
7. Carlson, L. A. and Butcher, R. W. In: Advances in Cyclic
    Nucleotide Research, Volume 1. P. Greengard, G. A. Robison
    and R. Paoletti. Raven Press, New York, 1972, p. 87.
8. Dorigo, P. , Gaion, R. M. Toth, E. and Fassina, G. Biochem.
    Pharmac. 22: 1949, 1973a.
9. Dorigo, P. , Prosdocimi, M. , Gaion, R. M. and Fassina, G.
    Abs. MP-34, pg. 37, Second Internat. Conference on Cyclic
    AMP, Vancouver, Canada, July 8-11, 1974.
10. Dorigo, P. , Visco, L. , Fiandini, G. and Fassina, G.
    Biochem. Pharmac. 22: 1957, 1973b.
11. Fain, J. N. Pharmacol. Rev. 25: 67, 1973.
12. Fassina, G. Life Sci. 5: 2151, 1966.
13. Fassina, G. Life Sci. 6: 825, 1967.
14. Fassina, G. and Dorigo, P. Adv. Exp. Med. Biol. 4: 117,
    1969.
15. Fassina, G. , Dorigo, P. , Badetti, R. and L. Visco.
    Biochem. Pharmac. 21: 1633, 1972a.
16. Fassina, G. , Dorigo, P. and Gaion, R. M. Third Internat.
    Symposium on Atherosclerosis, West Berlin, October 24-28,
    1973, Abs. 141.
17. Fassina, G. , Dorigo, P. and Gaion, R. M. Pharmac. Res.
    Commun. 6: 1, 1974a.
18. Fassina, G. , Gaion, R. M. , Bonazzi, F. and P. Dorigo.
    Second Internat. Conference on Cyclic AMP, Vancouver,
    Canada, July 8-11, 1974, pg. 36.
19. Fassina, G. , Dorigo, P. and Maragno, I. In: Adipose Tissue,
    Regulation and Metabolic Functions. B. Jeanrenaud and D.
    Hepp, eds. Georg Thieme Verlag and Academic Press, 1970,
    p. 88.
20. Fassina, G. , Dorigo, P. , Maragno, I. and Contessa, A. R.
    Giornale dell'Arteriosclerosi 7: 35, 1969.
21. Fassina, G. , Dorigo, P. , Perini, G. and Toth, E. Biochem.
    Pharmac. 21: 2295, 1972.
22. Fassina, G. , Maragno, I. and Dorigo, P. Biochem. Pharmac.
    16: 1439, 1967.

23. Harris, E. J. In: <u>Membrane Models and the Formation of</u>
    Biological Membranes. L. Bolis and B. A. Pethica, eds.
    North-Holland, Amsterdam, 1968, p. 247.
24. Havel, R. J. In: <u>Pharmacological Control of Lipid Metabolism,</u>
    W. L. Holmes, R. Paoletti and D. Kritchevsky, eds. Adv.
    Exp. Medicine and Biology 26, Plenum Press, New York,
    1972, p. 57.
25. Kinsky, S. C. Ann. Rev. Pharmac. 10: 119, 1970.
26. Khoo, J. C., Steinberg, D., Thompson, B. and Mayer, S. E.
    J. Biol. Chem. 248: 2823, 1973.
27. Korn, E. D. J. Biol. Chem. 215: 1, 1955.
28. Kuo, J. F. and P. Greengard. In: <u>Advances in Cyclic Nucleo-</u>
    tide Research. P. Greengard and G. A. Robison, eds. Raven
    Press, New York, 1972, p. 41.
29. Maragno, I., Dorigo, P. and Fassina, G. Biochem. Pharmac.
    20: 2149, 1971.
30. Paoletti, R. and Sirtori, C. In: <u>Proc. of the Internat. Symp.</u>
    on Atherosclerosis. D. A. Willoughby, F. Derom, V. Cicala
    and E. Malan. Carlo Erba Foundation, Milan, 1973.
31. Pressman, B. C. In: <u>Mitochondria Structure and Function.</u>
    L. Ernster and Z. Drahota, eds. Academic Press, New
    York, 1969, p. 315.
32. Rottenberg, H., Caplan, S. R. and Essig, A. In: <u>Membranes</u>
    <u>and Ion Transport</u>, Vol. 1. E. Bittar, ed. Wiley-Interscience,
    London, 1970, p. 165.
33. Shafrir, E. and Steinberg, D. J. J. Clin. Invest. 39: 310,
    1960.
34. Steinberg, D. In: <u>Pharmacological Control of Lipid Metabo-</u>
    <u>lism</u>. W. L. Holmes, R. Paoletti and D. Kritchevsky, eds.
    Adv. Exptl. Medicine and Biology 26. Plenum Press, New
    York, 1972, p. 77.
35. Strehler, B. L. and Totter, J. R. In <u>Methods in Biochem.</u>
    Analysis. D. Glick, ed. Vol. 1. Interscience, New York,
    1954, p. 341.
36. Wainio, W. <u>The Mammalian Mitochondrial Respiratory</u>
    <u>Chain.</u> Academic Press, New York, 1970.
37. Windmueller, H. G. and Spaeth, A. E. Arch. Biochem. Bio-
    phys. 13: 362, 1967.

MECHANISM OF ACTION OF HYPOLIPIDEMIC DRUGS

C. R. Sirtori, D. Torreggiani, and R. Fumagalli[*]

Center "E. Grossi Paoletti" for the Study of Metabolic Diseases and Hyperlipidemias, University of Milan; [*] Institute of Pharmacology and Pharmacognosy, University of Milan, Milan, Italy

Drugs may decrease serum lipid levels by impairing lipid absorption, lipoprotein synthesis or release, or by stimulating lipid or lipoprotein catabolism (45). Recent data point out, however, that agents such as clofibrate (CPIB), generally thought to act only by inhibiting lipid and lipoprotein synthesis and release (3), may also affect lipid absorption.

The present review will consider some of the more recent theories on CPIB's mechanisms of action, and their significance in terms of clinical efficacy and toxicity. We shall then examine the possibility of a pharmacological control of ethanol induced hyperlipidemias, which have clinical and social relevance in many areas of the world. Finally, data will be presented about a possible central mechanism of action of CPIB.

MECHANISM OF ACTION OF CPIB

CPIB exerts a variety of effects on the hepatic cells which have been thoroughly investigated both in vivo and in vitro. Some of these effects are listed in Table I.

Table I

Biochemical Effects of CPIB on Hepatic Cells

Increased:

α-GPDH
NAD/NADH
FFA Oxidation
Ac Acetyl CoA-Deacylase

Decreased:

HMG CoA reductase
Acetyl CoA carboxylase
Acyl CoA α-GP acyltransferase
TGFA release (?)

A typical effect of CPIB when added in vitro to liver slices is an increased oxygen consumption (52), which is likely to be related to an increased liver content of mitochondria (34) and peroxysomes (50). Mitochondria exhibit an increased NAD content and NAD/NADH ratio (40).

The enhanced mitochondrial activity is also expressed by α-glycerophosphate dehydrogenase (α-GPHD), which increases several fold in treated rats (52); this effect is similar to that induced by thyroid hormones, and is abolished by thyroidectomy. α-GPHD is, however, differently affected in the various animal species (27). Glycerol incorporation into triglycerides is therefore reduced (1), although a 5 mM concentration of CPIB is necessary for this effect to take place. Another possible explanation for the decreased triglyceride synthesis after CPIB is the inhibition of acyl CoA-α-glycerophosphate acyltransferase (35).

Other enzyme activities which are significantly reduced by CPIB are acyl CoA carboxylase (37) and β-hydroxy-methyl-glutaryl CoA reductase (4), while mitochondrial acetoacetyl CoA deacylase is increased (9). These latter two enzyme changes may significantly enhance ketogenesis. Although no change has been observed in the concentration of acetoacetate in the blood of treated rats (9), recent data by Wolfe et al (54) point out a marked increase of ketones

Table II

Arterial Concentrations of Ketone Bodies of Subjects
Treated with CPIB

	Acetoacetate	β-Hydroxybutyrate
	mol/ml	
Pre-treatment	0.16 ± 0.02	0.25 ± 0.03
Post-treatment	0.33 ± 0.04	0.40 ± 0.05

(from Wolfe et al., 1973)

in the arterial blood of both normal and hyperlipidemic patients treated with CPIB (Table II). These authors showed that the oxidation of FFA taken up by the liver is increased, although no change is observed in the fraction which is secreted as VLDL triglycerides.

Another observation by the same authors was that the effect of CPIB on splanchnic triglyceride production was different between normals and hypertriglyceridemic patients. Splanchnic trigly-ceride production was, in fact, increased in normals, where precursors other than FFA were utilized. On the other hand in hyper-triglyceridemic patients, production was unchanged and no source other than FFA was utilized. There was evidence in both groups of an improved extrasplanchnic clearance of VLDL-TG.

Data on lipolysis following CPIB are sometimes contradictory, possibly as a consequence of the drug's interference in the assay (42). CPIB lowers glycerol release from epididymal fat in vitro and antagonizes the lipolytic effects of noradrenaline, while cyclic AMP accumulation by adipocytes is reduced (10). These findings do not explain clinical data concerning catecholamine induced lipo-lysis in humans (31), although decreased cyclic AMP levels might promote, according to Tolman et al (51) increased lipoprotein lipase activity, which is part of the mechanism of action of CPIB.

Clinical studies have recently shown that CPIB interferes with sterol and bile acid absorption. An increased fecal loss of neutral steroids is readily seen in the majority of patients (26). This leads

Table III

Plasma Lipids Following CPIB and Colestipol

	Cholesterol (mg/dl)	Triglycerides (mg/dl)
Placebo powder	304 ± 11	130 ± 9
Colestipol	264 ± 7 °	150 ± 13
Placebo capsule	299 ± 12	124 ± 10
Clofibrate	264 ± 12 °	101 ± 10 °

Data from 26 patients
° p < 0.05 compared to placebo period
(from Dujovne et al., 1974)

to a reduction of the sterol pool size, and eventually to a reduction of plasma cholesterol levels. The 15-20% reduction of plasma cholesterol levels is probably an adequate explanation for the reduced cardiovascular mortality seen in English and American studies (6, 7, 33). A recent comparison between CPIB and an ion exchange resin, colestipol (16), indicated (Table III) that the effect of the two drugs on serum cholesterol was practically identical.

Aside from its own hypocholesteremic activity, CPIB has been successfully used in addition to purely intestinal drugs, such as cholestyramine (30) or neomycin (43) for the management of patients with severe hypercholesteremia. A possible mechanism, as pointed out by Grundy et al (26) may be related to an inhibition by CPIB of the increased sterol synthesis in the intestinal wall caused by the resin. CPIB, by its effects on HMG CoA-reductase, could, in fact, hinder the increased cholesterol production rate, which is seen in patients treated with bile-sequestrants.

This interpretation is however questioned in a recent study by Goodman et al (25). By measuring production and turnover rate of cholesterol in patients treated with an ion exchange resin, colestipol, they could indeed confirm that these were increased. However, upon adding CPIB to the regimen, the cholesterol production rate was hardly affected, not supporting the suggestion that CPIB may block the increased sterol synthesis. One may however note that the patients were mostly subjects with relatively mild hypercholesteremia, who generally do not exhibit an inadequate control over cholesterol biosynthesis. This would not be the case of homozygous or heterozygous type IIA patients, who have a complete or partial absence of the receptors for LDL apoprotein, which control sterol biosynthesis (8).

Recent studies on a possible hormonal effect of CPIB have pointed out that the drug may inhibit pancreatic insulin secretory response while maintaining or increasing glucagon secretion (17). These findings, confirmed in humans following arginine stimulation of pancreatic secretion (19), indicate that CPIB allows for an imbalance between insulin and glucagon to occur, thus favoring the hypolipidemic effect of glucagon (18).

Analyses of possible side effects of CPIB have included studies on alterations of bile composition in normal subjects. CPIB causes the concentration of biliary cholesterol to rise, and reduces bile acid levels, thus decreasing the rate of synthesis and the pool size of cholic acid (39). These data are consistent with an increased lithogenicity of bile. Similar data were obtained with estrogen-progestin combinations.

Reciprocal changes in plasma lipoproteins following CPIB treatment were described by Wilson and Lees (53). A decrease of VLDL cholesterol, according to these authors, is often followed by a reciprocal increase of LDL cholesterol, thus indicating the possible induction of hyperbetalipoproteinemia, a potentially more serious abnormality. Similar data have not been confirmed by other authors.

Our experience indicates that such an event is not commonly observed, and it is our impression that it should not be considered as a potentially dangerous consequence.

DRUGS AFFECTING ETHANOL INDUCED HYPERLIPIDEMIAS

A considerable interest has been recently devoted to ethanol as an agent inducing hyperlipidemia, especially because of the high incidence of abnormal lipid levels among alcoholics (12, 46). The effects of ethanol on lipid metabolism are well known.

Fatty liver is induced in normal rats by the administration of a single intoxicating dose of ethanol (36, 14) or of commercial alcoholic beverages (15); in these situations, plasma triglyceride concentration has been reported to be unaltered (23) or significantly increased (28). Increase of serum triglycerides has also been found after chronic ethanol feeding (5). Hypertriglyceridemia and plasma opalescence in intoxicated patients with a history of chronic alcoholism is also a frequent finding (2, 46).

Since elevated serum triglycerides may play a role in atherogenesis (11), the use of drugs able to prevent or correct alcohol-induced hypertriglyceridemia would be justified. Beta-benzal butyrate (BBA), an agent reported to reduce serum triglycerides in experimental animals (21) and in man (13), and one of its congeners, the diethylamide derivative (C_{11}), were therefore tested for their activity on an experimental model of ethanol induced hypertriglyceridemia in rats, and compared with CPIB and other hypolipidemic agents.

Ethanol was given ad libitum as a 10% solution in drinking water for three days. On the fourth day, a few hours before sacrifice, the rats received 5 g/kg of ethanol as a 50% solution by stomach intubation. The drugs tested, including CPIB, were administered once daily (300 mg/kg b. w.) by gastric intubation. The results are reported in Table IV.

Ethanol alone significantly increased serum triglycerides and both CPIB and C_{11} were effective against this type of hypertriglyceridemia, while BBA was ineffective.

This action of C_{11} was further confirmed in acutely induced alcoholic hypertriglyceridemia in rats and humans.

The activity of clofibrate on this test confirms previous results reported in the literature (32). The lack of activity of BBA on this kind of hypertriglyceridemia, contrasted with the efficacy of its diethylamide derivative. Since both drugs, as well as CPIB, were effective on fructose-induced hypertriglyceridemia (unpublished results), it is possible to speculate that the underlying mechanisms of these hypertriglyceridemias may be different.

Data by Puglisi et al (41) presented at the Symposium, indicated that hypoglycemic sulphonylureas may be potent inhibitors of ethanol induced hypertriglyceridemia.

Table IV

Effect of Clofibrate (CPIB), β-Benzal Butyrate (BBA)
and its Diethylamide Derivative (C_{11}) on Ethanol-Induced
Hypertriglyceridemia in Rats

	Serum Triglycerides mg/dl ± S. E.
Controls	60.3 ± 4.0
Ethanol	149.2 ± 22.0
Ethanol + CPIB	87.0 ± 6.0*
Ethanol + BBA	164.8 ± 16.5
Ethanol + C_{11}	58.5 ± 14.2*

Drugs were administered once daily for 4 days
(300 mg/kg, by stomach intubation)

* $p < 0.001$ as compared to ethanol alone

HYPOTHESIS ON A CENTRAL EFFECT OF CPIB

The possibility of an effect of CPIB on the central nervous
system has been raised by Spano et al (48). These authors examined
the ability of CPIB to displace tryptophan from its plasma binding
sites. Trytophan is, in fact, the only amino acid which is highly
bound to serum proteins (38). The tryptophan pool in brain is controlled by the unbound (free) fraction of serum tryptophan (24).
There is ample evidence that the rate of synthesis of 5-hydroxy-
tryptamine (5-HT) in brain is regulated principally by brain tryptophan (49).

Experiments in rats showed that CPIB (200 mg/kg b. i. d.
orally for 3 days) decreases total plasma tryptophan by about 70%,
while increasing the free fraction by 50%; brain tryptophan and 5-
hydroxyindoleacetic acid (5-HIAA) levels also increase by 50%
(Figure 1) (49). In man, the effect of a five day treatment with
CPIB (2,000 mg daily), was compared with a similar period of
placebo administration (48). CPIB again lowered total plasma
tryptophan by 50-70% in all subjects, while raising about 5-fold
the percentage of free amino acid.

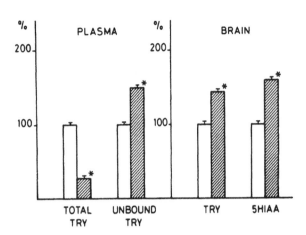

Figure 1: Percentage variations of (from l. to r.) total tryptophan, free tryptophan, tryptophan and 5-hydroxy-indoleacetic acid in plasma and brain of rats 6 hours after a single dose of clofibrate (200 mg/kg orally). All differences are statistically significant.

The meaning of an increased availability of free tryptophan for brain 5-HT synthesis, in terms of the hypolipidemic effect of CPIB, is not clear. One may however note that long acting salicylates, which also displace tryptophan (47), are potent hypolipidemic agents (29). Moreover, in a recent clinical trial on drugs for the treatment of nephrotic hyperlipidemia (44), the authors also evaluated l-tryptophan, on the grounds that the fasting serum levels of this amino acid are decreased in nephrotic patients (22). Surprisingly, the effect of daily l-tryptophan administration (0.4 g t. i. d.) was equivalent to that of CPIB (Table V).

Table V

Mean Percentage Decrease of Serum Lipids in
Patients with Nephrotic Hyperlipidemia

	Cholesterol	Triglycerides
Clofibrate[1]	34	34
Tryptophan[2]	38	36

[1] 0.5 g per g of serum albumin
[2] 0.4 g t. i. d.

From Schapel et al, 1974

SUMMARY

The mechanism of action of hypolipidemic agents may depend upon biochemical effects at the cellular level, or interference with lipoprotein synthesis or release, or to impaired lipid absorption.

Clofibrate exerts a variety of effects at every level. In humans mitochondrial oxidative potential is increased and extra-splanchnic clearance of VLDL-TG is improved. CPIB also interferes with sterol and bile acid absorption. Association of CPIB with ion exchange resins potentiates their hypocholesteremic effect; the mechanism is not clear, because the increased sterol production rate induced by the resins is apparently not affected by CPIB.

Recent studies on ethanol induced hypertriglyceridemia have pointed out that specific drugs may be particularly effective on this disorder. In particular, hypoglycemic sulphonylureas and the diethylamide derivative of β-benzal butyrate were the most effective agents when tested in the rat or in an acute test in humans.

A possible central effect of CPIB was described in our laboratory. We observed that this agent can displace plasma tryptophan from its albumin binding sites, thus increasing brain 5-HT synthesis. The significance of this finding is discussed on the basis of clinical data showing the hypolipidemic effect of tryptophan per se or of other drugs displacing tryptophan.

REFERENCES

1. Adams, L. L. , Webb, W. W. and Fallon, H. J. J. Clin. Invest. 50: 2339, 1971.
2. Albrink, M. J. and Klatskin, G. Ann. J. Med. 23: 26, 1957.
3. Avoy, D. R. , Swyryd, E. A. and Gould, R. G. J. Lipid Res. 6: 369, 1965.
4. Azarnoff, D. L. , Tucker, D. R. and Barr, G. A. Metabolism 14: 959, 1965.
5. Baraona, E. and Lieber, C. S. J. Clin. Invest. 49: 769, 1970.
6. Five-year study by a group of physicians of the Newcastle upon Tyne Region. British Medical J. 4: 767, 1971.
7. Report of a Research Committee of the Scottish Society of Physicians. British Medical J. 4: 775, 1971.
8. Brown, M. S. and Goldstein, J. L. Science 185: 61, 1974.

9.   Burch, R. E. and Curran, G. L.   J. Lipid Res. 10: 668, 1969.

10. Carlson, L. A. , Walldius, G. and Butcher, R. W.   Athero-
     sclerosis 16: 349, 1972.

11. Carlson, L.A. and Bottiger, L. E.   Lancet i: 865, 1972.

12. Chait, A. , February, A. W. , Mancini, M. , and Lewis, B.
     Lancet 8: 62, 1972.

13. Ciocia, D. and Cavalca, L. G. Arterioscler. 7: 1, 1969.

14. DiLuzio, N. R. and Zilversmit, D. B.   Am. J. Physiol. 199:
     991, 1960.

15. DiLuzio, N. R.   Quart. J. Stud. Alcohol 23: 557, 1962.

16. Dujovne, C. A. , Hurwitz, A. , Kauffman, R. E. and Azarnoff,
     D.L.   Clin. Pharmacol. Ther. 16: 291, 1974.

17. Eaton, R. P.   Metabolism 22: 763, 1973.

18. Eaton, R. P.   J. Lipid Res. 14: 312, 1973.

19. Eaton, R. P. and Schade, D. S.   Metabolism 23: 445, 1974.

20. Eccleston, D. , Ashcroft, G. W. and Crawford, T. B. B.   J.
     Neurochem. 12: 493, 1965.

21. Edwards, K. D. G. and Paoletti, R.   Med. J. Aust. 1: 474,
     1970.

22. Edwards, K. D. G. and Hawkins, M. R.   Austr. N. Z. J. Med.
     2: 104, 1972.

23. Elko, E. E. , Wooles, W. R. and DiLuzio, N. R.   Am. J.
     Physiol. 201: 923, 1961.

24. Gessa, G. L. , Biggio, G. and Tagliamonte, A.   Fed. Proc.
     31: 599, 1972.

25. Goodman, D. S. , Noble, R. P. and Dell, R. B.   J. Clin. In-
     vest. 52: 2646, 1973.

26. Grundy, S. M. , Ahrens, E. H. , Salen, G. , Schreibman, P. H. ,
     and Nestel, P. J.   J. Lipid Res. 13: 531, 1972.

27. Havel, R. J. and Kane, J. P.   Ann. Rev. Pharmacol. 13: 287,
     1973.

28. Hernell, O. and Johnson, O.   Lipids 8: 503, 1973.

29. Howard, A. N. , Hyams, D. E. , Everett, W. , Jennings, I. W. ,
     Gresham, G. A. , Bizzi, A. , Garattini, S. , Veneroni, E. ,
     and Miettinen, T. A.   European J. Pharmacol. 13: 244, 1971.

30. Howard, A. N. , Hyams, D. E. and Evans, R. C.   Adv. Exp.
     Med. Biol. 26: 179, 1972.

31. Hunningghake, D. B. and Azarnoff, D. L.   Metabolism 17: 588,
     1968.

32. Kahonen, M. T. , Ylikahri, R. H. and Hassinen, I.   Metabolism
     21: 1021, 1972.

33. Krasno, L. R. and Kidera, G. J.   J. Am. Med. Ass. 219:
     845, 1972.

34. Kurup, C. K. R. , Aithal, H. N. , and Ramasarma, T. Biochem. J. 116: 773, 1970.

35. Lamb, R. G. and Fallon, H. J. J. Biol. Chem. 247: 1281, 1972.

36. Malloy, S. and Bloch, J. L. Am. J. Physiol. 184: 29, 1956.

37. Maragoudakis, M. E. J. Biol. Chem. 244: 5005, 1969.

38. McMenamy, R. H. and Oncley, J. L. J. Biol. Chem. 233: 1436, 1958.

39. Pertsemlidis, D. , Panveliwalla, D. and Ahrens, E. H. Gastroenterology 66: 565, 1974.

40. Platt, D. S. and Cockrill, B. L. Biochem. Pharmacol. 15: 927, 1966.

41. Puglisi, C. , Caruso, V. , Conti, F. , and Sirtori, C. R. Presented at the Fifth International Symposium on Drugs Affecting Lipid Metabolism, Milan, Italy, 1974.

42. Ryan, W. G. and Schwartz, T. B. Metab. (Clin. Exp.) 14: 1243, 1965.

43. Samuel, P. , Holtzman, C. H. and Goldstein, G. Circulation 35: 938, 1967.

44. Schapel, G. J. , Edwards, K. D. G. and Neale, F. C. In: Progress in Biochemical Pharmacology, Volume 9, K. D. G. Edwards, editor. Karger, Basel, 1974, p. 82.

45. Sirtori, C. R. Fumagalli, R. and Paoletti, R. Adv. Exp. Med. Biol. 38: 171, 1973.

46. Sirtori, C. R. , Agradi, E. and Mariani, C. Pharmacol. Res. Comm. 5: 81, 1973.

47. Smith, H. G. and Lakatos, C. J. Pharm. Pharmacol. 23: 180, 1971.

48. Spano, P. F. , Szyszka, K. , Pozza, G. , and Sirtori, C. R. Res. Exp. Med. 163: 65, 1974.

49. Spano, P. F. , Szyszka, K. , Galli, C. L. , and Ricci, A. Pharmacol. Res. Comm. 6: 163, 1974.

50. Svoboda, D. and Azarnoff, D. L. J. Cell. Biol. 30: 442, 1966.

51. Tolman, E. L. , Tepperman, H. M. and Tepperman, S. Am. J. Physiol. 218: 1313, 1970.

52. Westerfeld, W. W. , Richert, D. A. , and Ruegamer, W. R. Biochem. Pharmacol. 17: 1003, 1968.

53. Wilson, D. E. and Lees, R. S. J. Clin. Invest. 51: 1051, 1972.

54. Wolfe, B. M. , Kane, J. P. , Havel, R. J. , and Brewster, H. P. J. Clin. Invest. 52: 2146, 1973.

NEWER HYPOLIPIDEMIC COMPOUNDS

David Kritchevsky

The Wistar Institute of Anatomy and Biology,
36th and Spruce Streets, Philadelphia, Pennsylvania

The inhibition of lipidemia can be achieved in several ways.
The most logical mechanism - interference with lipoprotein
metabolism (synthesis, release or catabolism) - has not been
approached in a rational manner. There are some effective
hypolipidemic drugs but their mechanisms of action are not clear
and the search for a more effective compound continues.

Since this discussion involves newer hypolipidemic drugs it
will not be possible to cover the entire spectrum of available
agents. Some of the newer agents have been discussed in a recent publication (1). This exposition will cover many of the newer
drugs and a few previously known compounds that are coming into
wider use.

The most widely used drug today is ethyl p-chlorophenoxy-
isobutyrate (Figure 1). This drug (also known as CPIB, clofibrate,
and Atromid-S) is an effective hypotriglyceridemic agent with a
somewhat lesser effect on serum cholesterol levels. However,
the success of CPIB has prompted a search among other aryloxy-
aliphatic derivatives.

One such compound, methyl clofenapate (Figure 1), exhibited
marked hypolipemic effects but has not been exploited further.
Craig and Walton (2) administered this compound to patients and
found it to lower cholesterol and triglyceride levels in Type II,
III, and IV lipoproteinemias. They also observed elevations in

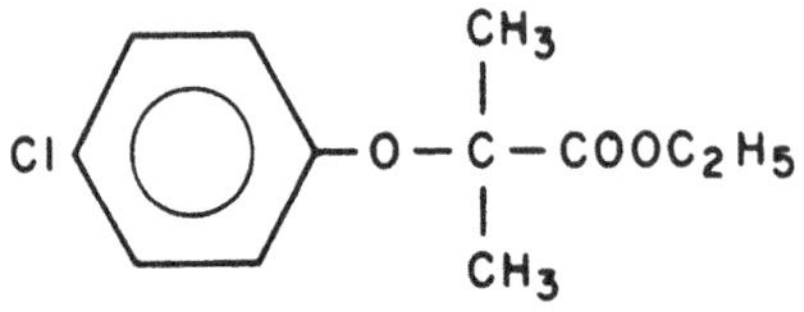

Clofibrate; CPIB

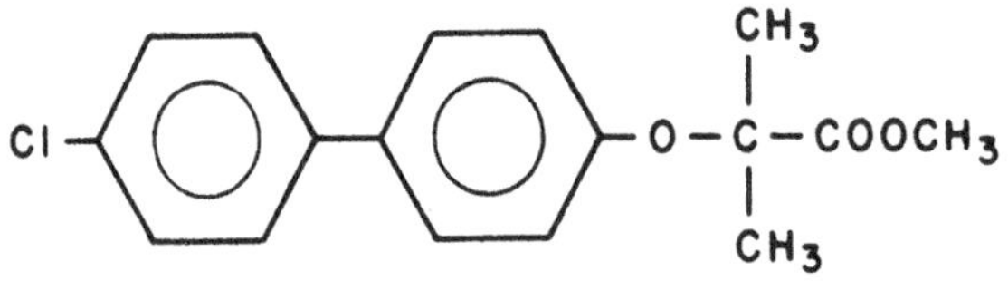

Methyl Clofenapate

Figure 1

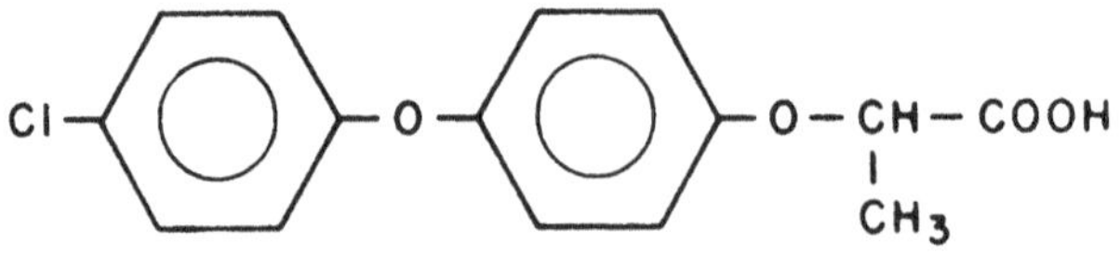

Figure 2

serum PBI (11%) and SGOT (77%).

Granzer and Nahm (3) have reported on 2-[4(4'-chlorophenoxy)-phenoxyl] propionic acid (HCG-004) (Figure 2), a compound of the aryloxyalkanoic acid type whose potency as a hypocholesteremic agent is 10.5 times that of clofibrate and whose potency as a hypotriglyceridemic compound is 26 times greater.

Imai and Shimamoto (4) have reported on 3[4-(1-ethoxy-carboxyl-1-methylethoxy) phenyl]-5(3 pyridyl)-1, 2, 4-oxadiazole (AT-308) (Figure 3 and Table 1). At a dosage of 0.03% of the diet this drug significantly lowers serum cholesterol levels of normal rats (by 18%); when added to a hypocholesteremic rat diet, at a level of 0.01% AT-308 reduces serum cholesterol by 36% (p < 0.05).

Another isobutyric acid derivative, 1, 1-bis [4'-1"-carboxy-1" methylpropoxy)-phenyl] cyclohexane (S-8527) (Figure 4) has been shown to have potent hypolipemic properties (5, 6). Table 2 summarizes its effects in rats. S-8527 had a slight positive effect on weight gain and was somewhat hepatomegalic, but not to the extent of CPIB. Thus the liver weight (as % body wt) was 4.01 for S-8527; 5.19 for CPIB and 3.64 in the controls.

Halofenate, 2-acetoamidoethyl (p-chlorophenyl) (m-trifluor-methylphenoxy) acetate (MK-185) (Figure 5) has been shown to lower serum triglycerides in rats (7, 8). In man it has been shown to lower serum triglycerides by 39% and serum uric acid by 44% after 40-48 weeks of treatment. Cholesterol levels were unaffected (9).

Probucol (DK-581) is 4, 4' (isopropylidenedithio) bis (2-6-di-t butylphenol) (Figure 6), is hyperlipidemic in the monkey, mouse and rat (10, 11) and when fed at the level of 1% of the diet this compound lessens the severity of atherosclerosis (0-4 scale) being 1.72 in the controls and 1.25 in rabbits fed DH-581 (12). Results on some clinical trials have been published (13-15), and a few of the results are summarized in Table 3. When fed for one year, DH-581 lowers both cholesterol and triglycerides by about 20%.

A new thiophenol derivative, DH 990 (Figure 7) has recently been reported to lower normal serum cholesterol levels in mice, rats and monkeys (16). This compound, 2-((3, 5-di-t-butyl-4-hydroxyphenyl)thio) hexanoic acid, when fed to rats at a level of

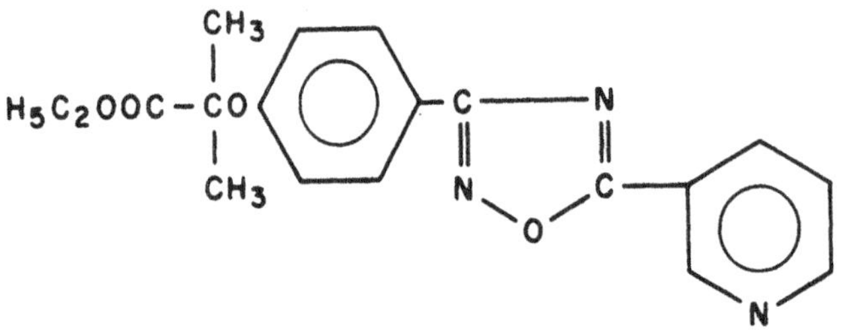

AT-308

Figure 3

Table 1

Influence of AT-308 on Cholesterol Levels in Rats*
(5 rats/gp; 7 days)

| Dosage (%) | Serum Cholesterol; mg/dl | |
	Normal Diet	Hypercholesteremic Diet
None	82 ± 3	240 ± 24
0.003	83 ± 4	200 ± 32
0.01	70 ± 4	154 ± 14a
0.03	67 ± 2b	137 ± 18b
0.10	64 ± 4b	125 ± 7c

*After Imai et al. (4).

a) $p < 0.05$; b) $p < 0.01$; c) $p < 0.001$.

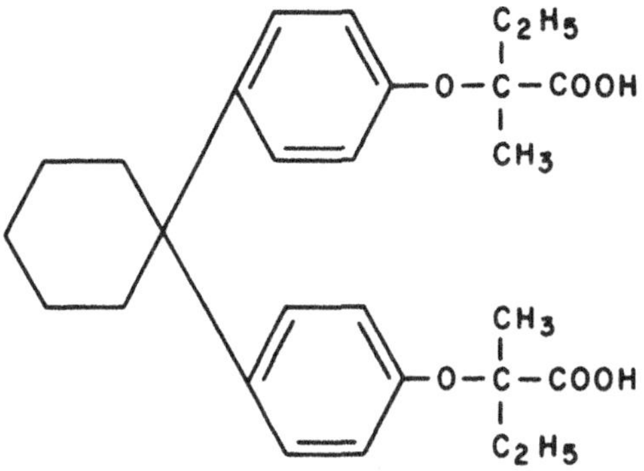

S-8527

Figure 4

Table 2

Influence of S-8527 (0.03% of Diet) on Cholesterol
Metabolism in Rats*

	S8527	Control	
Lipid Levels			
Cholesterol			
Serum (mg/dl)	30.5 ± 40	42.3 ± 3.1	p < 0.05
Liver (mg/100 g)	130 ± 8	136 ± 8	
Triglycerides			
Serum (mg/dl)	35.7 ± 6.4	65.0 ± 7.7	p < 0.02
liver (mg/100 g)	309 ± 92	489 ± 89	
Biosynthesis (% converted)			
$[1\text{-}^{14}C]$ acetate	0.71 ± 0.12	1.58 ± 2.6	p < 0.01
$[2\text{-}^{14}C]$ mevalonate	1.37 ± 0.10	1.98 ± 0.22	
% Oxidation of $[26\text{-}^{14}C]$ Cholesterol**			
$^{14}CO_2$/mg mitochondrial N	11.4 ± 1.9	8.7 ± 1.6	

*Data from three separate experiments.

**Using suitably fortified liver mitochondria.

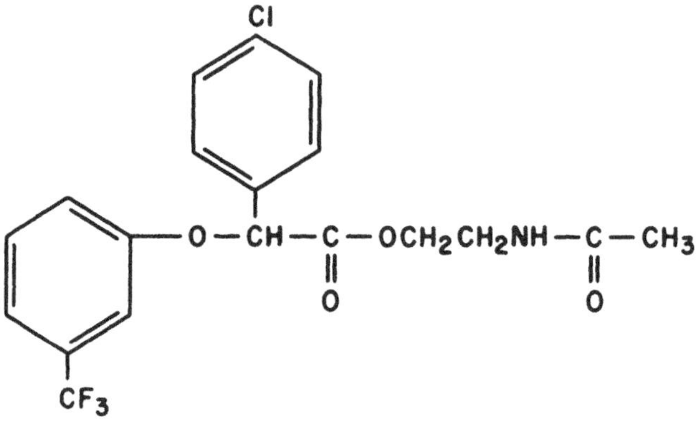

MK-185

HALOFENATE

Figure 5

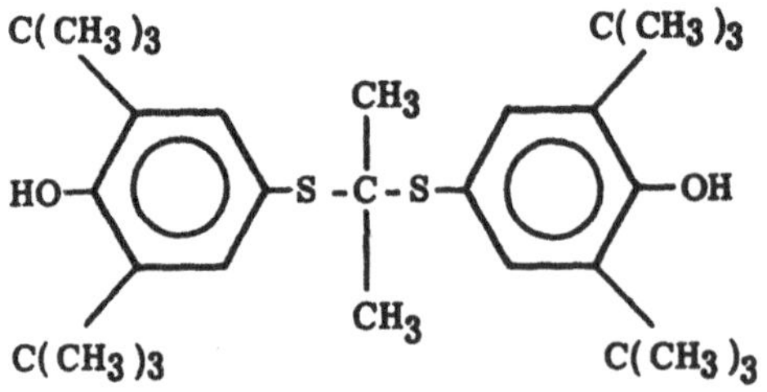

4,4'-(ISOPROPYLIDENEDITHIO)BIS
(2,6-DI-T-BUTYLPHENOL)

Figure 6

Table 3

Effect of Probucol (DH-581) on Serum Lipids in Man

No. of Patients	Duration (Wks)	Cholesterol, mg/dl			Triglycerides, mg/dl			Ref.
		Pre	Post	Δ%	Pre	Post	Δ%	
5	4	388	282	−27	117	139	+19	13
34	48	287	215	−25	172	160	− 7	14
50	52	329	263	−20	360	293	−19	15

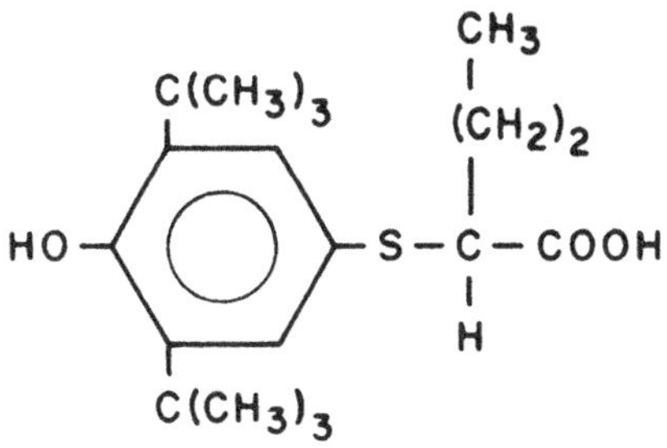

DH 990

Figure 7

0. 25% is hepatomegalic to the same extent as CPIB, and lowers
serum cholesterol and triglyceride levels by 28 and 80% respectively.

Another sulfur-containing compound, bis (hydroxyethylthio)
1, 10-decane (LL-1558) has been found to lower significantly
cholesterol levels in rats fed cholesterol and propythiouracil and
to inhibit atherosclerosis in cholesterol fed rabbits (17). In man,
LL-1558 reduces cholesterol, triglyceride and β-lipoprotein
levels in Type II and Type IV hyperlipoproteinemias (18). This
compound does not appear to be hepatotoxic in rats but does lead
to significant increases in liver weight and in the number of liver
peroxysomes seen under the electron microscope (19).

Yet another new sulfur derivative is WY-14643, [4-chloro-
(2, 3-xylidino)-2-pyrimidinylthio] acetic acid (Figure 8). Santilli
et al (20) have reported that at a dosage level of 1. 0 mg/day this
compound exerts a significant hypocholesteremic effect in rats.
In our laboratory, we have found that when administered to
cholesterol-fed rabbits at a level of 5 mg/day, WY-14643 significantly reduces the severity of atherosclerosis (Table 4).

Several other new hypolipemic compounds have recently been
reported. Tibric acid, 2-chloro-5-(cis-3, 5-dimethyl-piperidono-
sulfonyl) benzoic acid (Figure 9) reduces plasma lipids in normal
rats in doses as low as 5 mg/kg/day (21). The drug is also very
active in dogs.

Buchanan and Sprancmanis (22) have synthesized a series of
hypocholesteremic 5-methyltetrazole derivatives: two of them,
the 5-[bis (p-chlorophenoxy) methyl] and 5 {β-[4-(p-chlorophenyl)
phenoxy] methyl} derivatives (Figure 10) are especially active,
lowering cholesterol levels in normal rats by 47 and 30%, respectively.

Kaneda and Tokuda (23) isolated from mushrooms an active
hypocholesteremic principle that they named Lentysine. The
structure of this compound was identified as 2(R), 3(R) dihydroxy-
4 (9 adenyl) butyric acid (Figure 11) (24, 25) and it has been re-
named Eritadenine. Eritadenine lowers rat serum cholesterol,
triglycerides and phospholipids by 33, 39 and 27%, respectively,
when fed at a level of 4 mg/kg/day (26). Table 5 details a summary
of 23 experiments in rats. Although liver size is not greatly affected by the drug, liver lipid levels tend to increase. On a

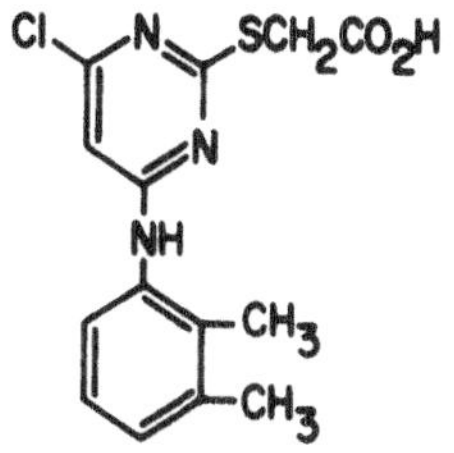

WY-14643

Figure 8

Table 4

Influence of WY-14643 and CPIB on Atherosclerosis
In Rabbits fed 2% Cholesterol and 6% Corn Oil for 8 Weeks

	Control	CPIB	WY-14643
Daily Dose (mg)	–	500	5
Cholesterol			
Serum (mg/dl)	1575 ± 233	1990 ± 171	2029 ± 368
Liver (g/100 g)	7.31 ± 0.55	4.41 ± 0.53	6.33 ± 0.66
Triglyceride			
Serum (mg/dl)	61 ± 10	97 ± 40	88 ± 15
Liver (g/100 g)	1.19 ± 0.11	0.84 ± 0.08	1.18 ± 0.13
Atherosclerosis			
Arch	2.3 ± 0.24	1.2 ± 0.21	1.5 ± 0.16
Thoracic	1.3 ± 0.17	0.9 ± 0.21	0.9 ± 0.15

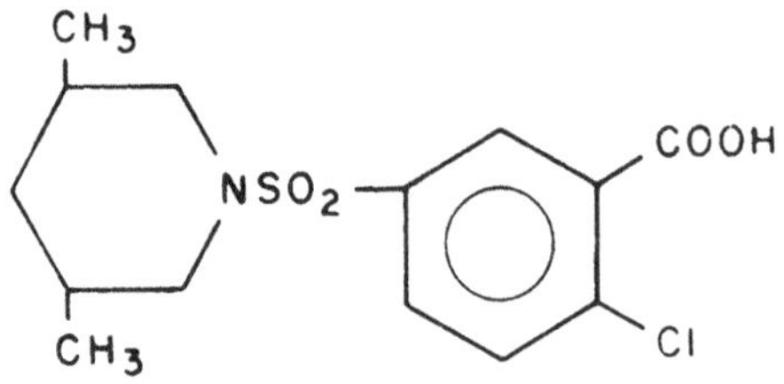

Tibric Acid

Figure 9

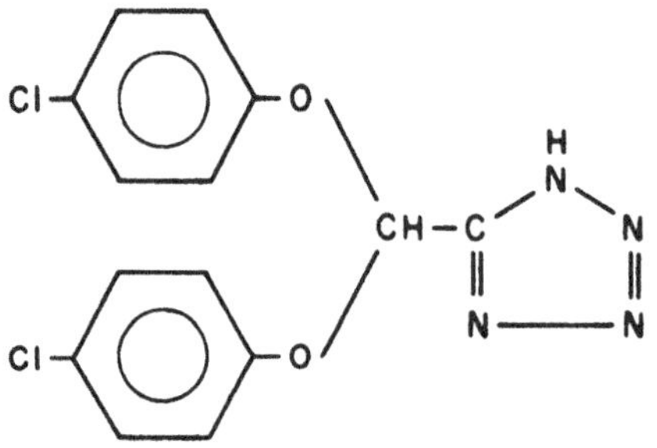

5 - [bis (p - chlorophenoxy) methyl] tetrazole

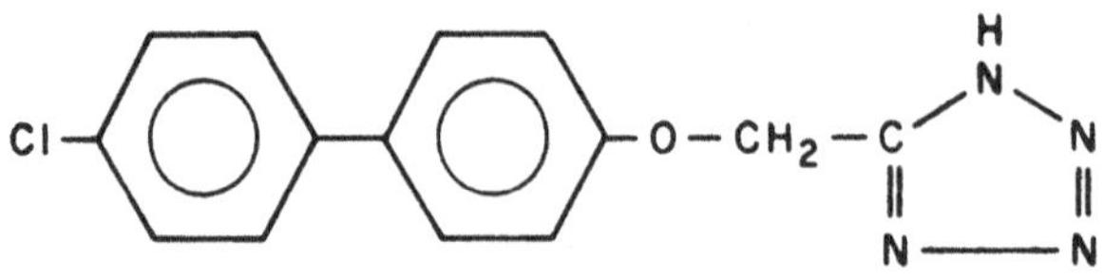

5 {β - [4 - (p - chlorophenyl) phenoxy] methyl} tetrazole

Figure 10

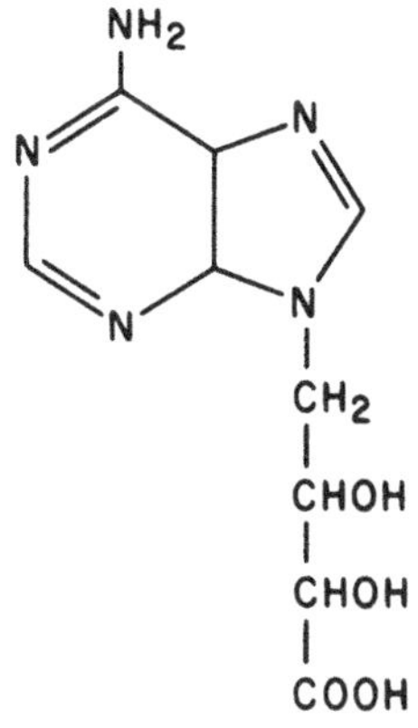

ERITADENINE

Figure 11

Table 5

Hypocholesteremic Effect of Eritadenine (Lentysine) in the Rat*
(Summary of 23 Experiments - 7 Day Feeding)

Drug	Serum lipids, mg/dl	
	Cholesterol	Triglycerides
None	79.3 ± 1.3	69.3 ± 4.0
Eritadenine (0.01%)	59.1 ± 1.0	50.4 ± 2.9

4 mg/kg/day dose liver cholesterol, triglyceride and phospholipid
levels increase by 8, 19 and 8%, respectively. Eritadenine does
not affect cholesterol biosynthesis from either acetate or meva-
lonate (27). One hypothesis regarding its mode of action suggests
redistribution of cholesterol between blood and tissues (27).

One type of hypocholesteremic drug whose mechanism of
action is understood is the kind that binds bile salts and thus
decreases cholesterol absorption. One such preparation has been
in use for some time. This material, called cholestyramine, is
a styrene-2% divinylbenzene copolymer to which are attached
quaternary ammonium groups. Its efficacy in treating hypercholesteremia is well documented (28-30). A new drug of a similar type is colestipol, an insoluble copolymer of tetraethylenepent-
amine and epichlorhydrin (31). In dogs, as little as 500 mg/kg/day
of colestipol reduces serum cholesterol and triglycerides by 15
and 20%, respectively, and increases fecal steroid excretion by
43% (32) (Table 6). When fed as 1% of the diet to rabbits maintained on an atherogenic diet, colestipol inhibits atherogenesis
by 27% (p < 0.05) (33). The drug has been studied in man by a
number of investigators (34-39) whose data are summarized in
Table 7. The studies have lasted between 9 weeks and 3 years
and all have shown drops in serum cholesterol levels which are
generally accompanied by increases in serum triglycerides.
Glueck et al (40) have compared colestipol and cholestyramine
therapy in a double crossover study and found them to be comparable.

Another bile salt sequestrant, secholex, has been tested alone
and in combination with clofibrate (41, 42). In Type IIa patients,
use of the resin alone didn't affect triglyceride levels but reduced
serum cholesterol by 20%. The combination of drugs lowered
cholesterol and triglyceride levels by 33 and 14%, respectively.
In Type IIb patients, the resin, when administered alone, reduced
serum cholesterol levels by 17% and triglycerides by 8%. The
combination therapy increased the hypolipemic effect with serum
cholesterol now being 26% lower and triglyceride levels falling
by 64%. The data are summarized in Table 8.

In the past year many new hypolipidemic agents have been
introduced. There are a number of variations on the clofibrate
theme. The appearance of many sulfur-containing preparations
has provided a type of compound in which there is considerable

Table 6

Serum and Fecal Lipids in Dogs Fed Colestipol*
(12 Months)

Colestipol (mg/kg/day)	Serum Lipids, mg/dl		Fecal Steroids µg/g feces	
	Cholesterol	Triglycerides	Acidic	Neutral
None	124	30	982	1616
500	106	24	2295	1423
1000	93	18	2869	1305
2000	76	15	2881	1219

*After Parkinson et al. (32).

Table 7

Influence of Colestipol in Serum Lipids in Man

No. Cases	Duration (Wks)	Cholesterol, mg/dl			Triglycerides, mg/dl			Ref.
		Pre	Post	Δ%	Pre	Post	Δ%	
14	52	292	252	-14	90	112	+24	34
22	26	362	334	- 8	100	131	+31	35
17	24	350	300	-14	165	175	+ 6	36
22	156	325	246	-24	125	167	+34	37
7	9	365	311	-15	179	272	+52	38
7	32	299	213	-29	210	160	-24	39

Table 8

Effect of Secholex on Serum Lipids*
(5 patients/group: 8 week treatment)

Lipoprotein Abnormality	Treatment	Serum Lipids, mg/dl			
		Cholesterol		Triglyceride	
		Before	After	Before	After
IIa	Secholex	316 ± 10	252 ± 15a	112 ± 8	115 ± 8
	Secholex + CPIB	283 ± 8	189 ± 8a	97 ± 13	83 ± 10
IIb	Secholex	321 ± 11	266 ± 14b	240 ± 17	220 ± 14
	Secholex + CPIB	277 ± 10	204 ± 8a	306 ± 38	111 ± 28

*After Howard and Evans (42).

a) $p < 0.001$; b) $p < 0.05$

interest. There has also been increasing substitution of aliphatic acids by isoxazole, imidazole and other azoxy ring compounds. Although not discussed here, some natural products have been found to possess hypocholesteremic properties, among them various sulfoxides from Cruciferae plants (43) and an extract of eggplant (44). As more is learned about lipoprotein assembly and degradation, it will become possible to assess accurately the mode of drug action and to design more effective drugs.

ACKNOWLEDGEMENT

This work was supported, in part, by USPHS grants HL-03299 and HL-05209 and a Research Career Award HL-0734 from the National Heart and Lung Institute.

REFERENCES

1. Kritchevsky, D. Lipids 9:97, 1974.
2. Craig, G. M. and K. W. Walton. Atherosclerosis 15: 189, 1972.
3. Granzer, E. and H. Nahm. Arzneimittel-Forschung 23: 1353, 1973.
4. Imai, Y. and K. Shimamoto. Atherosclerosis 17: 121, 1973.
5. Kritchevsky, D. and S. A. Tepper. Atherosclerosis 18: 93, 1973.
6. Toki, K., Y. Nakamura, K. Agatsuma, H. Nakatani and S. Aono. Atherosclerosis 18: 101, 1973.
7. Gilfillan, J. L., V. M. Hunt and J. W. Huff. Proc. Soc. Exp. Biol. Med. 136: 1274, 1971.
8. Kritchevsky, D. and S. A. Tepper. Proc. Soc. Exp. Biol. Med. 139: 1284, 1972.
9. Aronow, W. S., J. S. Vangrow, W. H. Nelson, J. Pagano, N. P. Papageorge's, M. Khursheed, P. R. Harding and M. Khemka. Current Therapeutic Res. 15: 902, 1973.
10. Barnhart, J. W., J. A. Sefranka and D. D. McIntosh. Am. J. Clin. Nutrition 23: 1229, 1970.
11. Kritchevsky, D. Fed. Proc. 30: 835, 1971.
12. Kritchevsky, D., H. K. Kim and S. A. Tepper. Proc. Soc. Exp. Biol. Med. 136: 1216, 1971.
13. Miettinen, T. A. Atherosclerosis 15: 163, 1972.
14. Polachek, A. A., H. M. Katz, J. Sack, J. Selig and M. L. Littman. Current Med. Res. and Opinion 1: 323, 1973.
15. Harris, R. J., Jr., H. R. Gilmore III, L. A. Bricker, I. M. Kiem and E. Rubin. J. Am. Geriatric Soc. 22: 167, 1974.
16. Renzi, A. A., D. J. Rytter, E. R. Wagner and H. K. Goersch. Abstracts 5th Symposium on Drugs Affecting Lipid Metabolism, p. 87, 1974.
17. Assous, E., M. Pouget, J. Nadaud, G. Tartary, M. Henry J. Duteil. Therapie 27: 395, 1972.
18. Rouffy, J. and J. Loeper. Therapie 27: 433, 1972.
19. Martin, E. and G. Feldmann, Path-Biol. 22: 179, 1974.
20. Santilli, A. A., A. C. Scotese and R. M. Tomarelli. Experientia, in press.
21. Pereira, J. N. and G. F. Holland. Abstracts 5th Symposium on Drugs Affecting Lipid Metabolism, p. 83, 1974.
22. Buchanan, R. L. and V. Sprancmanis. J. Med. Chem. 16: 174, 1973.
23. Kaneda, T. and S. Tokuda. J. Nutrition 90: 371, 1966.

24. Chibata, I., K. Okumura, S. Takeyama and K. Kotera. Experientia 25: 1237, 1969.

25. Kamiya, T., Y. Saito, M. Hashimoto and H. Seki. Tetrahedon Letters 53: 4729, 1969.

26. Takashima, K., K. Izumi, H. Iwai and S. Takeyama. Atherosclerosis 17: 491, 1973.

27. Takashima, K., C. Sato, Y. Sasaki, T. Morita and S. Takeyama. Biochem. Pharmacol. 23: 433, 1974.

28. Hashim, S. A. and T. B. Van Itallie. J. Am. Med. Assoc. 192: 289, 1965.

29. Fallon, H. J. and J. W. Woods. J. Am. Med. Assoc. 204: 1161, 1968.

30. Nazir, D. J., L. Horlick, B. J. Kudchodkar and H. S. Sodhi. Circulation 46: 95, 1972.

31. Parkinson, T. M., K. Gundersen and N. A. Nelson. Atherosclerosis 11: 531, 1970.

32. Parkinson, T. M., J. C. Schneider, Jr. and W. A. Phillips. Atherosclerosis 17: 167, 1973.

33. Kritchevsky, D., H. K. Kim and S. A. Tepper. Proc. Soc. Exp. Biol. Med. 142: 185, 1973.

34. Ryan, J. R. and A. Jain. J. Clin. Pharmacol. 12: 268, 1972.

35. Nye, E. R., D. Jackson and J. D. Hunter. New Zealand Med. J. 76: 12, 1972.

36. Sachs, B. A. and L. Wolfman. N. Y. State J. Med. 73: 1068, 1973.

37. Gross, L. and R. Figueredo. J. Am. Geriatrics Soc. 21: 552, 1973.

38. N. E. Miller, P. Clifton-Bligh and P. J. Nestel. J. Lab. Clin. Med. 82: 876, 1973.

39. Goodman, D. S., R. P. Noble and R. B. Dell. J. Clin. Invest. 52: 2646, 1973.

40. Glueck, C. J., S. Ford, Jr., D. Scheel and P. Steiner. J. Am. Med. Assoc. 222: 676, 1972.

41. Evans, R. J. C., A. N. Howard and D. E. Hyams. Angiology 24: 22, 1973.

42. Howard, A. N. and R. J. C. Evans. Atherosclerosis 20: 105, 1974.

43. Itokawa, Y., K. Inoue, S. Sasagawa and M. Fujiwara. J. Nutrition 103: 88, 1973.

44. Mitschek. G. H. A. Quart. J. Crude Drug Res. 10: 1550, 1970.

EXPERIMENTAL AND CLINICAL EVALUATION OF TWO

"ATROMID-S" ANALOGUES IN RELATION TO THEIR

DIFFERENTIAL MODES OF ACTION

M. C. Stone, J. M. Thorp* and J. S. Wain*

Research Unit, Leigh Infirmary, Leigh, Lancashire;
and *Research Department, Imperial Chemical Industries
Ltd., Macclesfield, Cheshire, United Kingdom

There is increasing evidence that plasma fibrinogen and some
of its partial breakdown products may play a critical role in the
initiation of atherosclerosis, the rheology of blood, and the availability of oxygen to the vessel wall and tissues. Pilgeram and
Pickart (1) suggested that the hepatic synthesis of fibrinogen is
related to the concentration of non-esterified fatty acids (FFA) in
plasma. It is recognized that acute tissue damage (surgery, myocardial infarction) is followed by an increase of FFA and (later)
of fibrinogen, with a sharp reduction of cholesterol-rich low-density lipoproteins (LDL).

Whether chronic changes in FFA are related to lipoprotein
synthesis or degradation, and to fibrinogen metabolism, is less
clear. The methods used to manipulate FFA mobilization are
generally relatively acute (e. g. fasting, heat, exercise, hormones,
drugs). Moreover, they are not devoid of other physiological and
metabolic effects, particularly on carbohydrate metabolism (2).
Atromid-S (clofibrate, CPIB), which reduces lipoproteins, fibrinogen and FFA, also has an effect on carbohydrate metabolism, most
readily seen as a reduction in liver glycogen (3).

We shall consider the properties of CPIB and two analogues.
These are equally effective in suppressing lipolysis in rat adipose

tissue, induced by a polypeptide in rat plasma (4, 5). They differ
in their effects on the binding of thyroxine to human albumin. The
pre-clinical evaluation of these compounds illustrates some of the
problems encountered in assessing potential hypolipemic drugs.
The clinical findings indicate some limitations of animal experiments in predicting hypolipemic activity in man. The results
enable us to draw tentative conclusions regarding the interrelationships between FFA, lipoproteins and fibrinogen.

EXPERIMENTAL FINDINGS

The structures of the three compounds to be considered are
shown in Figure 1. As indicated all occur in vivo as the free
acids. At the pH of plasma all are virtually completely ionized.
The free acid from clofibrate will be referred to as CPIB, that
from I. C. I. 55, 695 as I. C. I. 54, 856. At equimolar (ca. 0. 5mM)
concentrations relative to albumin, the fraction bound of each is:
CPIB (97%); I. C. I. 54, 856 (99. 8%); I. C. I. 55, 897 (99. 5%). The
enhanced persistence in vivo of the latter two compounds is probably largely due to their increased affinity for albumin.

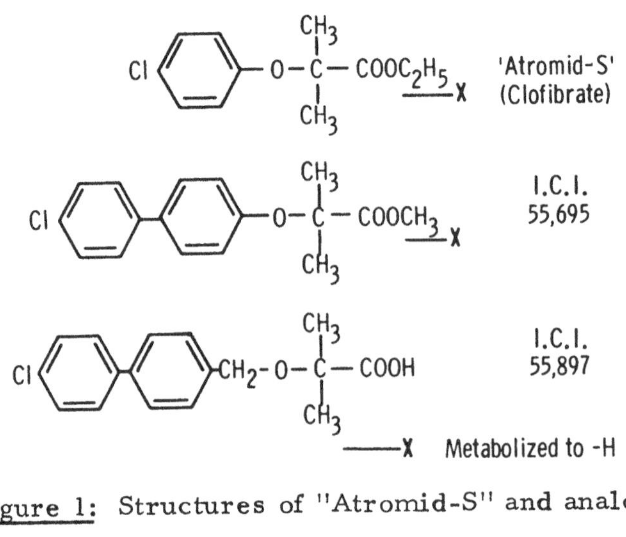

Figure 1: Structures of "Atromid-S" and analogues.

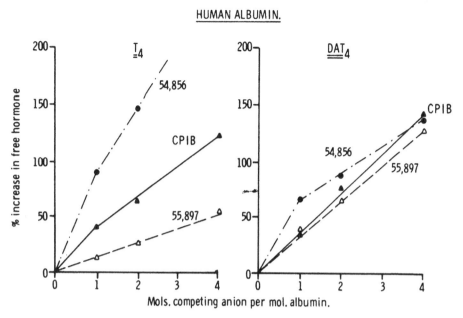

Figure 2: Effects of three compounds on binding of thyroxine (T_4) and desaminothyroxine (DAT_4) to human albumin in vitro.

The increased hypolipemic activity of I. C. I. 55, 695 in man (6, 7), compared with that of clofibrate, appeared to be related to an increased ability of the free acid to displace thyroxine (T_4) from human albumin (8). As shown in Figure 2, I. C. I. 55, 897 had significantly less effect than CPIB on the binding of thyroxine to albumin, whereas it appeared equiactive with both I. C. I. 54, 856 and CPIB in displacing desaminothyroxine (DAT_4) from albumin. The binding of DAT_4 to albumin models that of FFA.

Table 1 shows the comparative activity of the two compounds in the rat at doses giving similar serum concentrations. There is a selective loss of effects on liver weight and plasma cholesterol compared with plasma total esterified fatty acid (TEFA) and fibrinogen. The lower dose of I. C. I. 55, 897 required to achieve a given serum concentration reflects its longer half-life than that of CPIB.

TABLE 1

Effects of Administering CPIB and I. C. I. 55, 897

to Male Albino Rats for 14 Days

			CPIB	ICI 55,897
Drug concentration in serum		μg/ml	135.0	161.0
		mM	0.63	0.53
Drug % in diet			0.2	0.02
% Control		Growth	93	98
		Liver wt/body wt.	129	114
	Plasma	Cholesterol	54	83
		TEFA	72	81
		Fibrinogen	80	87

The differences in albumin bound fractions is of importance
in considering the relation between the toxicity of highly-bound
compounds and the concentration of the unbound fraction present,
at different total concentrations of drug. Figure 3 illustrates the
relationship between the free and total concentrations of a compound (having the indicated binding characteristics) to the albumin
of three species. The free concentration of the compound increases
more rapidly in relation to total drug level in the rat and dog than
in man. If doses chosen from chronic toxicological evaluation are
designed to produce a 3 to 4-fold multiple of the total concentration
regarded as "therapeutic" in the rat, the free concentration available for intra-cellular distribution may be increased by as much as
100-fold compared to the concentration at therapeutic doses in man.
It is presumably the free fraction which is more likely to be responsible for any toxicity, rather than the protein-bound drug.

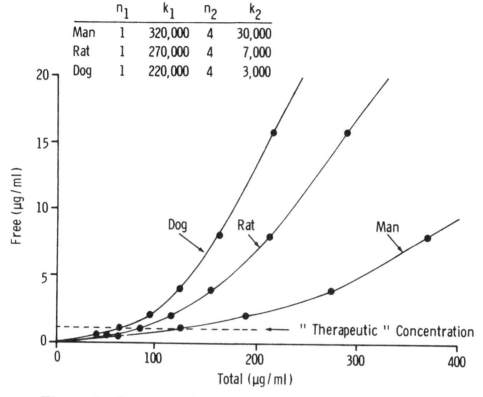

Albumin Concentration = 3.45%

	n_1	k_1	n_2	k_2
Man	1	320,000	4	30,000
Rat	1	270,000	4	7,000
Dog	1	220,000	4	3,000

Figure 3: Species differences in binding characteristics

Another factor to be considered in the pre-clinical evaluation of a compound is its metabolism and route of excretion. The latter may profoundly affect the nature of its activity and/or side-effects in different species. CPIB is excreted via the kidney both in the rodent and in man. I. C. I. 54,856 is excreted via the liver in the rodent, but via the kidney in man (6). Table 2 shows the disposition of I. C. I. 55,897 in different species. Note the switch from hepatic excretion in rat and dog to predominantly renal excretion (without entero-hepatic recirculation) in primates. As is often the case, there are varying differences in half-life between the sexes.

TABLE 2

Excretion and Persistence of I. C. I. 55,897

in Different Species

Species	Sex	Dose (mg/k)	Excretion (% dose)		Half-life (days)
			Faeces	Urine	
Rat	M	5	97	5	4
	F	5	82	4	6
Dog	M	10	87	2	<1
Marmoset	M	5	11	80	1.1
	F	5	11	93	0.5
Rhesus	M	10	19	78	<1
Man	M	1.5-2.5	-	66	2-5
	F	1-2	-	51	6-8

CLINICAL FINDINGS

After many years of laboratory and toxicological evaluation, we were eventually able to examine the effects of I. C. I. 55,897 in hyper-lipemic patients. One purpose of this trial was to test the validity of the hypothesis shown in Figure 4. Would a compound with selective effects on FFA release and transport regulate hepatic synthesis and peripheral levels of VLDL and LDL?

Thirteen patients with well-characterized lipoprotein abnormalities were treated with I. C. I. 55,897 for periods of 3-12 months. The doses used started at 50 mg daily, increasing to a maximum of 700 mg. Serum concentrations of I. C. I. 55,897 were monitored continuously. The results for 12 patients are shown in Table 3. The compound tended to increase cholesterol and LDL. There were small and variable reductions in total esterified fatty acid (TEFA) and VLDL. VLDL response was much less than that achieved by

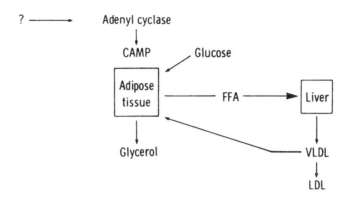

Figure 4: A widely held hypothesis.

TABLE 3

Mean Responses of Hyperlipemic Patients to

Treatment with I. C. I. 55,897

Lipoprotein type (sex)		II A (M)	II A (F)	II B (M)	IV (M)	All
No. of patients		2	2	3	5	12
Mean plateau drug concentration (µg / ml)		216	192	218	251	227
Cholesterol	Initial	348	375	331	214	292
	% change	+4.3	+18.9	+12.7	+20.9	+14.8
Total ester fatty acid	Initial	25	22	33	35	30.7
	% change	-12.0	+4.5	-12.0	-17.1	-12.7
LDL	Initial	683	742	591	347	530
	% change	+6.3	+18.7	+16.5	+30.0	+19.6
VLDL	Initial	209	183	436	492	379
	% change	-24.8	+10.9	-2.5	-10.2	-8.7
Fibrinogen	Initial	354	353	306	374	350
	% change	-33.9	-32.0	-18.3	-33.4	-29.4

CPIB, at concentrations in serum a half those of I. C. I. 55, 897.
A similar lack of response was found in one Type III patient who
had previously shown a typically dramatic lipoprotein response to
treatment with "Atromid-S".

We considered whether the lack of lipoprotein response could
be due to a chance selection of "non-responders, " or to sex-de-
pendent metabolic differences.   That this seems unlikely is illustrated by the findings in one patient, previously treated with the
"Thyroxine-specific" I. C. I. 55, 695 (Table 4).   This had reduced
cholesterol and LDL.   However, I. C. I. 55, 897, at more than
double the concentration in serum, increased both lipid fractions.
These observations may be of interest to workers attempting to
establish correlations between structure and activity based on
in vitro techniques.

TABLE 4

Responses to Treatment with I. C. I. 55, 695 and

I. C. I. 55, 897 of a Type IIA Patient (F, 58 yr)

Treatment		ICI 55,695	ICI 55,897
Dose (mg / day)		10	150
Drug concn. in serum (μg / ml)		75	186
Cholesterol (mg / 100 ml)	Initial	475	443
	Final	330	542
	% change	-30	+22
LDL (mg / 100 ml)	Initial	960	910
	Final	660	1,060
	% change	-31	+17

TABLE 5

Effects of I. C. I. 55, 897 at Two Drug Levels

in the Same Group of 12 Patients

Variables	Control level	Effects (% control) at mean ICI 55,897 concentrations of:	
		58 μg / ml	180 μg / ml
Fibrinogen	325	90	78
E.S.R.	7.3	95	89
Uric acid	7.6	90	80
Alkaline phosphatase	81	108	108
SGOT	14.4	94	83
ICDH	6.5	101	93
CPK	53	99	119

In marked contrast to its lack of hypolipemic activity, I. C. I. 55, 897 significantly reduced plasma fibrinogen (Table 3). This reduction averaged 29% from an initial level of 350 mg/dl. The relationship between pre-treatment levels and response is discussed later. The dependence of the fibrinogen response on the serum concentration of I. C. I. 55, 897 is shown in Table 5. Similar drug-level dependent reductions of E. S. R., uric acid and SGOT occurred. Of interest is the fact that alkaline phosphatase and SGOT showed small changes in opposite directions to those usually observed with "Atromid-S" and I. C. I. 55, 695. We believe these to be directly related to the mechanism of action of these compounds. Isolated increases of CPK occurred at the higher dosages in some patients, but were not sustained, remained within the "normal range" of the individual, and were not accompanied by other subjective or objective abnormality.

How does the effect of I. C. I. 55,897 compare with that of
CPIB or I. C. I. 55,695? Figure 5 shows pre- and post-treatment
levels of fibrinogen in the patients. With one exception, in whom
no change occurred, all are lower after treatment, the regression
line indicating that the response is greater the higher the pre-
treatment level, and that there is a level, (about 230 mg/dl) at
which no response would be expected. Figure 6 shows similar
regression lines for two drug levels of I. C. I. 55,897, for I. C. I.
55,695 and for CPIB. This suggests that the slope of the line is
a function of drug concentration, and is probably independent of
structural differences between these three compounds. Note that
all 4 trials give an intercept with the zero-effect (45) line at about
250 mg/dl. This may represent the "physiologically normal" level
of plasma fibrinogen. We suggest that these responses represent
a relatively non-specific effect (in this series) on the release and/
or transport of FFA. This is accompanied by a parallel reduction
in fibrinogen synthesis by the liver.

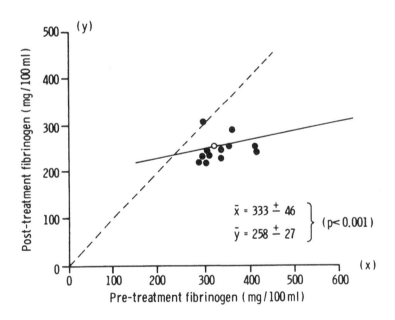

Figure 5: Effect of I. C. I. 55,897 (mean dose 4.9 mg/k; serum
concentration 0.7 mM) on fibrinogen in man.

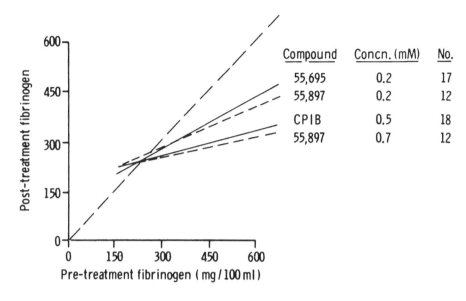

Figure 6: Comparison of effects of three oxyisobutyrates on plasma fibrinogen in man.

CONCLUSIONS

The differential activities of the three compounds considered confirm the validity of the in vitro model. Thus differential effects on the binding of thyroxine to albumin are precisely equivalent to relative hypolipemic activity in man. Conversely, similarity of effects on DAT_4 (FFA) binding to albumin are equated with similarity of fibrinogen responses. These findings support the view that the mode of action of "Atromid-S" involves a selective localization of thyroxine into liver, and an extrahepatic suppression of lipolysis and FFA mobilization (9).

What evidence is there for a relationship between FFA and fibrinogen in man? Hoak et al (10) have shown that triiodothyronine induces equivalent increases (60-70%) of both FFA and fibrinogen. Neither is suppressed by simultaneous administration of the β-adrenergic antagonist propanolol. Benaim et al (11) found a linear relationship between FFA and fibrinogen in patients with

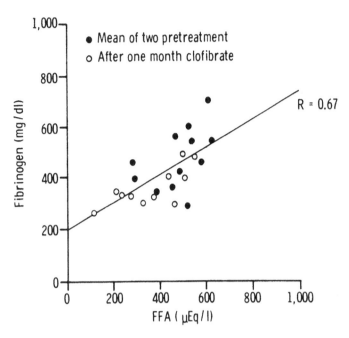

Figure 7: Correlation between resting FFA and fibrinogen in angina patients.

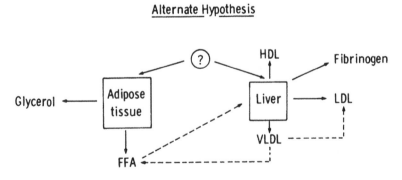

Figure 8: An alternate hypothesis for the role of FFA.

angina. This was maintained, at lower levels, after one month of treatment with clofibrate (Figure 7). It is of interest that the intercept at the ordinate occurs at 200 mg/dl of fibrinogen. This is of the same order as the "zero-effect" intercepts shown in Figure 6.

These observations suggest an alternate hypothesis (Figure 8) to account for the differential effect of hormones or drugs on lipo- lysis and FFA on the one hand, and hepatic synthesis of lipoproteins and fibrinogen on the other. Compounds of the albumin-bound oxy- isobutyrate series may cause differential and independent responses of adipose tissue lipolysis and of hepatic synthesis of lipoproteins or fibrinogen. This may occur through a purely extra-cellular effect on the distribution of thyroid hormones and FFA. It is also possible that they interfere at the cell membrane with the effects of FFA themselves, or of a common mediator (? polypeptide) which regulates metabolic activity of both adipose tissue and liver.

What, if any, is the clinical significance of a compound able to reduce fibrinogen? Dormandy et al (12) found that clofibrate re- duced blood viscosity and plasma fibrinogen in patients with inter- mittent claudication. A proportion of patients showed evidence of clinical improvement. A similar mechanism may account for the improvement in peripheral blood flow in hyperlipoproteinemic type III patients treated with clofibrate (13).

The prognostic significance of a raised fibrinogen concentra- tion has received relatively little attention. Hart et al (14) found a correlation between sequelae and fibrinogen in insulin-requiring diabetics, but no correlation with lipoproteins. A 3-year follow- up of total mortality in this group of patients has recently been completed (15). Of the characteristics studied at entry, only age and fibrinogen showed significant segregation of subsequent mor- tality (Table 6). In this group of patients there was no significant correlation between age and fibrinogen. The mean age of those with fibrinogen less than 300 mg/dl was 49.8 ± 17.7 years, and total mortality 18.5%. The mean age of those with fibrinogen greater than 300 mg/dl was 54.4 ±14.5 years, and total mortality 35.3%.

Wardle et al (16) found that eleven out of twenty-six diabetic patients with a plasma fibrinogen over 400 mg/dl sustained a major cardiovascular event within two years. Bottiger and Carlson (17)

TABLE 6

Mortality (all causes) in 3-year Follow-up of 116 Diabetics

Related to Characteristics at Screening

Characteristic	Group	% Mortality	χ^2	p
Age	<50	10.4	10.19	<0.01
	≥50	36.8		
Sex	Female	35.6	0.57	NS
	Male	23.0		
Capillary fragility	Normal	23.4	0.25	NS
	Abnormal	27.5		
Sequelae	Absent	20.0	2.28	NS
	Present	32.1		
LDL	<500	27.6	0.18	NS
	≥500	24.1		
VLDL	<180	26.6	0.04	NS
	≥180	25.0		
Fibrinogen	≤300	18.5	4.22	<0.05
	>300	35.3		

found a 2-1/2-fold increase in infarction rate between the lowest and highest quintiles of E. S. R. (correlated with fibrinogen) in a 9-year follow-up of asymptomatic men.

It is an open question whether "enhanced" effects of novel compounds on LDL and/or VLDL, if unaccompanied by any action on HDL or the FFA/fibrinogen axis, are likely to be of clinical efficacy. Only long-term trials to determine the effect of such compounds on the incidence of cardiovascular morbidity and mortality can answer this question. If appropriate measurements are note made at screening and follow-up the mechanism of any successful intervention will remain obscure.

REFERENCES

1. Pilgeram, L. O. and Pickart, L. R.   J. Atheroscler. Res. 8: 155, 1968.
2. Barrett, A. M. and Thorp, J. M.   Br. J. Pharm. Chem. 32: 381, 1968.
3. Platt, D. S. and Thorp, J. M.   Biochem. Pharmacol. 15: 915, 1966.
4. Thorp, J. M. and Barrett, A. M.   Prog. Biochem. Pharmacol. 2: 337, 1967.
5. Barrett, A. M.   Br. J. Pharm. Chem. 26: 363, 1966.
6. Thorp, J. M.   In: Atherosclerosis: Proceedings of the Second International Symposium (R. J. Jones, editor), p. 541, 1970.
7. Craig, G. M.   Atherosclerosis 15: 265, 1972.
8. Thorp, J. M.   Excerpta Medica Int. Congr. Series 254: 98, 1971.
9. Thorp, J. M.   Excerpta Medica Int. Congr. Series 283: 90, 1973.
10. Hoak, J. C., Wilson, W. R., Warner, E. D., Theilem, E. O., Fry, G. L. and Benoit, F. L.   J. Clin. Inv. 48: 768, 1969.
11. Benaim, M. E., Dewar, H. A. and Thorp, J. M.   In preparation.
12. Dormandy, J. A., Gutteridge, J. M. C., Hoare, E. and Dormandy, T. L.   Br. Med. J. 4: 259, 1974.
13. Zelis, R., Mason, D. T., Braunwald, E. and Levy, R. I.   J. Clin. Inv. 49: 1007, 1970.
14. Hart, A., Thorp, J. M. and Cohen, H.   Postgrad. Med. J. 48: 435, 1971.
15. Hart, A., Cohen, H. and Thorp, J. M.   Unpublished observations.
16. Wardle, E. N., Piercey, D. A. and Anderson, J.   Postgrad. Med. J. 49: 1, 1973.
17. Bottiger, L. E. and Carlson, L. A.   In: Early Phases of Coronary Heart Disease -Skandia Symposia 1972.   J. Waldstrom, T. Larsson, and N. Ljungstadt, editors, p. 158.

Approaches to Treatment
of Hyperlipidemias

PATHOGENESIS OF HYPERLIPIDEMIAS,

CLUES TO TREATMENT?

Daniel Steinberg, M. D. , Ph. D. , David B. Weinstein,
Ph. D. , Thomas E. Carew, Ph. D.

Division of Metabolic Disease, Department of Medicine,
School of Medicine, University of California, San Diego,
La Jolla, California

Other papers presented at this Symposium have dealt with
specific recent developments in treatment of hyperlipidemia by
dietary, pharmacologic and surgical intervention. There continues
to be a high level of interest and research activity in these areas.
What we would like to do today is to present a speculative discussion
of where we may be heading with regard to modes of intervention,
pharmacologic and otherwise. There have been rapid and impressive advances in recent years in our understanding of lipoprotein
structure, lipoprotein metabolism and of the enzymes involved in
the latter. Do these new findings inform us with regard to new
opportunities in the management of hyperlipidemia?

As we learn more about the metabolism and ultimate fate of
lipoproteins, particularly their metabolism by peripheral tissues
(including the artery), we can begin to ask possibly important
questions about our yardsticks for evaluating therapy. Currently
we rely almost exclusively on steady-state plasma lipid levels.
Because a given intervention is successful in decreasing steady-
state plasma lipoprotein levels does not necessarily mean that it
represents good management of arteriosclerosis and its complications. This is a concern recently expressed nicely by Dr. Donald
B. Zilversmit (1) and shared by many of us. If it is correct that
metabolism of lipoproteins in peripheral tissues, perhaps including
arterial tissue, is quantitatively significant (2, 3) then one can

Table I

A CLASSIFICATION OF SOME THEORETICALLY FEASIBLE
APPROACHES TO THE REDUCTION OF SERUM LIPID LEVELS

I.   Decrease the rate of production and secretion of lipoproteins into the serum.

   A.   By reducing the availability of the component parts needed for the
production of lipoproteins — glycerides, phospholipids, cholesterol,
cholesterol esters or lipoprotein-protein.

      1.   By reducing dietary intake or reducing absorption:

         a.   Of the constituents themselves [β -sitosterol; cholestyramine]

         b.   Of the precursors of these constituents

         c.   Of the cofactors required for their synthesis

      2.   By reducing endogenous (hepatic) synthesis from lower molecular
weight precursors

         a.   By interfering directly with enzymatic reactions involved in
the biosynthesis [triparanol and other inhibitors of cholesterol
synthesis; puromycin and other inhibitors of protein synthesis]

         b.   By accelerating alternative pathways that complete for the
intermediates or precursors in the biosynthesis.

         c.   By interfering with the synthesis of cofactors essential for the
biosynthesis.

         d.   By accelerating the breakdown and/or excretion of cofactors.

      3.   By interfering with delivery of precursors from the periphery (e.g.
free fatty acids) [nicotinic acid; ? clofibrate]

      4.   By accelerating degradation [thyroid hormone and analogues]

      5.   By accelerating excretion [cholestyramine]

Table 1 (cont.)

B. By interfering directly with the process of lipoprotein manufacture and/or delivery into the serum [?clofibrate; ?colchicine]

    1. By offering analog molecules that disrupt lipid micelle formation or make the lipoproteins difficult to transport out of the cell.

    2. By otherwise disrupting the system (as yet undefined) for amalgamation of the component parts of lipoproteins.

    3. By interfering with the system (as yet undefined) for transporting lipoproteins from liver to serum.

II. Increase the rate of removal of lipoproteins from the serum.

    A. By increasing the rate of degradation of individual components of the lipoproteins.

        (Note that there may be different mechanisms at play determining the rate of degradation of lipid or protein components as they exist in the tissues, on the one hand, and after they have been incorporated into the serum lipoproteins on the other.)

    B. By modifying the structure of the lipoproteins in such a way as to reduce their life-time in the serum.

    C. By stimulating systems responsible for removal of lipoproteins from the serum [heparin and heparinoids; ?clofibrate]

[Reproduced with permission from Advances in Pharmacology, Vol. 1, (S. Garattini and P.A. Shore, eds.), Academic Press, New York, 1962, p. 81]

conceive of intervention modes that decrease plasma lipoprotein
levels yet <u>favor</u> deposition of lipids in the arterial wall. This is
certainly not a new concern but it is one that may nag at us more
persistently as more and more newer agents enter the therapeutic
arena, especially when their mode of action is uncertain.

APPROACHES TO THE MANAGEMENT OF HYPERLIPIDEMIA

In 1962 in the course of writing a reveiw on the then relatively
new field of chemotherapeutic management of hyperlipidemia, I
tried to list a catechism of all the theoretical ways one might
intervene for the correction of hyperlipoproteinemia (Table 1) (4).
In many instances it was, in retrospect, quite fanciful. However,
some of the approaches suggested that indeed fanciful at that time,
in view of our then limited understanding of lipoprotein structure
and metabolism, are beginning to enter or may very soon enter
the realm of the pharmacologically feasible. The classification
proposed was couched in terms of lipoprotein secretion and degradation but there was not much to say about intervention <u>directly</u>
modifying lipoprotein metabolism. Instead, the bulk of what could
be said then and of the work done over the intervening (no pun intended) years has dealt with approaches directed at modifying the
metabolism of one or another component moiety of the lipoproteins.
Indeed, most of the drugs in current use can be fit into a niche in
Section 1A, as shown in the brackets added to Table 1.

Section 1B proposed intervention directly on the process of
lipoprotein manufacture and/or delivery into the serum. At the
time there were no drugs known to be in that category. With the
deeper understanding we now have of the mechanisms involved in
lipoprotein biosynthesis and secretion (5) it may be possible soon
to deliberately screen for and evaluate agents that affect these
processes. We know that the apoproteins are synthesized in the
rough endoplasmic reticulum in the liver and that they move on
by way of the smooth endoplasmic reticulum in the liver to the
Golgi apparatus, arriving there pretty much completed. However,
much remains to be learned about the biology of the Golgi apparatus
and of the processes involved, for example, in the packaging of
VLDL molecules into secretory vesicles. They are evidently
transported within such vesicles to the cell surface for discharge
into the space of Disse. If we knew the details of these processes,
would it be reasonable to expect to be able to interfere specifically

with them and yet not alter the many other vital functions of the
hepacytes? I think the answer may be yes. I say that in part because I am so impressed by the dramatic - and dramatically
specific - effects of orotic acid in the rat. As you know, orotic
acid added to an adenine-poor diet will result in the almost complete disappearance of VLDL and LDL from rat plasma (6). Yet
these animals, other than developing a fatty liver, appear to carry
on quite nicely in other respects. The synthesis and secretion of
other proteins made in the liver seems to go on unimpaired. The
exact mechanism of action of orotic acid is not known, nor is it
known why the effect is species specific. Nevertheless, the im-
plication is that some aspect of lipoprotein biosynthesis and
secretion is sufficiently unique to allow intervention that can affect
it without adversely affecting other functions.

INTERVENTION AFFECTING LIPOPROTEIN BIOSYNTHESIS

Interference with protein biosynthesis in a totally nonspecific
way would not appear to be a likely approach; one would of course
anticipate unacceptable side effects. Even if intervention affected
only secreted proteins but failed to discriminate among them, the
spectrum of effects might be too broad (e. g. changes in fibrinogen
levels). While one should not rule out completely the possibility
of intervention that need not be qualitatively totally specific but is
at least quantitatively selective, the ideal approach must be quite
specific.

Recent observations in our laboratory give some further basis
for believing that lipoprotein synthesis and secretion may be sufficiently unique and different from the synthesis and secretion of
other proteins to allow intervention limited largely to lipoprotein
production (7). Dr. Weinstein set out to study lipoprotein synthesis
by isolated hepatocytes. Wanting to have a cell line that could be
grown and thus provide multiple dishes of identical cells for study,
he explored the use of fetal rat liver cells prepared by methods
like those developed by Leffert and Paul (8). Using this technique,
one can derive hepatocyte cultures that grow for up to three weeks,
going through three or four cell cycles. These cells demonstrated
several characteristic properties of the growing hepatocyte, namely,
secretion of albumin, secretion of α-1- fetoprotein and the ability
to synthesize arginine from ornithine and thus grow in an arginine-
deficient medium. Upon incubation with labeled amino acids, the

cells synthesized and secreted labeled proteins into the medium
at a high rate. However, they did not appear to secrete lipoproteins that could be identified as serum lipoproteins. There was
a small amount of radioactivity present in protein with density
1.063 - 1.21 but immunochemical studies showed that this was not
related to any of the circulating rat serum lipoproteins.

In view of this negative result, we had to ask whether fetal rat
liver simply lacked a significant capacity for lipoprotein secretion.
However, tissue slices prepared from fetal rat liver did secrete
lipoproteins which were shown to be immunochemically identical
with normal circulating rat lipoproteins. In fact, as much as 15%
of the radioactivity in secreted proteins found in the medium was
attributable to lipoproteins. In this respect, the fetal rat liver is
not qualitatively different from adult rat liver (9). Why, then, did
the isolated cells in culture fail to synthesize and secrete lipoproteins? The plating efficiency for the fetal hepatocytes is very
low, so we had to consider the possibility that we were selecting
a subpopulation of liver cells and that these particular cells were
incapable of secreting lipoproteins. The other possibility was that
contact with the plastic surface in some way inhibited lipoprotein
synthesis and/or secretion, or that the conditions for cell culture
lacked some essential stimulus for lipoprotein synthesis and
secretion.

Dr. Weinstein then turned to studies of Morris hepatoma 7777.
Slices of this tumor had been reported to synthesize and secrete
lipoproteins (10) and this was readily confirmed (with immunochemical characterization of the secreted lipoproteins). Then
cells derived from the same hepatoma but grown in monolayer
culture were studied. These cells in monolayer made and secreted
almost no lipoprotein. In this case there was little ambiguity with
regard to the question of selection because the tumor cells, of
course, grow very nicely and the yield from plating was always
very high - at least 40%. Thus, it appears that the cells in monolayer culture secrete proteins other than the lipoproteins very
actively and total synthesis of cell protein occurs very rapidly.
However, there seems to be something unique, perhaps, about
the secretion of the lipoproteins so that it is selectively deleted
or suppressed in monolayer culture. In the present context, these
observations again suggest that lipoprotein biosynthesis and secretion is enough different from the biosynthesis and secretion of
other hepatic proteins that one might theoretically intervene specifically and leave the patient in good condition otherwise.

In recent years, we have seen a great deal of research by cell biologists on intracellular transport. We are now beginning to understand microtubules and microfilaments and their role in the secretion of proteins and protein hormones (11). Drugs that disrupt these systems (e. g. colchicine, vinblastine and cytochalasin B) have provided powerful tools for the study of these processes in a variety of secretory cells. It has been shown that colchicine does indeed inhibit lipoprotein secretion (12, 13). However, albumin secretion is also inhibited i. e. the effect seems not to be specific with respect to lipoprotein secretion. Is it possible that drugs can be found that will slow down the process of lipoprotein secretion without affecting secretion of other hepatic products? The answer depends on whether the process of moving lipoprotein-containing vesicles is indeed different from the process of moving albumin or other secreted proteins through the cytoplasm of the liver cell and out into the plasma compartment.

INTERVENTION AFFECTING LIPOPROTEIN DEGRADATION

In 1962, there was little information available as to how lipoproteins were removed from the plasma compartment. Of the possibilities listed in our speculative classification (Table I, section II), the only one about which much could be said was the role of heparin in the clearance of chylomicrons and VLDL (IIC). The fate of LDL and HDL was essentially unknown at that time. We are only now beginning to see some light on this problem of lipoprotein catabolism. We begin to see that the basic metabolic error in most, but probably not all, of the genetically determined hyperlipoproteinemias lies in systems for removal of lipoproteins from the plasma compartment (see reference 14 for review). We do not intend to review those studies here; much of it has been covered in other sections of these Proceedings. We only want to make a few remarks about the potential and also the hazard of approaches designed to increase the rate of removal of lipoproteins from the plasma compartment.

The central and vital question is whether uptake of lipoproteins (or of their component parts) into arterial wall shares the same properties as removal of lipoproteins by other tissues. If it does, then anything we do to increase the rate of removal of lipoproteins from the plasma may increase the rate of their uptake into the arterial wall as well. That, obviously, may not be good. On the

other hand, if the fundamental process in the artery differs qualitatively, then we may indeed be able to reduce the concentration
of lipoproteins that the artery "sees" by facilitating uptake in
other body tissues and thus reducing plasma concentration.

The development by Ross of a method for culturing smooth
muscle cells derived from the artery (15) has made it possible
to study the question of lipoprotein uptake by these cells in culture.
Bierman, Stein and Stein (16) have already reported that these
cells take up and degrade both HDL and VLDL. We have been
particularly interested in the metabolism of LDL by peripheral
tissues in view of the results of Sniderman et al (3) suggesting
that most of the removal of LDL occurs in peripheral tissues
rather than in the liver. The studies of Brown and Goldstein show
that fibroblasts can degrade LDL and, most importantly, that a
defect in this mechanism may underly familial essential hypercholesterolemia (17). If arterial tissue shares the ability of other
peripheral tissues to remove LDL, then interventions that increase
the rate of removal of LDL might actually accelerate atherogenesis!

As shown in Figure 1, swine aortic smooth muscle cells do
take up LDL at a significant rate (18). They also degrade the
apoprotein moiety converting ^{125}I-labeled LDL to fragments soluble in trichloroacetic acid (TCA) (Figure 2). Very little TCA-
soluble radioactivity remained associated with the cells at any
time. As in fibroblast cultures (19, 20), the presence of cholesterol
in the medium suppressed cholesterol synthesis by pig smooth
muscle cells and so did the addition of LDL itself to the medium
(Table II). Whereas HDL has little effect on cholesterol synthesis
in human fibroblast cultures (17), it suppressed acetate incorporation into cholesterol by about 30% in our smooth muscle cell cultures. Degradation of LDL has also been observed by Stein and
Stein in Jerusalem using cultured rat aortic smooth muscle cells
and rat LDL (21).

At least quantitatively, two peripheral cell types that have been
studied - fibroblasts and smooth muscle cells - behave similarly
in regard to LDL catabolism and the feedback effect of LDL on
cholesterol synthesis. Are all peripheral cells going to behave
in a life fashion? Are the peripheral tissues importantly involved
in LDL removal or not? If, as has been suggested by some
investigators (22, 23), the liver is the primary site of LDL removal,
and if the mechanism for its removal in the liver is very different

Table II

INHIBITION OF STEROL SYNTHESIS BY LDL AND CHOLESTEROL IN SWINE SMOOTH MUSCLE CELLS

Addition to medium	$I-[^{14}C]$-acetate incorporation relative to that in lipoprotein-free medium
	(%)
Fetal calf serum	42
Lipoprotein-free fetal calf serum	100
Lipoprotein-free fetal calf serum:	
+ 5 µg LDL-cholesterol/ml	50
+ 20 µg LDL-cholesterol/ml	26
+ 40 µg LDL-cholesterol/ml	19
Lipoprotein-free fetal calf serum:	
+ 5 µg cholesterol/ml	68
+ 20 µg cholesterol/ml	38
+ 40 µg cholesterol/ml	35

Swine smooth muscle cells were grown to 50% monolayers in Dulbecco's modified Eagle's medium containing 10% fetal calf serum. Maximum sterol synthesis rates were attained by shifting the clutures to medium containing 10% lipoprotein-free fetal calf serum for 18 hr. Swine low density lipoprotein (expressed as µg LDL cholesterol) or free cholesterol (in 10 µg ethanol) were added to the cultures and sterol synthesis rates were measured by $I-[^{14}C]$-acetate incorporation during the sixth and seventh hour after the addition of lipoprotein or cholesterol.

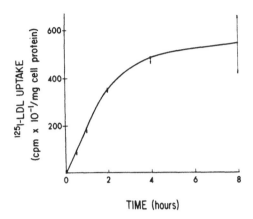

<u>Figure 1:</u> Swine smooth muscle cells incubated with medium containing 10% lipoprotein-free fetal calf serum plus 10 μg ^{125}I-LDL protein/ml medium.   Ordinate shows total radioactivity associated with cells after specified time of incubation at 37° C. Cell associated radioactivity was trichloroacetic acid precipitable (> 95%) and predominantly in protein (less than 22% extractable by chloroform-methanol).   Maximum uptake at 8 hr is equivalent to 1.5 μg LDL protein/mg cell protein.

from that in peripheral tissues, then intervention that increases the rate of removal of LDL may be a safe way to correct hyper-betalipoproteinemia. If, on the other hand, most of the removal of LDL occurs in the periphery, as suggested by our own work (2, 3), and if arterial tissue indeed shares properties of the other peripheral tissues, then any intervention that increases rates of LDL removal requires very careful evaluation.

A similar argument can be made with regard to methods of intervention that increase the rates of removal of VLDL or chylomicrons. Zilversmit has stated the problem very clearly (1). As he points out, the <u>process</u> of removal, if it includes the production of lipoprotein degradation products that enhance atherogenesis, may be detrimental even while accomplishing the nominal purpose of decreasing plasma lipoprotein levels.

PORTACAVAL SHUNT

In closing we want to discuss briefly a dramatic new approach to therapy - the portacaval anastomosis as performed by Starzl and

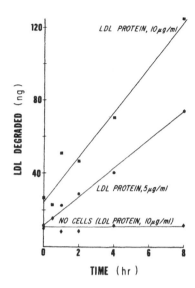

Figure 2: Degradation of ^{125}I-LDL to non-iodide trichloroacetic
acid (TCA) soluble products by swine smooth muscle cell cultures.
Cells incubated with 5 µg/ml and 10 µg/ml LDL protein released
labeled split products into medium in an approximately linear
fashion. Simultaneous control plates incubated with no cells present
showed no increase in non-iodiode TCA-soluble radioactivity with
time.

coworkers (24). An end-to-side anastomosis of the portal vein to
the inferior vena cava was carried out in the case of a 12 year old
girl with homozygous familial hypercholesterolemia. She had
already had a myocardial infarction, suffered intractable angina,
and had congestive heart failure with rather severe aortic stenosis.
Coronary angiograms revealed almost total occlusion along the
entire length of both main arteries and the circumflex branch was
not visualized at all. Her cholesterol levels ranged from 600 to
800 mg% and had failed to respond to any of the diet and drug regimens tried. Average life expectancy in cases of this kind is about
20 years and this girl's prognosis was grave indeed, justifying
radical measures.

After surgery, the patient's cholesterol level fell progressively
and by six months had dropped from about 700 to 300 mg%. Her

xanthomata melted away to practically nothing and her angina
quickly disappeared. Sixteen months postoperatively, a coronary
angiogram now showed all three major vessels and the lumens
were obviously widened generally, although some localized con-
strictions remained (T. E. Starzl, personal communication). The
murmur of aortic stenosis had disappeared and the measured
pressure gradient across the aortic valve had dropped from 50 mm
Hg to 10 mm Hg! This is perhaps the most clear-cut and dramatic
example of objectively demonstrated regression of human atherosclerosis.

How does it work? We have reported that hepatectomy causes
an increase in the fractional rate of LDL removal from plasma in
swine and dogs (3). The mechanism involved is not known but must
relate either to alterations in the LDL or in the cellular processes
effecting uptake. The portal vein is, of course, anastomosed to
the vena cava in these animals. Could shunting alone somehow
bring about a similar improvement in the "efficiency" of LDL
removal?

From the exciting findings of Brown and Goldstein we know
that the fibroblasts of homozygous Type II patients - and I believe
they examined the fibroblasts from Starzl's patient also - lack the
high-affinity receptors for LDL and therefore lack both the feed-
back control of sterol synthesis found in normal fibroblasts and also
the ability to take up and degrade LDL at low concentrations of the
lipoprotein (17, 20). If the high-affinity receptor is a specific membrane protein it is unlikely that the number of such receptors can
be increased, certainly not if the genetic information is lacking.
On the other hand, the cellular events that internalize LDL from
the low-affinity sites, which even the homozygotes seem to have
(20), might very well be modifiable. For example, the shunt
procedure presumably increases peripheral blood concentrations
of a number of substances including bile acids, insulin, glucagon,
intestinal hormones and so on. By interaction with cell membranes,
these materials might enhance inhibition of LDL. Such an effect
should be revealed by an increase in the fractional removal rate of
LDL and possibly other serum proteins. Our laboratory has tested
this possibility by measuring fractional catabolic rate of LDL in
swine before and after creation of a portacaval shunt (25). As
shown in Table III, there was no consistent change in LDL degradation rate as a result of the shunting procedure. There was a fall
in plasma cholesterol levels in the immediate postoperative period

Table III

FRACTIONAL CATABOLIC RATE (FCR) OF ^{125}I-LDL
IN SWINE BEFORE AND AFTER PORTACAVAL SHUNTING

Pre-shunt FCR	Post-shunt FCR
(hr^{-1})	(hr^{-1})
0.051	0.060 (5 days)
0.060	0.064 (7 days)
0.060	0.079 (8 days)
0.054	0.056 (13 days)
0.056	0.057 (14 days)

Fractional catabolic rate (FCR) is the fraction of the plasma LDL pool irrever-

sibly removed in 1 hr. The data show a small change in FCR in animals

studied 5 - 8 days post-shunt; by 13 - 14 days the pre- and post-shunt values

do not differ significantly. Interval between shunting and repeat determina-

tion of FCR given in parentheses.

and 4 months later levels were still about 20% below control
values. However, FCR was normal, indicating a decrease in
total LDL flux.

It is difficult to say whether or not one should expect in a
normal animal changes like those that may occur in the homozygous
Type II patients. For this reason, it is only possible to offer a
tentative interpretation of these results. What they suggest is that
the basic response to the shunting is a decrease in the rates of
LDL production rather than an increase in the rates of LDL removal. Immediately on creation of a shunt, the total blood flow
to the liver drops. Although there is some compensatory increase
in hepatic artery flow, the best estimates are that total flow is

reduced by about 50%. Thus, the flow of free fatty acids and other substrates to the liver may be drastically reduced and output of VLDL might be expected to drop. Moreover, Starzl and his co-workers noted substantive changes in the subcellular structure of the liver in the patient after shunting, including a marked decrease in the amount of the rough endoplasmic reticulum. Whether the changes reflect only reduction in total blood flow, or , also, shunting of hormones and nutrients around the liver is of some importance in suggesting avenues of approach. A basic question is that of whether pharmacologic means can be found to similarly alter hepatic lipoprotein production. We have already discussed reasons for believing that lipoprotein production is indeed a highly specialized and sensitive hepatic function. If the shunt produced a somewhat selective inhibition of lipoprotein production, should it not be possible to do the same thing non-invasively?

CONCLUSION

As our concepts of lipoprotein metabolism evolve, the ways in which we can think about intervention - drugs, diet or surgery - must also evolve. Ten years ago, except for the use of heparin, most of our thinking centered on the metabolism of component lipids in the lipoproteins - mainly cholesterol - or lipids contributing to the synthesis of lipoproteins - mostly free fatty acids (FFA). Now we have a broader stage on which to work and perhaps we can approach the problem of regulating the metabolism of the lipoproteins themselves. Our approaches over the next years will probably draw as much on cell biology as on biochemistry.

REFERENCES

1. Zilversmit, D. B. Circulation Res. 33: 633, 1973.
2. Steinberg, D. , Carew, T. , Chandler, J. G. and Sniderman, A. D. In: Regulation of Hepatic Metabolism (F. Lindquist and N. Tygstrup, eds.), Academic Press, New York, 1974, p. 144.
3. Sniderman, A. D. , Carew, T. E. , Chandler, J. G. and Steinberg, D. Science 183: 526, 1974.
4. Steinberg, D. In Advances in Pharmacology, Vol. 1, Academic Press, New York, 1962, p. 59.
5. Margolis, S. and Capuzzi, D. In Blood Lipids and Lipoproteins: Quantitation, Composition and Metabolism (G. J. Nelson, ed.), Wiley-Interscience, New York, 1972, p. 825.

6. Standerfer, S. B. and Handler, P. Proc. Soc. Exper. Biol.
    Med. 90: 270 (1955); Windmueller, H. G. J. Biol. Chem.
    239: 530, 1964.

7. Weinstein, D. B. and Engelhorn, S. Fed. Proc. 33: 1479, 1974.

8. Leffert, H. and Paul, D. J. Cell Biol. 52: 559, 1972.

9. Marsh, J. B. and Whereat, A. F. J. Biol. Chem. 234: 3196,
    1959; Radding, C. M. and Steinberg, D. J. Clin. Invest. 39:
    1560, 1960.

10. Narayan, K. and Morris, H. P. FEBS Letters 27: 311, 1972.

11. Olmsted, J. B. and Borisy, G. G. Ann. Rev. Biochem. 42:
    507, 1973.

12. Stein, O. , Sanger, L. and Stein, Y. J. Cell. Biol. 62: 90,
    1974.

13. Le Marchand, Y. , Singh, A. , Assimacopouls-Jeannet, F. ,
    Orci, L. , Rouiller, C. and Jeanrenaud, B. J. Biol. Chem.
    248: 6862, 1973.

14. Steinberg, D. Proc. Third International Symposium on Athero-
    sclerosis, 1973, Berlin, W. Germany, Springer-Verlag, in
    press.

15. Ross, R. J. Cell Biol. 50: 172, 1971.

16. Bierman, E. L. , Stein, O. and Stein, Y. Circulation Res. 35:
    136, 1974.

17. Brown, M. S. and Goldstein, J. L. Proc. Nat. Acad. Sci.
    (U. S. A.) 71: 788, 1974.

18. Weinstein, D. , Carew, T. E. and Steinberg, D. Circulation
    (Suppl. III) 50: 270, 1974.

19. Williams, C. D. and Avigan, J. Biochim. Biophys. Acta 260:
    413, 1972.

20. Brown, M. S. , Dana, S. E. and Goldstein, J. L. J. Biol. Chem.
    249: 789, 1974.

21. Stein, O. and Stein, Y. Circulation Res. , in press.

22. Hay, R. V. , Pottenger, L. A. , Reingold, A. L. , Getz, G. S.
    and Wissler, R. W. Biochem. Biophys. Res. Commun. 44:
    1471, 1971.

23. Eisenberg, S. , Windmueller, H. G. and Levy, R. I. J. Lipid
    Res. 14: 446, 1973.

24. Starzl, T. E. , Chase, H. P. , Putman, C. W. and Porter, K. A.
    Lancet II: 940, 1973.

25. Carew, T. E. , Saik, R. P. , Johansen, K. H. , Dennis, C. A.
    and Steinberg, D. Circulation (Suppl. III) 50: 183, 1974.

SERUM LIPOPROTEIN COMPOSITION IN DIFFERENT TYPES OF HYPERLIPOPROTEINEMIA

Lars A. Carlson

King Gustaf V Research Institute, Karolinska Hospital, Stockholm, Sweden

DEFINITION OF TYPES OF HYPERLIPOPROTEINEMIA

At present the six types of hyperlipoproteinemia (HLP) defined in the WHO memorandum (1) as an extension of the typing system of Fredrickson et al (2) is in common use. According to this memorandum the diagnosis of a type of HLP is based upon "elevation" of one or more of the following lipoprotein (LP) classes: chylomicrons, very low density LP (VLDL) and low density LP (LDL). This may seem simple and clear but there are many difficulties involved. One major problem is to define "elevated." This definition may certainly vary depending on its purpose, which for example can be clinical (diagnostic, treatment), epidemiological, genetic, physiological, etc. The definition of "normal" and "elevated" may furthermore vary with factors such as age, sex, season, etc. Whatever the purpose is for definition of normal values we prefer to use the statistical method with construction of cumulative frequency curves for reasons discussed in detail elsewhere (3). With these curves it is easy to find the lipid level corresponding to a given percentile of the control (normal) population. In the study to be described we have for clinical purpose used the upper 90th percentile as an upper "normal" limit, values above are then considered elevated.

MATERIAL AND METHODS

The material comprises all male cases referred to the Lipid Clinic, Department of Geriatrics, Uppsala University from September 27, 1971 to January 31, 1973. The reason for these dates are that the laboratory set-up of this new department was ready in September, 1971 and the same method for LP analysis was used until the end of January, 1973 at which time the methodology was changed. Cases with secondary HLP, subjects on lipid lowering regimens and cases with acute illnesses were excluded. The material thus comprises a number of clinical categories: control subjects, asymptomatic accidentally discovered HLP, various atherosclerotic manifestations with and without HLP. LP of fasting sera were separated in the preparative ultracentrifuge into the very low (VLDL), the low (LDL) and the high density (HDL) LP classes by centrifugation at d=1.006 and d=1.063 as described in detail elsewhere (4). These LP fractions were analyzed for their content of cholesterol and triglycerides (4). Agarose gel lipoprotein electrophoresis was performed according to Noble (5) on whole serum and on the top and bottom fraction obtained after centrifugation at d=1.006. With these techniques two lipoprotein "variants" can be seen as described elsewhere (4). In the top fraction containing VLDL this LP has the characteristic pre-β-mobility. However, in addition a slower moving LP can be seen in about 20-30% of all cases (3). The mobility of this LP is often slightly more than that of the β LP and it has been called LPB (Late Pre Beta) (5). In the bottom fraction containing LDL and HDL usually only the β (LDL) and α (HDL) LP bands are seen. However also in about 20% an additional band with pre-β mobility is seen. This band has been called SPB (Sinking Pre Beta) (6).

This report describes LP values in the 609 men fulfilling the above criteria. Of these 107 (18%) had LPB and 73 (12%) SPB.

INFLUENCE OF THE DEFINITION OF NORMAL LIMITS ON THE DISTRIBUTION OF TYPES OF HYPERLIPOPROTEINEMIA

As might be anticipated the level of the cut off points for defining "elevated" will influence the frequencies of the various types of HLP. Table 1 shows the effects of choosing the cut off point at either the 85th or 90th percentile of a control population. At the lower value less subjects were of course "normal." The

Table 1

Percentile	90%	85%
Upper "normal" LP value		
LDL cholesterol mg/100 ml	210	200
VLDL triglycerides mmol/l	1.8	1.4
	n	n
Type of HLP		
Normal	281	208
II A	54	54
II B	12	33
III	11	12
IV	65	116
V	6	6

Number of men with various types of HLP in the sample of 429 men without any LP variants. Two cut off points were used, the upper 90th and 85th percentile for control men (3).

more interesting effects of choosing the lower level was that particularly the number of subjects with type II B and IV HLP increased two-to threefold. This clearly shows that not only the proportion of normal and HLP in the population but also the proportion of the various types of HLP is greatly influenced by the definition of "elevated." The inevitable fact that one has to set fixed limits for "elevated" is one of many drawbacks of the present system for classification of HLP.

LIPOPROTEIN COMPOSITION IN THE VARIOUS TYPES OF HYPERLIPOPROTEINEMIA

The concentration of cholesterol and triglycerides in the three main LP classes are given in Table 2 for the various types of HLP when no LP "variants" were present. Here and in the following the upper "normal" limit was chosen at the 90th percentile of a control material (3). Type II A was thus present when LDL cholesterol was above 210 mg/100 ml, type IV when VLDL triglycerides were above 1.8 mmol/l, type II B when both these criteria were present, type III when VLDL triglycerides were above 1.8 mmol/l and floating β-LP was seen and type V when VLDL was elevated and chylomicrons were present ("standing test").

A number of LP abnormalities were present besides those inherent in the definition of each type of HLP. Thus type II A exhibited a raised VLDL cholesterol causing the ratio cholesterol/triglycerides to be slightly increased. Also LDL triglycerides were increased above the normal group. HDL lipids of type II A showed no deviations from the pattern of the normal group.

All types with elevated VLDL triglycerides had the same kind of abnormal pattern for HDL: increase in its triglyceride content and decrease in cholesterol. These types also showed a rise in LDL triglycerides.

The composition of VLDL, LDL and HDL in the various types of HLP were further analyzed by comparing the relation between their cholesterol and triglyceride content to the relation between these lipids seen in control subjects (3). Figure 1 shows that for VLDL the most abnormal relation existed for type III. In correspondence with previous reports (7) type III VLDL had a high

Table 2

Concentration of triglycerides (TG, mmol/l) and cholesterol (Chol, mg/100 ml) in the three serum LP classes, VLDL, LDL and HDL, in different groups of hyerplipoproteinemia. Only sera without LP variants. Mean ± SEM.

Group[1]	n	VLDL TG	VLDL Chol	VLDL Chol/TG[2]	LDL TG	LDL Chol	HDL TG	HDL Chol
N	281	1.02±.02	20±.5	19	0.51±.01	155±2	0.24±.01	48±1
II A	54	1.15±.05	24±1^{xxx}	21^{xx}	0.70±.02^{xxx}	246±6	0.27±.01	46±1
II B	12	2.73±.26	52±4^{xxx}	19	0.79±.03^{xxx}	229±3	0.28±.02^{x}	39±2^{xxx}
III	11	3.66±.98	125±21	34^{xxx}	0.66±08	128±19	0.30±.02^{xx}	38±2^{xxx}
IV	65	3.10±21	53±4^{xxx}	17^{x}	0.57±.02	149±5	0.30±.01	38±1^{xxx}
V	6	33.0±13.7	394±125^{xxx}	12^{xxx}	0.65±.07^{x}	70±21	0.38±.04^{xxx}	20±4^{xxx}

Underlined values indicate the lipoprotein which by definition of the type is elevated. For VLDL TG this value was 1.80 mmol/l and for LDL cholesterol 210 mg/100 ml.

1. N = normolipoproteinemia, other symbols referring to types of hyperlipoproteinemia according to ref (1).

2. Ratio Chol/TG

x, xx and xxx indicate that the difference against group N was significant at the 5, 1 and 0.1% level.

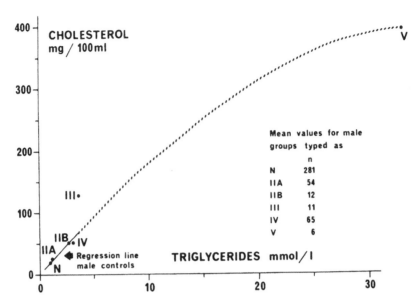

Figure 1: Relation between the cholesterol and triglyceride content of VLDL in the various types of HLP without LP variants. The mean value for each type is given.

cholesterol content in relation to its triglyceride content. For groups N, II A, II B and IV the relation in VLDL was near normal. Type V had a lower ratio cholesterol/triglycerides than the controls. However since the cholesterol and triglyceride content of type V is far outside that of the controls one cannot extrapolate from the controls into the region of type V. Furthermore with the technique used in the LP analysis type V VLDL contain chylomicra which are known to have a lower cholesterol/triglyceride ratio than VLDL.

The normolipoproteinemic group (N) had a LDL composition close to the relation for the controls (Figure 2). Also for type II B the average composition was fairly close to that of the controls, while type II A had a somewhat more cholesterol rich LDL. The relation between cholesterol and triglycerides in LDL for types III, IV and V, particularly the latter, were characterized by

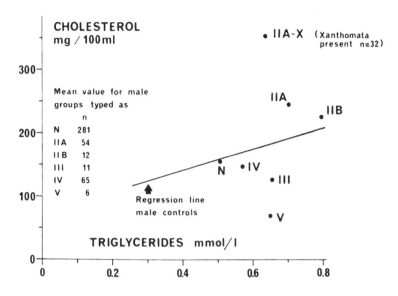

Figure 2: Relation between the cholesterol and triglyceride content
of LDL in the various types of HLP without LP variations. The
mean value for each type is given. In addition the mean value for
a group of patients with type II A-X (see text) is given.

falling below the line for the normal LDL composition i. e. a rich-
ness of triglyceride.

For HDL (Figure 3) going from type II A to type V there was
an increasing deviation from the normal relation between cholesterol and triglycerides. As this suggested that both the decrease
in HDL cholesterol as well as the increase in HDL triglycerides
were quantitatively related to the VLDL concentration these HDL
parameters were plotted against the VLDL triglyceride level in
Figures 4 and 5. That there exists very strong quantitative relationships is evident from these figures, HDL cholesterol decreasing and HDL triglycerides increasing with increasing VLDL
triglyceride concentration.

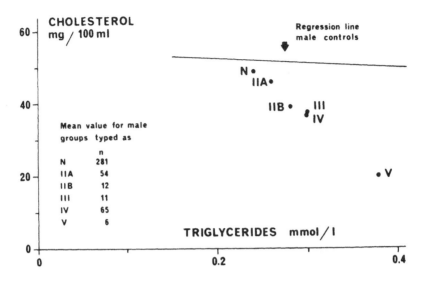

<u>Figure 3:</u> Relation between the cholesterol and triglyceride content of HDL in the various types of HLP without LP variants. The mean value for each type is given.

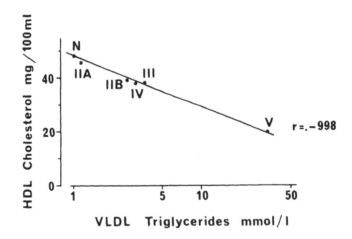

<u>Figure 4:</u> Relation between the concentration of VLDL triglyceride and the cholesterol content of HDL for the various types of HLP. The regression line and the correlation coefficient are indicated.

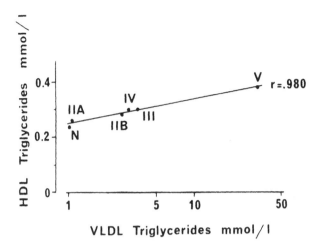

<u>Figure 5</u>: Relation between the concentration of VLDL triglyceride and the triglyceride content of HDL for the various types of HLP. The regression line and the correlation coefficient are indicated.

LIPOPROTEIN COMPOSITION IN THE VARIOUS TYPES OF HYPERLIPOPROTEINEMIA IN THE PRESENCE OF LPB (Late Pre Beta)

There are two main features which are characteristic for the LP composition of <u>all</u> groups both normo- and hyperlipoproteinemia when LPB was present (Table 3). The <u>first</u> is an increased cholesterol content of VLDL which leads to a raised ratio cholesterol/triglycerides in this LP. The <u>second</u> is an elevation of LDL triglycerides. These features of LPB have been described before both in normal male subjects (3) and in men with HLP (8). LPB LP may be the cholesterol rich so called "intermediary particles" which are degradation products of chylomicra and VLDL (77).

Table 3

Concentration of triglycerides (TG mmol/1) and cholesterol (Chol, mg/100 ml) in the three serum LP classes, VLDL, LDL and HDL, in different groups of hyperlipoprotenemia. Sera containing the LBP (late pre-β LP). Mean ± SEM.

Group [1]		VLDL			LDL		HDL	
		TG	Chol	Chol/TG [2]	TG	Chol	TG	Chol
N	59	1.07±.05	28±2^{xxx}	26^{xxx}	0.63±.02^{xxx}	166±3^{xx}	0.28±.01^{xxx}	47±1
II A	19	1.34±.08	37±3^{xxx}	28^{xxx}	0.82±.05^{xx}	235±4	0.30±.02^{x}	45±2
II B	4	2.83±.11	73±4^{xx}	26^{xx}	0.96±.08^{x}	234±8	0.33±.05	39±3
IV	25	3.01±.25	69±6^{xx}	23^{xxx}	0.73±.04^{xxx}	162±6	0.28±.01	39±2

Underlined values indicate the lipoprotein which by definition of the type is elevated. For VLDL TG this value was 1.8 mmol/1 and for LDL cholesterol 210 mg/100 ml.

1. N = normolipoproteinemia, other symbols referring to types of hyperlipoproteinemia according to ref (1).

2. Ratio Chol/TG

The values for each group were tested against the values for the corresponding group without LPB LP (Table 1).

x, xx and xxx indicate that the difference was significant at 5, 1 and 0. 1% level.

LIPOPROTEIN COMPOSITION IN THE VARIOUS TYPES
OF HYPERLIPOPROTEINEMIA IN THE PRESENCE OF SPB
(Sinking Pre Beta)

In contrast to LPB the presence of SPB had no major influence on the LP composition except a tendency for slightly higher cholesterol concentration in HDL (Table 4). This may be due to the presence of SPB in our HDL fraction which contains all LP with d<1.063. If SPB is identical with the LP carrying the LP (a) antigen one would expect this to be the case as this LP is found in the 1.05-1.12 g/ml density fraction of plasma (9).

THE COMMON TYPE II A AND THE UNCOMMON (II A-X)

In this material none of the men who's serum was assigned type II A HLP had tendinous xanthomata. In the text book descriptions of type II A great emphasis is put on the so called familial hypercholesterolemia which goes with often multiple tendinous xanthomata. In the Uppsala and Stockholm region this well-defined genetic disease is rare while moderate hypercholesterolemia of the type II A pattern is common. From the LP point of view there are characteristic differences between the common and moderate type II A and the one with tendinous xanthomata here called II A-X. To illustrate these LP differences I have compiled the data from all type II A-X I have seen at the Lipid Clinic, Department of Medicine, Karolinska Hospital since 1960. Table 5 shows that the most pronounced difference between the common type II A and type II A-X is the much higher LDL cholesterol in II A-X. The composition of LDL is also different with regard to the relation cholesterol/triglycerides as seen in Figure 2. II A-X had a much more cholesterol rich LDL LP. This probably reflects a greater proportion of LP with S_f 0-12 above S_f 12-20.

There were also differences in VLDL between II A-X and the common type II A. Both the triglyceride and cholesterol content was lower in II A-X sera. However, the triglyceride content was proportionally lower than the cholesterol. Thus the VLDL of type II A-X were more cholesterol rich than the VLDL of common II A.

These results show that there are not only clinical differences between II A-X HLP and the common type II A HLP but also both quantitative as well as qualitative differences in LDL and VLDL.

Table 4

Concentration of triglycerides (TG, mmol/1) and cholesterol (Chol, mg/100 ml) in the three serum LP classes, VLDL, LDL and HDL, in different groups of hyperlipoproteinemia. Sera containing the SPB (sinking pre-β).   Mean ± SEM.

Group[1]		VLDL			LDL		HDL	
		TG	Chol	Chol/TG[2]	TG	Chol	TG	Chol
N	45	0.94±.06	17±1	18	0.49±.02	165±4	0.25±.01	51±1ˣˣ
II A	13	1.07±.11	23±3	21	0.68±.04	229±5	0.26±.01	45±2
II B	5	2.79±.42	46±6	16	0.74±.04	226±6	0.31±.02	46±3ˣ
IV	10	2.49±.19ˣ	45±4	18	0.57±.04	165±3	0.25±.02	42±2

Underlined values indicate the lipoprotein which by definition of the type is elevated.   For VLDL TG this value was 1.8 mmol/1 and for LDL cholesterol 210 mg/100 ml

1. N = normolipoproteinemia, other symbols referring to types of hyperlipoproteinemia according to ref (1).

2. Ratio Chol/TG

The value for each group was tested against the values for the corresponding group without SPB LP (Table 1).

x and xx indicate that the different against group N was significant at the 5 and 1% level.

Table 5

Concentration of triglycerides (TG, mmol/l) and cholesterol (Chol, mg/100 mg) in the three LP classes VLDL, LDL and HDL in the common type II A and in the uncommon, called II A-X. Mean ± SEM.

Group	n	VLDL			LDL		HDL	
		TG	Chol	Chol/TG	TG	Chol	TG	Chol
II A	54	1.15 ± .05	24 ± 1	21	0.70 ± .02	246 ± 6	0.27 ± .01	48 ± 1
II A-X	32	0.53 ± .09 xxx	18 ± 2 xx	34 xxx	0.63 ± .03	355 ± 13 xxx	0.20 ± .01 xxx	50 ± 2

xx and xxx indicates that the difference between II a and II A-X were significant at the 1 and 0.1% level.

SUMMARY

Fasting serum lipoproteins (LP) were separated into VLDL, LDL and HDL by ultracentrifugation and the content of cholesterol and triglycerides analyzed in each LP class in 609 consecutive men attending a lipid clinic.

The effect of using different cut off points in the definition of HLP was discussed. It was pointed out that by using lower values for the cut off points there is not only an increase in the number of subjects with hyperlipoproteinemia (HLP) but also shifts in the proportions between the various types of HLP, particularly with increase in the amount of types IIB and IV.

In addition to the LP abnormalities inherent in the definition of each type of HLP other LP abnormalities were observed. Thus type IIA HLP had cholesterol rich VLDL with an increased ratio cholesterol/triglycerides. The types of HLP with increased VLDL triglycerides had characteristic changes in both LDL and HDL. For LDL its triglyceride content was increased and HDL showed a lowering of its cholesterol content and a rise in triglycerides. These changes were more pronounced the higher the VLDL tri- glyceride concentration was.

Both normo- and hyperlipoproteinemic subjects having the second pre-β LP on agarose gel electrophoresis of the VLDL fraction called LPB (Late Pre Beta) had two characteristic LP features. VLDL had an increased cholesterol/triglyceride ratio. LDL had a raised triglyceride content. The relation of LPB to so called intermediary particles was discussed.

When the SPB (Sinking Pre Beta) LP variant was present this had negligible effects on the LP composition.

Type IIA was present in 14 percent of the 609 men. None had tendinous xanthomata. The LP pattern of this common type IIA was compared to the LP pattern of the uncommon type IIA where tendinous xanthomata are present, called IIA-X. Type IIA-X had much higher LDL cholesterol and in relation to the triglyceride content a more cholesterol rich LDL. Furthermore type IIA-X had lower VLDL lipids than the common type IIA, but type IIA-X was more cholesterol rich. The differences in clinical appearance as well as in quantitative and qualitative LP composition between the common type IIA and type IIA-X makes it important to separate these two types of HLP from each other.

ACKNOWLEDGEMENT

This work was supported by grants from the Swedish Medical Research Council (19X-204).

REFERENCES

1. Beaumont, J. L. , Carlson, L. A. , Cooper, G. R. , Fejfar, Z. , Fredrickson, D. S. and Strasser, T. Bull. Wld. Hlth Org. Org. Mond. Sante 43: 891, 1970.
2. Fredrickson, D. S. , Levy, R. I. and Lees, R. S. New England J. Med. 276: 34, 94, 148, 215, 273; 1967.
3. Carlson, L. A. and Ericsson, M. Atherosclerosis 21, in press.
4. Carlson, K. J. Clin. Path. 26, Suppl. 5: 32, 1973.
5. Noble, R. P. J. Lipid Res. 9: 693, 1968.
6. Ellefson, R. D. , Jimenez, B. S. and Smith, R. C. Mayo Clinic Proc. 46: 328, 1971.
7. Hazzard, W. R. , Porte, D. and Bierman, E. L. Metabolism 21: 1009, 1972.
8. Carlson, K. and Carlson, L. A. Scand. J. Clin. Lab. Invest., in press.
9. Wiegandt, H. , Lipp, K. and Wendt, G. G. Physiol. Chem. 349: 489, 1968.

DIET IN THE MANAGEMENT OF HYPERLIPIDEMIC PATIENTS

M. Mancini[1], E. Farinaro[3], C. O. Moro[2], L. Di Marino[1],
R. Rubba[1], A. Postiglione[1], and P. Oriente[3]

[1] Centro per le Malattie Metaboliche e l'Arteriosclerosi,
Semeiotica Medica, II Facolta di Medicina e Chirugia,
Universita di Napoli; [2] Clinica Medica, I Facolta di
Medicina, Universita di Napoli; [3] Clinica Medica,
II Facolta di Medicina, Universita di Napoli

INTRODUCTION

Hyperlipidemia (HL) is a metabolic abnormality of growing
interest to the medical profession because it is generally recognized that it signifies increased risk of cardiovascular complications.

Fasting HL may be _primary_ or _secondary_ to diabetes mellitus,
hypothyroidism, chronic renal disease, etc. When not secondary
to such other diseases, it is related, in the genetically susceptible
person, to habitual pattern of eating and drinking.

Various types of HL or hyperlipoproteinemia (HLP) have been
identified in man based on the distribution of lipoproteins in plasma
as evaluated by electrophoresis, ultracentrifugation or ultrafiltration
(8, 29, 27). The classification in five types of HLP proposed by
Fredrickson (8), slightly modified by a WHO committee (4), is
currently the most popular and has stimulated a wide and interesting
discussion (5)

Although there continues to be much research attention to the
unresolved question of application of these classifications, the

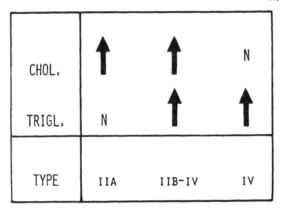

Figure 1

chemical measurement of serum cholesterol and triglyceride
concentration is at present the simplest and the most useful way,
clinically, to delineate HLP in order to prescribe an optimal
treatment.   By this easy routine procedure most cases of HL
can be divided into three broad categories (Fig. 1):

1.   with elevated serum cholesterol only, corresponding to
type IIA HLP;

2.   with combined elevation of serum cholesterol and triglyceride, corresponding to type IIB and severe type IV HLP;

3.   with elevated serum triglyceride only, corresponding to
mild type IV HLP.

In general, in regard to the choice of treatment for a patient
presenting with HL a preliminary distinction between primary
and secondary forms is necessary, the latter being in part amena-
ble to control by correction of the underlying disease.

In primary HL, however, therapy is possible only with regard
to environmental - that is nutritional - factors, because knowledge
of the underlying pathogenetic derangement is still almost non-
existent.

In the practical management of primary HL, one must decide
whether to prescribe lifelong treatment with one or more drugs,
or alternatively to try to change life habits, particularly diet, in
order to lower blood lipid levels.   In our opinion, whenever possible, the latter is a preferable decision.

A sound treament for HL must: normalize blood lipid concentration on a long-term basis; be well accepted for an indefinite
period of time; be without unwanted side effects; and be relatively
inexpensive.

Dietary treatment fulfills these requirements in most cases.
In the last 10 years we have prescribed two slightly different diets
for the management of most of the HL seen in our lipid clinic:

1. a diet for patients presenting with hypercholesterolemia
as the main lipid abnormality therefore classifiable phenotypically
as type IIA and IIB patients;

2. a diet for patients whose lipid elevation is primarily in
the triglycerides, due to a marked increase of prebetalipoproteins,
therefore classifiable, on a probability basis, as type IV patients.

We will not discuss in this presentation the diets that must be
used for type I, III and V HLP because they are less frequent and
form a very small proportion of all cases of HLP seen in a lipid
clinic.

Although - as we will see - both diets that we have used lower
serum cholesterol and triglyceride at the same time, we shall
refer to the former as the cholesterol-lowering (CL) and to the
latter as the triglyceride-lowering (TL) diet.

The composition of the CL diet is shown in Table I. Detailed
menus with many possible variants for this diet have already been
published (21). The diet is set at four calorie levels. The 1200-
1500 kcal scheme can be utilized for lowering serum lipids and
body weight at the same time, whenever necessary. The 1800-
2000 kcal diet is used when body weight is within an acceptable
range.

The diet has a relatively high protein content (21-28% of total
calories), is moderate in carbohydrate (41-49%) and fats (26-31%),
and low in saturated fats and cholesterol (< 300 mg/day).

From the qualitative point of view it should be noticed that:

- the proteins are of high nutritive value, being mainly of animal sources, in particular fish and white meats (chicken, for
example);

Table I

CHOLESTEROL LOWERING ("CL") DIET FOR PATIENTS
WITH TYPE IIA AND IIB HYPERLIPIDEMIA

NUTRIENT	1200 Cal.		1500 Cal.		1800 Cal.		2000 Cal.	
	g	%	g	%	g	%	g	%
Proteins	85	28	95	26	101	23	105	21
Carbohydrates	123	41	180	48	213	49	240	48
monosaccharides		11		9		8		7
disaccharides		6		5		5		4
polysaccharides		24		34		36		37
Fats	42	31	44	26	58	29	70	31
polyunsaturated		13		12		12		14
saturated		6		5		5		4
P/S	2.2		2.4		2.7		3.1	
cholesterol	0.263		0.263		0.263		0.263	

- the carbohydrates are mainly polysaccharides from starchy foods such as bread, pasta, rice, potatoes and vegetables;

- the fats are those containing a minimum of saturated and a maximum of polyunsaturated fatty acids (F. A.), so that the percent of total calories derived from saturated F. A. is between 4% and 6%, from polyunsaturated F. A. 12-15% and P/S ratio becomes the highest possible. This is obtained by avoiding fatty meats such as beef and pork, butterfat and hard margarines, cream and fat milk, fatty cheese, and by substituting for these items lean meats, de-fatted milk and cheese, and by using oils rich in polyunsaturated F. A. for cooking, baking, salads, etc.

The composition of the TL diet is shown in Table II. For this diet, too, detailed menus have been published (22). Similar to the CL diet, this diet has also been set at four calorie levels. The 1200-1500 kcal schemes are particularly useful when hypertrigly-ceridemia is associated with adiposity, as is very often the case.

As mentioned these two diets are very similar in composition (Table III). The protein content, in fact, is virtually identical. The diets are both very low in cholesterol (285 mg/day) and in saturated fatty acids (3-6% of total calories). The only difference is a lower content of carbohydrates in the TL diet (37-43% of total calories, almost exclusively polysaccharides) and, consequently, a higher content of total fats (30 to 42%), particularly those rich in polyunsaturated fatty acids. Alocholic beverages are completely excluded in the TL diet.

Comparing the practical instructions for the TL diet with those for the previously described CL diet, only a few additional recom-mendations are necessary for patients needing the TL diet. Indeed they should avoid - as diabetics do - sugar and sweets in general, reduce the consumption of fruit and compensate for these restric-tions with larger use of polyunsaturated oils.

When compared to other fat-controlled diets used by other workers in the U. S. A. and Scandinavian countries, our CL diet ap-pears moderately low in total fats, very low in saturated F. A. and cholesterol and only relatively high in polyunsaturated F. A. The TL diet has a higher proportion of polyunsaturated F. A. (Table IV).

Table II

TRIGLYCERIDE LOWERING ("TL") DIET FOR PATIENTS
WITH TYPE IV HYPERLIPIDEMIA

NUTRIENT	1200 Cal.		1500 Cal.		1800 Cal.		2000 Cal.	
	g	%	g	%	g	%	g	%
Proteins	86	29	95	25	95	22	99	20
Carbohydrates	125	41	158	43	158	37	185	38
monosaccharides		6		4		3		3
disaccharides		4		4		4		3
polysaccharides		31		35		30		32
Fats	41	30	54	32	78	41	92	42
polyunsaturated		13		12		17		20
saturated		3		6		4		4
P/S	2.6		3.7		4.6		5.4	
cholesterol	0.258		0.258		0.258		0.258	

Table III

COMPOSITION OF THE 2000 CALORIE
"CL" AND "TL" DIETS

NUTRIENT	"CL"	"TL"
	(% total cal.)	
PROTEINS	21	20
FATS	31	42
sat.F.A.	4	4
cholesterol	263°	258°
CARBOHYDRATES	48	38
simple sugar	11	6

°mg/day

PATIENTS AND METHODS

From a group of over 100 patients who were referred to us
with primary HL and who received detailed dietary instructions
as described above, 64 have been followed up with monthly examinations (Table V). This is, therefore, a group of selected cases of
mild HL that were referred by other physicians to our lipid clinic
in Naples for specialized treatment.

Thirty-one presented hypercholesterolemia due to hyperbetalipoproteinemia as the only lipid abnormality, classified as type
IIA HLP. Eleven of these presented clinical and electrocardiographic evidence of IHD. No one presented xanthomas. Patients
with extensive tuberous and tendinous xanthomas have been, in
fact, always considered separately as they are very resistent to
treatment in general and need intensive combined dietary and
pharmacological therapy.

Nineteen presented hypercholesterolemia and hypertriglyceridemia due to the combined increase of beta and pre-beta lipoprotein
as shown by electrophoresis. They were classified, therefore, as

Table IV

SERUM LIPID LOWERING DIETS USED IN LONG-TERM STUDIES*

Reference	Diet Designation	Tot.fat %Cal.	Satur. %Cal.	Polyuns. %Cal.	Cholest. (mg/day)
National Diet-Heart	B - B^a- BC C - C - E^a	29-38	5-7	10-22	117-266
Stamler	"CPEP"	30	10	10	300
Turpeinen et al.	----	31	8	11	229
Rinzler	"Prudent"	32	8	10	400
Dayton et al.	----	39	9	16	365
Leren	----	39	8	21	264
Mancini et al.	"CL"	26-31	4-6	12-14	263
Mancini et al.	"TL"	30-42	3-6	12-20	263

*Modified from Brown H.B. in: Atherosclerosis, Proceedings of II Intern. Symp.
Jones R.J. Editor, Springer-Verlag, Berlin 1970.

Table V

64 PATIENTS TREATED BY LIPID LOWERING DIET (M±SEM)
(pretreatment values)

TYPE	AGE (yr.)	CHOL. (mg/dl serum)	TRIG.	B.W.I.
II A (22M,9F)	48 + 2	329 + 10	111 + 6	1.10 + .03
II B (17M,2F)	48 + 2	316 + 13	235 + 16	1.13 + .03
IV (14M)	44 + 2	296 + 18	603 + 61	1.14 + .04

(M=males, F=females, BWI=body weight index)

type IIB hyperlipoproteinemic patients. Six of them presented clinical and electrocardiographic evidence of IHD.

Fourteen were patients with marked hypertriglyceridemia caused by an increased plasma concentration of prebetalipoproteinemia and, therefore, classified as having type IV HLP. None of these were alcoholics. In five of these patients clinical and electrocardiographic signs of IHD were detected.

All the patients were well motivated for dietary prescription; in fact some of them were relatives of IHD patients and many of them reported clinical signs of IHD.

Body weight of our patients is shown as body weight index (BWI). This index is calculated by the equation:

$$\frac{\text{body weight (kg)}}{\text{height (cm)} - 100}$$

On the average the patients were slightly overweight, especially the type IV patients, but only a proportion of them had a BWI > 1.10: 13 out of 31 IIA: 8 out of 19 IIB and 6 out of 14 type IV patients.

   Clinical examination, chest x-ray, ECG and routine screening
laboratory tests were performed initially in each patient. Blood
lipids were measured in duplicate in the fasting state at least
twice before treatment and regularly every 1-2 months during
treatment. Serum cholesterol was determined manually according
to Abell and Kendall (1). Serum triglyceride determinations were
performed by a modification of the manual method of Van Handel
and Zilversmit (30). Serum lipoproteins were examined in all
the patients by electrophoresis on cellogel (25) (Chemetron,
Milano, Italy) and in special cases by ultracentrifugation according
to Hatch and Lees (9).

   Dietary history was taken by a dietician, initially to assess
the habitual diet of each subject and subsequently at 1-2 month
intervals, to ascertain adherance to the prescribed diet. Detailed
dietary instructions were given on these occasions.

Table VI

CALORIES, CARBOHYDRATES AND FATS OF CUSTOMARY
DIET OF 16 PATIENTS TREATED BY LIPID-LOWERING DIETS
(percent range of total calories)

	II A (3M, 2F)	II B (4M, 2F)	IV (5M)
	2230-2700	2570-3420	1560-3550
Carbohydrates	53-57	47-63	49-62
simple sugar	10-20	10-19	5-28
starch	25-36	35-46	22-46
Fats	23-32	22-32	24-39
sat.F.A.	6-7	4-10	4-8
poly-uns.F.A.	1-2	1-5	1-2
Wine (ml)	100[a]	200-400[b]	100-500[c]

a) in 2M;   b) in 4M, 1F; c) in 2M

RESULTS

The composition of the customary diet of a randomly selected subsample of our patients, calculated on the basis of dietary history, is shown in table VI. When the patients do follow the prescribed lipid-lowering diets described the main change in nutrient intake, besides the exclusion of alcohol, is in the quality of dietary fat in CL diet, and in both the quality of fat and the amount of simple sugars in the TL diet.

In patients with exclusive hypercholesterolemia classified as type IIA, a significant reduction of serum cholesterol is evident after the first month of treatment by CL diet. After two months the decrease is greater. On average it was reduced from a base-line level of 329 mg/dl to a mean level of 265 mg/dl. Serum triglycerides, within normal range initially, show a slight change during treatment, the mean level falling from 111 to 93 mg/dl. Simultaneously body weight is slightly reduced, especially in overweight patients.

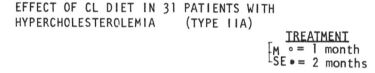

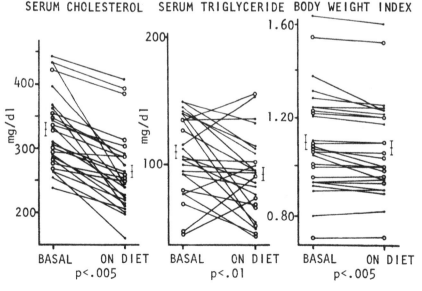

Figure 2

EFFECT OF CL DIET IN 19 PATIENTS WITH HYPERCHOLESTEROLEMIA
COMBINED WITH HYPERTRIGLYCERIDEMIA (TYPE II B)

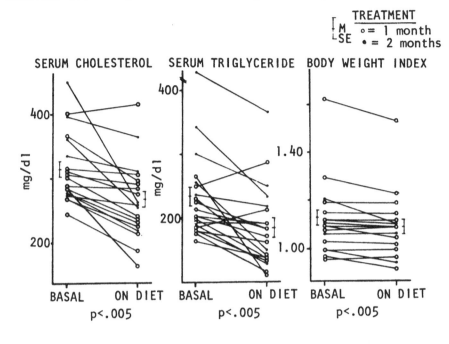

Figure 3

Patients with hypercholesterolemia and moderate hypertriglyceridemia classified as type IIB, when treated by the CL diet,
showed a clear reduction of serum cholesterol and triglyceride.
Within two months of treatment, serum cholesterol was decreased
to a mean value of 266 mg/dl. This value is lower than the 95th
percentile of the serum cholesterol values of a comparable normal
population in Naples (15). Serum triglycerides were lowered to a
mean concentration of 184 mg/dl. At the same time a decrease
in body weight was obtained (Figure 3).

In patients who presented a predominant hypertriglyceridemia,
due to marked hyperprebetalipoproteinemia, as shown by an electrophoretic pattern of type IV, the TL diet produced remarkable changes
in blood lipid concentration within two months of treatment. Serum
triglyceride level, the main lipid abnormality, was decreased

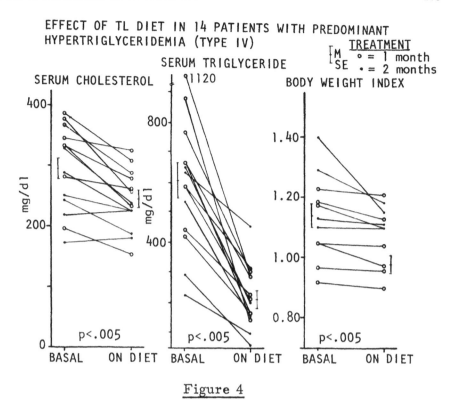

Figure 4

markedly and reduced from 603 mg/dl to a mean value of 219 mg/dl.
Serum cholesterol concentration was also simultaneously decreased
from 296 mg/dl to a mean value of 244 mg/dl. In this group body
weight showed the greatest reduction (Figure 4).

Table VII summarizes the percent decrease of serum lipids
and body weight in normal weight versus overweight patients in
the three different HL groups.

Serum cholesterol was reduced by 20% in type IIA and 17% in
type IIB patients irrespective of initial body weight and of the
greater weight loss in the overweight patients. In type IV patients
serum cholesterol was decreased by 19% when BWI was higher
than 1.10 and by 15% when it was lower than 1.10.

Table VII

SERUM LIPIDS AND BODY WEIGHT DECREASE IN HYPERLIPIDEMIC PATIENTS ON DIET FOR 1-2 MONTHS (percent of pretreatment values)

TYPE	BWI > 1.1			BWI < 1.1			A L L		
	CHOL	TG	BW	CHOL	TG	BW	CHOL	TG	BW
II A	20**	9	3.6**	20**	9	1.0*	20*	9*	2.3**
II B	17**	30**	2.7***	17**	15*	1.4*	17**	21***	2.0***
IV	19*	72*	7.1**	15	56*	2.1	17**	63***	4.8**

Significance * p< .05   ** p< .005

TG=serum triglyceride; CHOL=serum cholesterol; BW=body weight in kg; BWI=body weight index.

CHOLESTEROL-LOWERING EFFECT OF CL DIET IN
20 PATIENTS WITH HYPERCHOLESTEROLEMIA
(TYPE IIA AND IIB)

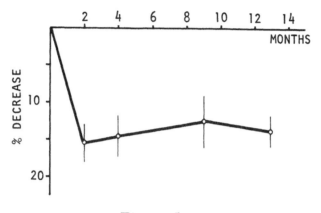

Figure 5

LIPID-LOWERING EFFECT OF TL DIET IN 6 PATIENTS WITH
PREDOMINANT HYPERTRIGLYCERIDEMIA (TYPE IV)

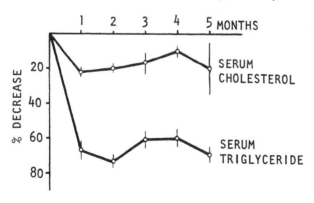

Figure 6

Serum triglycerides were only slightly reduced (by 9%) in type IIA patients regardless of the initial BWI. In type IIB and type IV subjects with elevated concentration of serum triglycerides, the greatest reductions of this lipid fraction were obtained when the BWI was above 1.10 and weight loss more pronounced.

The blood lipid lowering effect is maintained as long as the patients follow the CL or TL diet with good adherence. As shown in Figure 5, the hypercholesterolemic effect of CL diet persisted when 20 hypercholesterolemic patients (IIA and IIB) were treated by diet for over one year.

Similarly, 6 type IV patients retained lower blood cholesterol and triglyceride values, during 5 months of good adherence to the TL diet (Figure 6).

DISCUSSION AND CONCLUSION

The vast literature of the last 20 years demonstrates the possibility of lowering serum cholesterol levels in man by a diet adequate in total calories and low in saturated fatty acids and cholesterol. Our data obtained in free living well motivated individuals, followed up as outpatients, are in keeping with these conclusions. The lipid-lowering diets that we used are acceptable long-term to a majority of patients. This is understandable when one considers that they are not experimental diets but are very similar to the customary diet of entire populations, as for instance, those of the Mediterranean area. Besides calorie restrictions prescribed, if obesity coexisted, the change that we have produced in nutrient intake in our patients was mainly confined to the quality of dietary fats and to the total amount of simple sugar.

The mechanism of action of the lipid lowering diets is not as yet very clear. One of the most interesting explanations is the increase in fecal excretion of neutral sterols and bile acids when serum cholesterol concentration decreases as a consequence of isocaloric substitution of saturated by polyunsaturated F. A. in the diet (17, 20, 28, 31).

More recently the relationship between nutrient intake and serum triglyceride concentration in man has been elucidated and the reduction of total calories, simple sugars, saturated fatty acids, cholesterol and alcohol has been emphasized for lowering blood lipids in the common cases of hypertriglyceridemia (14, 16, 19, 22).

The mechanism by which glyceride metabolism is affected by changing diet composition also has not yet been well elucidated, although some explanations have been advanced (14, 23, 24, 26).

A relevant observation is that the dietary substitution of saturated fatty acids with an equicaloric amount of polyunsaturated F. A. has a lowering effect not only on plasma cholesterol but also on plasma triglyceride concentration (2, 3, 16, 18, 19, 23).

Certainly the beneficial effect that has been observed with alcohol withdrawal in patients with type IV hypertriglyceridemia (6) does suggest that consumption of alcohol should be avoided by hypertriglyceridemic patients.

The extent to which a diet can lower blood lipids varies from patient to patient, depending on the type of HLP, previous customary diet and adherence to prescribed diet (11).

The effectiveness of an appropriate diet in lowering serum lipid concentration, amply confirmed by various authors (7, 10, 12, 13) cannot be ignored whenever the problem of treating hyperlipidemic patients arises.

Only in a minority of cases dietary regulation is not sufficient to bring blood lipid concentration within a desirable range. This happens in cases of severe hypercholesterolemia (the very rare homozygous or some cases of heterozygous type IIA HPL with serum cholesterol well above 400 mg/dl) or with cases of marked hypertriglyceridemia (the rare type I and V, and some type IV HPL with serum triglyceride well above 1000 mg/dl). These are certainly conditions that must be treated - after a dietary trial - by addition to the diet of one or more hypolipidemic drugs. It is clear that even in instances of this sort, the diet plays an important role in the long-term correction of HLP.

REFERENCES

1. Abell, L. L. , Levy, B. B., Brodie, B. B. , and Kendall, F. E.
    J. Biol. Chem. 195: 357, 1952.

2. Ahrens, E. H. , Jr. , Hirsch, J. , Insull, W. , Tsaltas, T. T. ,
    Blomstrand, R. and Peterson, M. L. Lancet 1: 943, 1957.

3. Anderson, J. T. Am. J. Clin. Nutr. 20: 169, 1967.

4. Beaumont, J. L. , Carlson, L. A. , Cooper, G. R. , Fejfar, Z. ,
    Fredrickson, D. S. and Strasser, T. Bull. World Health
    Org. 43: 891, 1970.

5. Carlson, L. A. Fifth International Symposium on Drugs
    Affecting Lipid Metabolism, Milan, 1974, Abstract, p. 37.

6. Chait, A. , Mancini, M. , February, A. W. and Lewis, B.
    Lancet 2: 62, 1972.

7. Evans, D. W. , Turner, S. M. , and Ghosh, P. Lancet 1:
    172, 1972.

8. Fredrickson, D. S. , Levy, R. I. and Lees, R. S. New England
    J. Med. 276: 32, 1967.

9. Hatch, F. T. and Lees, R. S. Adv. Lipid Res. 6: 1, 1968.

10. Hegsted, D. M. , McGandy, R. E. , Meyers, M. L. and Stare,
    F. J. Am. J. Clin. Nutr. 17: 281, 1965.

11. Keys, A. , Anderson, J. T. and Grande, F. Metabolism 14:
    766, 1965.

12. Keys, A. , Anderson, J. T. and Grande, F. Am. J. Clin.
    Nutr. 19: 175, 1966.

13. Kuo, P. T. J. A. M. A. 20: 87, 1967.

14. Kuo, P. T. and Basset, D. R. Ann. Int. Med. 59: 495, 1963.

15. Lewis, B. , Chait, A. , Oakley, C. , Krikler, P. , Carlson,
    L. A. , Ericsson, M. , Bosey, J. , Mancini, M. , Oriente, P. ,
    Paggi, E. , Micheli, H. , Malczewski, B. , Weisswange, A.
    and Pometta, D. Third Internat. Symposium on Athero-
    sclerosis, West Berlin, 1973, Abstract, # 109.

16. Lewis, B. , Mancini, M. , Ishiwata, J. and Mattock, M.
    Fifth Annual Meeting of the European Society for Clinical
    Investigation, Scheveningen, 1971, Abstract, # 69.

17. Lewis, B. Postgrad. Med. J. 35: 208, 1959.

18. Mancini, M. , Oriente, P. , Varriale, E. and DiMarino, L.
    Via Metabolica dell'Aterogenesi, Symp. Pathophysiol. Nutr.
    and Clin. Diet. , R. Patron, Bologna, 1972, p. 421.

19. Mann, J. I. , Truswell, A. S. and Manning, E. B. South
    African Medical J. 46: 827, 1972.

20. Moore, R. B. , Anderson, J. T. , Taylor, H. L. , Keys, A.
    and Frantz, I. D. J. Clin. Invest. 47: 1517, 1968.

21. Moro, C. O. , Mancini, M. , Cuzzupoli, M. , DiMarino, L. and Caputo, V. Quad. Nutr. 28: 31, 1968.

22. Moro, C. O. , Mancini, M. and DiMarino, L. Quad. Nutr. 30: 93, 1970.

23. Nestel, P. J. , Carrol, K. F. and Havenstein, N. Metabolism 19:1, 1970.

24. Nestel, P. J. J. Clin. Sci. 31: 31, 1966.

25. Oriente, P. In: Human Hyperlipoproteinemias. R. Fumagalli, G. Ricci and S. Gorini, editors. Plenum, New York, 1973.

26. Reaven, C. M. , Hill, O. B. , Gross, E. C. and Farquhar, J. W. J. Clin. Invest. 44: 1826, 1965.

27. Stone, M. C. and Thorp, J. M. Clin. Chim. Acta 14: 812, 1966.

28. Spritz, N. , Ahrens, E. H. and Grundy, S. J. Clin. Invest. 44: 1482, 1965.

29. Strisower, E. H. , Adamson, G. , and Strisower, B. Am. J. Med. 45: 488, 1968.

30. Van Handel, E. and Zilversmit, D. B. J. Lab. Clin. Med. 52: 152, 1957.

31. Wood, P. D. S. , Shioda, R. and Kinsell, L. W. Lancet 2: 604, 1966.

THE PARTIAL ILEAL BYPASS OPERATION IN TREATMENT OF THE HYPERLIPIDEMIAS

Henry Buchwald, M. D. , Ph. D. , Richard B. Moore, M. D. , and Richard L. Varco, M. D. , Ph. D.

University of Minnesota Medical School, Minneapolis, Minnesota

We performed the first human partial ileal bypass operation specifically for cholesterol reduction on May 29, 1963 (1). Currently other institutions, in the United States and in Europe, have initiated test programs to study this method of cholesterol lowering (2-11, *).

Prior to a discussion of the clinical results it may be important to review the laboratory antecedents, as well as the metabolic studies in cholesterol dynamics designed to provide an understanding of the procedure: The original experiments with the partial ileal bypass technique were carried out from 1962-1964. Studies in White New Zealand rabbits, pigs and, by retrospective analysis, in patients who had undergone ileal resections for causes other than carcinoma (e. g. incarcerated hernia), showed that both the cholesterol absorption from the intestinal tract and the whole blood cholesterol concentration were markedly and significantly (statistically) reduced, without concomitant weight loss, following diversion or loss of substantial lengths of distal small intestine (12, 13). Additional studies demonstrated that although the entire small intestine is capable of cholesterol absorption, with normal bowel continuity preferential cholesterol uptake occurs in the

---

*Streuter, personal communication; Morgan and Moore, personal communication.

distal half of the small bowel (14). Transit time in the small
intestine also strongly influences quantitative cholesterol absorption (13). In addition, we demonstrated that bypass of the distal
one-third of the small bowel interferes with the enterohepatic
bile acid cycle and results in a loss of bile acids in the feces at
a rate at least three-fold that of normal (15). Thus, the partial
ileal bypass operation alters body cholesterol homeostasis by:
(1) a direct drain on the body cholesterol pool and (2) an indirect
drain on the cholesterol pool through forced conversion of
cholesterol to its metabolic end-product bile acids, in order to
maintain the stressed bile acid reservoir.

In 1965, we reported the development in the rabbit of an
animal model with a reproducible 50% myocardial infarction attack rate (16). Utilizing this preparation, we showed, both in
adult (17) and in infant (18) rabbits, that partial ileal bypass prevents hypercholesterolemia and atherosclerosis despite consumption of a severely atherogenic (2% cholesterol by weight) diet.
The operation, in rabbits with established hypercholesterolemia
and atherosclerosis, returns whole blood cholesterol values to
below normal, reduces cholesterol xanthomata accumulations,
and arrests and reverses the atherosclerotic process, even though
the animals remain on the 2% cholesterol diet. For the infant
rabbit, loss of absorption from the bypassed segment does not
interfere with structural growth or normal body weight gain.

These findings have been confirmed in other species: Scott,
et al (19) in the dog and Shepard, et al (20) in the Rhesus monkey.
Indeed, Scott and co-workers have shown that the partial ileal
bypass operation will achieve twice the circulating cholesterol
reduction that is achieved by a 1.5 mg/kg daily of cholestestyra-
mine in the Rhesus monkey (21). These investigators demonstrated that with all animals on the same atherogenic regimen, the
average serum cholesterol concentration for the non-treated monkeys was 803 mg%, the cholestyramine treated animals 418 mg%,
and the partial ileal bypass animals 175 mg%. There was a significant difference in the protection afforded against the development
of atherosclerotic lesions on comparison of the aortas of the partial
ileal bypass treated monkeys and the cholestyramine animals, with
lesions nearly as severe as those found in the untreated animals
in the animals on cholestyramine and essentially no lesions in the
partial ileal bypass group. In studies with the white Carneau
pigeon (22), birds with naturally occurring atherosclerosis, par-

tial ileal bypass not only arrested the progression of aortic atherosclerosis but resulted in demonstrable atherosclerotic plaque regression, without interfering with avian growth and weight gain.

These laboratory experiments have been complemented by human cholesterol dynamics studies utilizing radioisotope methods (23, 24). We have shown that cholesterol absorption is reduced 60% following partial bypass. There is a 3. 8-fold increase in total fecal steroid excretion, with a much greater increase in bile acids (4. 9-fold) than in neutral steroids (2. 7-fold). This state of reduced cholesterol absorption and increased steroid excretion has been maintained for years of follow-up testing. Compensatory cholesterol and bile acid absorptive adaptation by the functioning small intestine apparently does not occur.

In order to compensate for the increased loss of cholesterol and bile acids in the feces, body cholesterol synthesis has been demonstrated to increase 5. 7-fold (23, 24). Concomitantly, the cholesterol turnover rate has been demonstrated to increase markedly (23, 24). The net result of these dynamic mechanisms is a reduction in the total exchangeable cholesterol pool by about one-third at one year following partial ileal bypass in hypercholesterolemic patients (23, 24). This lowering is reflected in both the freely miscible cholesterol pool (plasma, red blood cells, liver, intestinal mucosa) and the less freely miscible cholesterol pool (depot fat, muscle, organs). The less freely miscible cholesterol pool includes cholesterol in the arterial walls. Loss of cholesterol from this pool can, therefore, reflect a loss of cholesterol from atherosclerotic plaques.

OPERATIVE TECHNIQUE

It is essential to differentiate the jejuno-ileal bypass for obesity from the partial ileal bypass operation for the hyperlipidemias by primary intent of the procedures, resultant weight reduction versus no weight reduction, moderately severe versus mimimal side effects, and unique associated complications for jejunoileal bypass compared to no unique complications associated with partial ileal bypass. The reason for these marked differences resides in the operative technique employed. Jejuno-ileal bypass involves a better than 90% small bowel bypass with two anastomosis. The partial ileal bypass is a much briefer and simpler operation consisting of a single anastomosis, end-to-side ileocecostomy, 200 cm from the ileocecal valve (a one-third small bowel bypass); closure of the proximal end of the bypassed segment; and closure of all mesenteric defects.

EFFECT ON CHOLESTEROL CONCENTRATION

We have currently operated upon 140 patients and 126 have been carefully followed and re-evaluated for three months to eleven years. In our experience, the circulating cholesterol concentration is reduced an average of 41% from the pre-operative post-dietary baseline after partial ileal bypass (25, 26). In the series reported by investigative groups elsewhere in the United States and in Europe, the mean cholesterol concentration reduction after dietary therapy has been virtually identical to our own finding; namely, about 40% (2-10, *). The cholesterol lowering effect of the operation is neither uniform nor is it precisely predictable for each person. The range of cholesterol response after dietary therapy has varied from 5% to 79%. The operation has proven effectiveness in lowering the cholesterol concentration in all of the hyperlipoproteinemic types. We have achieved the standard 40% cholesterol lowering response in individuals (primarily, type IIA patients) who were refractory to dietary and to drug therapy. In a cohort of severe type II hypercholesterolemic individuals, it has been demonstrated that dietary management in combination with partial ileal bypass produced an average 53% cholesterol level lowering from the pre-treatment baseline (27).

We have operated upon eight pre-pubertal children with type IIA hypercholesterolemia and have achieved essentially comparable results (28). To date, the least impressive responders have been the type IIA homozygous young people. Yet, Balfour and Kim (11) reported two homozygous children followed for three years, with sustained cholesterol reductions of 42% and 33%.

Thus, we can state that the partial ileal bypass procedure alone can lower the cholesterol concentration an average of 40% and in combination with dietary management can essentially halve the circulating cholesterol concentration. How is this

*Streuter, personal communication; Morgan and Moore, personal communication.

reflected in comparison to the average cholesterol levels in the United States? The average cholesterol concentration of middle-aged men in the United States is about 250 mg%; the average pre-operative cholesterol concentration for individuals in our patient series has been over 330 mg%. Following partial ileal bypass, better than 80% of these subjects have circulating cholesterol levels below 250 mg% and better than 50% have levels below 200 mg% (25, 26).

EFFECT ON TRIGLYCERIDE CONCENTRATION

The partial ileal bypass operation has demonstrated effectiveness in lowering triglyceride levels following maximum type specific dietary therapy (25, 26). This effect has primarily been achieved in the type IV hypertriglyceridemic patients. In our experience with this group of individuals, we have seen an average 53% triglyceride level reduction from the post-dietary preoperative baseline. Triglyceride lowering has also been achieved by the partial ileal bypass operation in the type IIB patients, those individuals with a hypertriglyceridemia accompanying their dominant hypercholesterolemia. On the other hand, a small paradoxical increase in triglyceride levels has been noted in the type IIA patients, i.e. in those hypercholesterolemic individuals with low or normal preoperative triglyceride concentrations. The average triglyceride level, however, in the IIA subgroup has remained within the accepted normal range. To this time, a satisfactory explanation for this phenomenon in the type IIA patients has not been offered.

MORTALITY AND MORBIDITY

Our in-hospital, or operative, mortality has been confined to one patient, who died on the fourth postoperative day from a myocardial infarction; he had sustained three myocardial infarctions prior to his partial ileal bypass operation. Thus, our in-hospital mortality has been less than 1%, the presence of co-existing coronary artery disease in many of these patients not withstanding. Prolongation of hospitalization beyond one week has occurred in only 2% of these patients and was due to wound infections, pulmonary emboli, or other serious postoperative complications. Bowel obstruction requiring re-operation, early

or late, developed in four of our total of 140 cases. We have not
had a single instance of intussusception of the proximal end of
the bypassed segment or obstruction secondary to an internal
hernia caused by inadequate closure of the rotational mesenteric
defect.

Analysis of long-term survival in our patient experience has
been encouraging (26). Comparing our survival data to the statistics compiled by a group at the Mayo Clinic (29) for patients
surviving a myocardial infarction and local controls, reveals
that the partial ileal bypass patients' survival parallels that of
the controls. Though this is not a statistically rigorous comparison, the partial ileal bypass patients seem to fare significantly
better than the Mayo Clinic group with a myocardial infarction.

SIDE EFFECTS

Diarrhea is the one annoying side effect experienced by the
majority of individuals after partial ileal bypass (4-6, 9, 25, 26, *).
This diarrhea is, as a rule, self-limited. Within one year, approximately 90% of individuals undergoing partial ileal bypass
have five bowel movements or less daily, while on no bowel
control medications.

Vitamin B_{12} absorption is either severely impaired or totally
lost immediately following partial ileal bypass (30). After several
years, however, absorptive adaptation for vitamin B_{12} seems to
occur in about one-half of these individuals (31, **). We believe
it is prudent not to rely on this absorptive adaptation and we prescribe parenteral vitamin B_{12} supplementation, 1,000 micro-
grams intramuscularly every two months, for all partial ileal
bypass patients. This regimen is continued indefinitely.

Nutrient malabsorption has not been described following partial ileal bypass; no essential long-term weight change occurs (25).
Contrary to the jejuno-ileal bypass operation for obesity, electrolyte changes do not occur with the limited one-third intestinal

---

* Brown, personal communication; Miettinen, personal communication; Streuter, personal communication.

** Coyle et al, unpublished data.

bypass. Neither have the complications of liver failure, hepatic fatty infiltration, arthritic phenomena, and nephrolithiasis, which at times can result after jejuno-ileal bypass, every been described following partial ileal bypass.

CLINICAL OBSERVATIONS

A postoperative decrease in size, or even disappearance, of periorbital xanthelasma, subcutaneous xanthomata and tendon xanthomata, especially of the plantar extensor tendons, has been described (6, 32). This finding may indicate that other tissue stores of lipid, possibly in arterial atherosclerotic plaques, have been mobilized and excreted from the body.

Of 61 patients with angina pectoris present prior to partial ileal bypass, 40 (66%) experienced improvement or total remission postoperatively (26). In certain of these patients, there has been a concomitant improvement in excercise tolerance, free of the development of ischemic ST-T changes, on the treadmill exercise electrocardiogram. Others have reported similar findings (2, 5, 9, *). These findings may be indicative of an improvement in circulatory hemodynamics and/or tissue oxygen availability. Possible evidence to support this hypothesis can be found in an in vitro experiment, utilizing rabbit blood, which demonstrated that oxygen extraction from blood with a high cholesterol content is significantly less than from blood with a low cholesterol content (33).

SERIAL ARTERIOGRAPHY

We have and are measuring coronary plaque lesions, by serial coronary arteriography, in our partial ileal bypass patients. To date, our study indicates an apparent non-progression rate of coronary artery disease in 55% of patients followed for up to three years (34, 35). This statistic compares quite favorably with the data of a patient series followed by serial coronary arteriography and not treated by partial ileal bypass (36). Apparent coronary arteriographic evidence of true plaque regression was noted in three of

---

* Streuter, personal communication.

our partial ileal bypass patients (35). We are not aware of
another report of human arteriographic plaque regression.

CONCLUSIONS

Partial ileal bypass is, today, the single most effective means
available for lowering the plasma lipids, in particular the plasma
cholesterol concentration. The cholesterol lowering effect of this
procedure is universally lasting; response escape or rebound of
lipid levels has not occurred. The operation is safe. In addition,
the obligatory benefits of this mode of therapy make it attractive
as a therapeutic alternative, especially in a young and asymptomatic population. We do not advocate this operation as the treatment of choice for all hyperlipidemic individuals. It may be the
treatment of choice for certain patients with hyperlipidemia.

ACKNOWLEDGEMENT

This work was supported by grants from the National Heart
and Lung Institute, HL-11901 and HL-06314; Minnesota Heart
Association; and a Special State of Minnesota Legislative Appro-
priation.

REFERENCES

1. Buchwald, H. : Circulation 28(II): 649, 1963
2. Fritz, S. H. , Walker, W. J. : Am. Surg. 32: 691, 1966
3. Lewis, L. A. , Brown, H. B. , Page, I. H. : Circulation 38(6):
    128, 1968
4. Strisower, E. H. , Kradjian, R. , Nichols, A. V. , Coggiola, E. ,
    Tsai, J. : J. Atheroscl. Res. 8: 525, 1968
5. Swan, D. M. , McGowan, J. M. : Am. J. Surg. 116: 81, 1968
6. Helsinger, N. , Jr. , Rootwelt, K. : Nord. Med. 82: 1409, 1969
7. Rowe, G. G. , Young, W. P. , Wasserburger, R. H. : Circulation
    40(III): 22, 1969
8. Miettinen, T. : In: Proceedings Second International Sympo-
    sium on Atherosclerosis, edited by Jones, R. J. , New York,
    Springer Verlag, 1970, p.304
9. Sodal, G. , Gjertsen, K. T. , Schrumpf, A. : Acta. Chir.
    Scan. 136: 671, 1970

10. Clot, J. P. , Rouffy, J. , Loeper, J. , Mercadier, M. :
    Chirurgie 97: 57, 1971
11. Balfour, J. F. , Kim, R. : JAMA 227: 1145, 1974
12. Buchwald, H. , Gebhard, R. : Am. J. Physiol. 207: 567, 1964
13. Buchwald, H. : Circulation 29: 713, 1964
14. Gebhard, R. L. , Buchwald, H. : Surgery 67: 474, 1970
15. Buchwald, H. , Gebhard, R. : Ann. Surg. 167: 191, 1968
16. Buchwald, H. : J. Atheroscler. Res. 5: 407, 1965
17. Buchwald, H. : Surgery 58: 22, 1965
18. Buchwald, H. , Moore, R. B. , Bertish, J. , Varco, R. L. :
    Ann. Surg. 175: 311, 1972
19. Scott, H. W. , Jr. , Stephenson, S. E. , Jr. , Younger, R. ,
    Carlisle, R. B. , Turney, S. W. : Ann. Surg. 163: 95, 1966
20. Shepard, G. H. , Wimberly, J. E. , Younger, R. K. , Stephenson,
    S. E. , Jr. , Scott, H. W. , Jr. : Surg. Forum 19: 302, 1968
21. Younger, R. K. , Shepard, G. H. , Butts, W. H. , Scott, H. W. ,
    Jr. : Surg. Forum 20: 101, 1969
22. Gomes, M. M. , Kottke, B. A. , Bernatz, P. , Titus, J. L. :
    Surgery 70: 353, 1971
23. Moore, R. B. , Frantz, I. D. , Jr. , Buchwald, H. : Surgery
    65: 98, 1969
24. Moore, R. B. , Frantz, I. D. , Jr. , Varco, R. L. , Buchwald,
    H. : In: Proceedings of the Second International Symposium
    on Atherosclerosis, edited by Jones, R. J. , New York,
    Springer-Verlag, 1970, p. 295.
25. Buchwald, H. , Moore, R. B. , Varco, R. L. : Circulation 49
    (I): I-1, 1974
26. Buchwald, H. , Moore, R. B. , Varco, R. L. : Ann. Surg. ,
    in press.
27. Buchwald, H. , Moore, R. B. , Lee, G. B. , Frantz, I. D. , Jr. ,
    Varco, R. L. : Arch. Surg. 97: 275, 1968
28. Buchwald, H. , Varco, R. L. : Surgery 68: 1101, 1970
29. Juergens, J. L. , Edwards, J. E. , Achor, R. W. , Burchell,
    H. B. : Arch. Int. Med. 105: 444, 1960
30. Buchwald, H. : Am. J. Dig. Dis. 9: 755, 1964
31. Nygaard, K. , Helsinger, N. , Rootwelt, K. : Scand. J. Gast.
    5: 349, 1970
32. Buchwald, H. : Derm. Dig. 9: 65, 1970
33. Steinbach, J. H. , Blackshear, P. L. , Jr. , Varco, R. L. ,
    Buchwald, H. : J. Surg. Res. 16: 132, 1974
34. Baltaxe, H. , Amplatz, K. , Varco, R. L. , Buchwald, H. :
    Am. J. Roentg. 105: 784, 1969.

35. Knight, L., Scheibel, R., Amplatz, K., Varco, R. L.,
     Buchwald, H.: Surg. Forum 23: 141, 1972
36. Bemis, C. E., Eber, L. M., Kemp, H. G., Gorlin, R.:
     Circulation 43(II) 47, 1971

Drugs and Thrombosis

THE ACTIVATION AND INHIBITION OF FIBRINOLYSIS

Francis J. Castellino, Lloyd A. Schick, William J. Brockway and James M. Sodetz

The Department of Chemistry, Program in Biochemistry and Biophysics, The University of Notre Dame, Notre Dame, Indiana

The mechanism of activation of the single chain proenzyme, plasminogen, to the two-chain disulfide linked protease, plasmin, is catalyzed by several activators. Any study of this mechanism must include the fact that at least two peptide bonds are cleaved in the activation process (1-3). Although most activators of plasminogen are proteases; the bacterial activator, streptokinase, possesses no proteolytic activity. Therefore, it becomes pertinent to inquire as to how two inactive proteins, i.e. plasminogen and streptokinase, can supposedly interact and result in the proteolytic cleavages required to convert plasminogen into plasmin. In this regard, it was found that streptokinase could form a 1:1 complex with human plasmin and this complex could directly activate plasminogen; a reaction that neither protein could catalyze independently (4-6). Further, this same activator complex was formed whether human plasmin or human plasminogen was used as one of the starting materials (6).

It has been known for several years that compounds related to Σ-amino caproic acid were inhibitors of fibrinolysis. The mechanism of action of these synthetic inhibitors has been speculated. Alkjaersig et al (7) demonstrated that Σ-amino caproic acid inhibits the conversion of plasminogen to plasmin, thus manifesting its antifibrinolytic activity. Other theories suggest that Σ-amino caproic acid alters the structure of the fibrin, resulting in a diminished capacity for dissolution by plasmin (8, 9) and that Σamino caproic acid binds to plasminogen in a 1:1 stoichiometry (11) resulting in a well characterized conformational alteration in plasminogen (7, 11-13). Whether this alteration in plasminogen has anything to do with the antifibrinolytic activity of Σamino caproic acid is not known at this time.

MATERIALS AND METHODS

The preparation and purity of all materials used as well as all the techniques used can be found in related manuscripts from this laboratory: plasminogen preparation, determination of $S^o_{20,w}$ (12); streptokinase preparation, plasmin assays and active site titrations, polyacrylamide gel electrophoresis and sucrose density centrifugation techniques (14); amino terminal amino acid sequence analysis (15); isothermal fluorescence polarization measurements (13).

RESULTS AND DISCUSSION

When the single chain plasminogen (Pg a) is activated by streptokinase (SK) or urokinase (UK) and the resulting plasmin (Pm b) is reduced, carboxymethylated and subjected to gel filtration in denaturing buffers, 3 polypeptide chains can be resolved. A heavy chain (H b) of molecular weight 62,000; a light chain (L) of molecular weight 24,000 and a peptide (P) of dodecyl sulfate gel electrophoretic systems, in the presence and absence of mercaptoethanol, show that the heavy chain is linked by disulfide bond(s) to the light chain. Further, the amino terminal peptide is not covalently linked to the remainder of the molecule. The amino terminal amino acid sequences of Pg a and the three plasmin chains are shown in Table I. In this case, data is given for rabbit Pg a and the component rabbit plasmin chains. These results can be extrapolated to the human system with very little changes. Carboxyl terminal analyses show that the carboxyl terminus of plasminogen a as well as the plasmin light chain is asparagine. Clearly then, the peptide must be split from the amino terminus of plasminogen and the light chain is derived intact from the carboxyl terminus of plasminogen. The heavy chain results from the amino terminus of plasminogen, minus the peptide released.

Table I

Amino Terminal Amino Acid Sequences of Rabbit Plasminogen
and the Component Plasmin Chains[a]

Sequence no.	Amino acid present in			
	Pg a	H b	L	P
1	glu	met	val	glu
2	pro	tyr	val	pro
3	leu	leu	gly	leu
4	asp	X	gly	asp
5	asp	glu	X	asp
6	tyr	X	val	tyr

[a]Abbreviations used: Pg a, native plasminogen; H b, L and P
represent the plasmin heavy, light and peptide chains,
respectively.

In an attempt to understand the mechanism of activation of
human plasminogen by streptokinase, we have examined the α-N-
tosyl-L-arginine methyl ester (tos-arg-OMe) esterolytic, caseinolytic and plasminogen activator activities of plasmin (Pm) as
a function of SK concentration. These results are shown in
Figure 1. Clearly, the esterolytic activity is unaffected by SK
whereas the caseinolytic activity decreases as a function of added
SK and extropolates to zero proteolytic activity at ratios of 1:1,
SK to Pm. Although the general proteolytic activity of plasmin
decreases with increasing SK addition, the plasminogen activator
activity of Pm shows a parallel increase as a function of added
SK. This activity again is maximal at ratios of 1:1, SK to Pm.
The interpretation at this point is that Pm and SK for a 1:1 complex
and this complex, although possessing little proteolytic activity,
appears to be specific for activation of Pg. Thus, Pg may be
activated to Pm by streptokinase in the presence of a small amount
of Pm contaminant according to the above considerations.

Although the above activation can certainly occur, it does not
explain the fact that activation of human Pg by SK can occur if all
contaminating Pm is specifically inactivated by diisopropylfluorphosphate or similar reagents, prior to addition of SK (16). An
important experiment which sheds some light on this point is shown

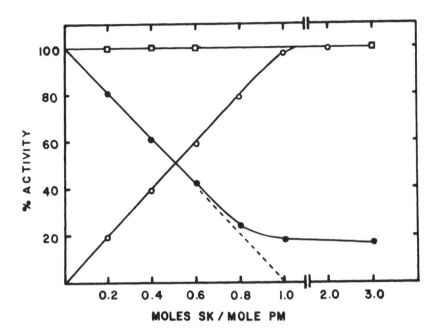

Figure 1: Activity of human plasmin at 25° toward ( ), tosarg-
OMe; (O), azocasein; and (O), bovine plasminogen as a function
of added streptokinase. All methods are described in ref. 14.

in Figure 2. Here, we have mixed human Pg with a 10-fold excess of the plasmin and trypsin actylating agent, p-nitrophenyl-
p'-guanidino benzoate (NphBzoGdn). This reagent forms an
instantaneous acyl-enzyme complex, with a corresponding release
of p-nitrophenolate, with the plasmin active site. This inactive
acyl-enzyme is a relatively stable species (17). To the mixture
of Pg and NphBzoGdn we added a stoichiometric amount of SK.
Immediately, upon addition of SK, 0.85 moles of p-nitrophenolate
were released per mole of Pg initially present; indicating the
presence of an active site. All further proteolysis was naturally
stopped. Neither Pg nor SK independently catalyzed the release
of p-nitrophenolate from this compound. The sodium dodecyl
sulfate gel of the protein components present in this experiment,
shown in gel 3 in Figure 2, indicate that only Pg and SK are present. Thus the formation of an active site in an SK· Pg complex
accompanies the addition of SK to Pg. This is the earliest active
site formed. However, if equal molar quantities of SK and Pg are
incubated for 10 minutes, prior to addition of NphBzoGdn (gel 4 in
Figure 2), again 0.80 moles of p-nitrophenolate are released per

mole of initial Pg. However, in this case the protein components are Pm and an altered for of SK. This shows that the initial active site in the SK· Pg complex will catalyze the formation of Pm from Pg within the complex.

We have established the fact that the active site within the SK· Pg complex resides on the Pg moiety (18). This was done

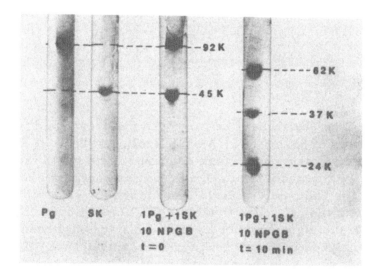

Figure 2: Sodium dodecyl sulfate-mercaptoethanol gel electro-phoretic analysis of the effect of stoichiometric addition of SK to human Pg. The first two gels show the starting materials, viz. , Pg and SK, used for these experiments. Gel 3 represents the ex-periment in which 1 molar equivalent of Pg was incubated with 10 molar equivalents of NphBzoGdn (NPGB), immediately followed by addition of 1 molar equivalent of streptokinase. The solution was incubated for 10 min prior to analysis. One mole of active site per initial mole of Pg was found. Gel 4 represents the ex-periment in which the same molar amounts of SK and Pg were incubated for 10 minutes, followed by addition of 10 molar equivalents of NPGB. Again, one mole of active site was found per mole of initial Pg. The numbers along each band on these gels represents the molecular weight of the bands under denaturing conditions.

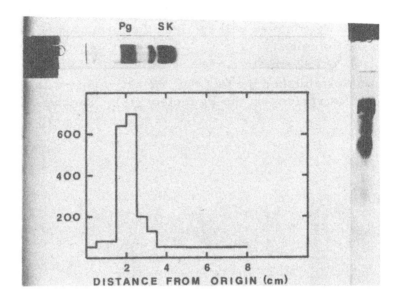

Figure 3: The acylation of human Pg in the presence of stoichiometric levels of SK by $[^{14}C]$-AmSMeBzoNph at 25°. A duplicate
unreduced and unstained sodium dodecyl sulfate gel to that shown
horizontally alligned was sliced and the radioactivity eluted from
the gel. The radioactivity level determined for each slice, is
alligned with the gel. Positive identification of the radioactive
band as plasminogen (and not plasmin) was accomplished by similar gels analyzed in the presence of mercaptoethanol. This gel
is shown vertically on the extreme right. This gel could not be
analyzed for radioactivity since mercaptoethanol deacylates
plasminogen.

by preparing a radioactive derivative, p-nitrophenyl p-(amidino-
thiomethyl)benzoate (AmSMeBzoNph), of NphBzoGdn, which acts
very similarly to NphBzoGdn. We found, that when SK is added
to a mixture of Pg and $[^{14}C$-AmSmeBzoNph, all the radioactivity
is present in the Pg moiety of the complex. This clearly establishes the hypothesis that an active site is induced in Pg following
addition of SK. The results which led to this conclusion are shown
in Figure 3.

At this point, we can forward a mechanism for the SK induced
activation of HPg. This is shown in Figure 4. Here, in the initial
step SK and Pg form a complex (SK· Pg) which results in a

rearrangement of the Pg moiety such than an active site is induced in the complex (SK·Pg'). This complex can autocatalytically yield an SK·Pm complex, which can also form from SK + Pm. The complexes (SK·Pg)' and (SK·Pm) are called plasminogen activator complexes since, when present in catalytic amounts, lead to activation of all remaining plasminogen to plasmin. By this mechanism catalytic levels of SK will activate human Pg to Pm by formation of a small level of activator complexes. It is of further interest to determine which activator complex is the major activator of Pg. Our studies (14, 18), as well as those of Markus (19, 20) indicate that the (SK·Pg)' complex is probably the major activator.

It is now necessary to prove that all the above complexes can indeed form. We have established (14) that an SK·Pg' complex forms when SK is added to a mixture of human Pg and NphBzoGdn and that an SK· Pm complex is formed when SK is added to human Pg, followed by addition of NphBzoGdn, after 10 minutes. Further, we have established that SK will complex with human Pm or diisopropylfluorphosphate treated human Pm. Thus, all necessary complexes can in fact form, lending credence to the above described mechanism.

We have been involved in the last few years in the characterization of the conformational changes induced in plasminogen by agents such as Σ-amino caproic acid (Σ-ACA or ΣAHx) and

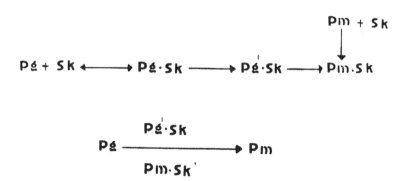

Figure 4: The proposed mechanism for the activation of plasmino-gen by streptokinase. Refer to text for abbreviations.

Table II

Alteration in the $S_{20,w}^o$ Value of Human Plasminogen
by Molecules of the ε-ACA Class

		$S_{20,w}^o$		
Agent	Pg species	N^a	I^b	$K_{Diss.}^c$
t-AMCHA	Human	5.72 S	4.83 S	8×10^{-5} $\underline{M}$
	Rabbit	5.70 S	4.79 S	1.6×10^{-4} $\underline{M}$
ε-ACA	Human	5.72 S	4.78 S	4.5×10^{-4} $\underline{M}$
	Rabbit	5.70 S	4.80 S	3.1×10^{-3} $\underline{M}$
$\underline{L}$-lysine	Human	5.72 S	4.78 S	6.8×10^{-2} $\underline{M}$
	Rabbit	5.70 S	4.81 S	9.0×10^{-2} $\underline{M}$

[a]Native plasminogen in 0.05 $\underline{M}$ tris·HCl, 0.1 $\underline{M}$ NaCl, pH 8.0.

[b]Altered plasminogen in 0.05 $\underline{M}$ tris·HCl, 0.1 $\underline{M}$ ligand, pH 8.0.

[c]At 25°C.

trans-4-aminomethylcyclohexane-1-carboxylic acid ($\underline{t}$-AMCHA).
These compounds are known to inhibit the streptokinase induced
activation of human Pg to Pm (7, 21). We have characterized the
conformational alteration by sedimentation velocity analysis (12)
and isothermal fluorescence polarization measurements (13).
Further, we have shown that the conformation alteration in Pg
induced by these agents is directly due to the binding of these
agents to Pg. A list of the effects of Σ-ACA and $\underline{t}$-AMCHA on
the $S_{20,w}^o$ values of two species of Pg are shown in Table II.
Further, $K_{Diss.}$ values for these agents to each Pg, obtained by
titration of the $S_{20,w}^o$ values (12) are also given in Table II.
Clearly, the comparative effectiveness of these agents as ligands
for each Pg is: t-AMCHA > Σ-ACA > L-lysine. This series also
is identical as the series displaying the effectiveness of these
agents as fibrinolytic inhibitors. Hydrodynamic parameters,
obtained by rotational and translational measurements, of the
conformational alterations produced in human Pg by Σ-ACA and

Table III

Hydrodynamic Parameters for Human Plasminogen (HPg) Obtained by Translational and Rotational Measurements

Species	ρ_h (nsec) [b] 25°	ρ_h/ρ_o [c]	$f/f_{(min)}$ [d]
HPg	262 ± 10	3.69	1.41
HPg + ε-ACA[a]	156 ± 8	2.20	1.75
HPg + t-AMCHA[a]	160 ± 8	2.25	1.75

[a]Buffers contained levels of ligand which saturated the Pg binding site for these compounds (ref. 12). [b]Refers to the mean harmonic rotational relaxation time. Calculated as described in ref. 12. [c]The value of ρ_o is calculated from $\rho_o = 3\eta V/RT$; where ρ_o is the mean harmonic rotational relaxation time of a sphere of the same apparent molar volume of plasminogen. The molar volume (V) of human plasminogen is 58,360 cm^3/mole. [d]Calculated from $f/f_{(min)} = D^o_{max}/D^o$. D^o_{max} was calculated as described in ref. 13. D^o for HPg was calculated based on the known molecular weight and $S^o_{20,w}$ value of HPg.

t-AMCHA are summarized in Table III. Briefly, the fact that the f/f_{min} values for Pg, obtained from translational hydrodynamic measurements, increase upon saturation of the binding site on Pg for these compounds, demonstrates that binding of Σ-ACA and t-AMCHA leads to a more asymmetric structure in Pg. However, the fact that the rotational relaxation times (ρ_h), or the ratio of ρ_h/ρ_o, decreases upon binding of these agents to Pg demonstrates that this more asymmetric conformation is also internally more flexible than the native Pg conformation. Thus, the structure of Pg in the presence of these compounds is more flexible and more asymmetric compared to native Pg.

The streptokinase induced conversion of Pg to Pm occurs in several distinct steps, and it is not fully understood what the influence of these antifibrinolytic compounds is on each of the steps. In other words, the exact effect of the altered Pg conformation (induced by these compounds) on its ability to interact with SK to form the Pg activator complexes and on its ability to become a substrate for the Pg activator (in terms of each of the two bonds cleaved in Pg) are not fully understood. In addition, the fact that these antifibrinolytics are direct competitive inhibitors of the enzymatic activity of both Pm, (SK·Pg)' and (SK·Pm) probably greatly contribute to their antifibrinolytic effects at high concentrations (22).

ACKNOWLEDGEMENTS

These studies were supported by grants HL-13423 and HL-15747 from the N. I. H. as well as grants from the Indiana and American Heart Associations. F. J. C. is the recipient of a Research Career Development Award (HL-70717) from the N. I. H.

REFERENCES

1. Robbins, K. C., Bernabe, P., Arzadon, L. and Summaria, L. J. Biol. Chem., 248: 7242, 1973.
2. Wiman, B. and Wallen, P. Eur. J. Biochem. 36: 25, 1973.
3. Sodetz, J. M., Brockway, W. J., Mann, K. G. and Castellino, F. J. Biochem. Biophys. Res. Comm., in press.
4. Blatt, W. F., Segal, H. and Gray, J. L. Thromb. Diath. Haemorrh. 11: 393, 1964.
5. Ling. C. -M., Summaria, L. and Robbins, K. C. J. Biol. Chem. 240: 4213, 1965.
6. Ling, C. -M., Summaria, L. and Robbins, K. C. J. Biol. Chem. 242: 1419, 1967.
7. Alkjaersig, N., Fletcher, A. P. and Sherry, S. J. Biol. Chem. 234: 832, 1959.
8. Maxwell, R. E. and Allen, D. Nature 209: 211, 1966.
9. Maxwell, R. E., Nawrocki, J. W. and Nickel, V. S. Thromb. Diath. Haemorrh. 19: 117, 1968.
10. Okamoto, S. Keio J. Med. 8: 211, 1959.
11. Abiko, Y., Iwamota, M. and Tomikawa, M. Biochim. Biophys. Acta 185: 424, 1969.
12. Brockway, W. J. and Castellino, F. J. Arch. Biochem. Biophys. 151: 194, 1972.
13. Castellino, F. J., Brockway, W. J., Thomas, J. K., Liao, H. -t. and Rawitch, A. B. Biochemistry 12: 2787, 1973.

14. Schick, L. A. and Castellino, F. J. Biochemistry 12: 4315, 1973.
15. Castellino, F. J., Siefring, G. E., Jr., Sodetz, J. M. and Bretthauer, R. K. Biochem. Biophys. Res. Comm. 53: 845, 1973.
16. McClintock, D. K. and Bell, P. H. Biochem. Biophys. Res. Comm. 43: 694, 1971.
17. Sodetz, J. M. and Castellino, F. J. Biochemistry 11: 3167, 1972.
18. Schick, L. A. and Castellino, F. J. Biochem. Biophys. Res. Comm. 57: 47, 1974.
19. Reddy, K. N. N. and Markus, G. J. Biol. Chem. 247: 1683, 1972.
20. Reddy, K. N. N. and Markus, G. J. Biol. Chem. 249, 4851, 1974.
21. Brockway, W. J. and Castellino, F. J. J. Biol. Chem. 246: 4641, 1971.
22. Brockway, W. J., Ph. D. thesis, University of Notre Dame, 1974.

THE ROLE OF LIPIDS IN THE TISSUE FACTOR PATHWAY

OF BLOOD COAGULATION

Yale Nemerson

Department of Internal Medicine, Yale University
School of Medicine, New Haven, Connecticut 06510,
USA

When blood is shed from a vein, collected into a glass tube
and allowed to clot spontaneously, fibrin will form in about 15 or
20 minutes. On the other hand if small amounts of various tissues
but particularly lung, brain, and placenta are added to this blood,
it will clot in something of the order of 12 to 20 seconds. The
fact that blood clots at all when withdrawn from the body is due
to the initiation of a complex series of reactions involving many
proteins, calcium ions and phospholipids. When no tissue extracts are added and the blood is allowed to simply clot spontaneously the initial reaction involves the activation of Factor XII
or Hageman factor and the entire series of events which then
follows is referred to as the intrinsic system. When tissue factor is added in the form of acetone powders of whole tissues or
as a more purified preparation, the initiating event is the formation of a complex between tissue factor and a plasma protein
Factor VII. The reactions which then lead to the formation of
fibrin are called the extrinsic system or the tissue factor pathway
of blood coagulation.

Both pathways of coagulation converge at a point in which
Factor X, a plasma zymogen, is proteolytically converted to its
active enzyme, Factor X_a. Before describing the events involved
in the tissue factor pathway I shall summarize the reactions of
the intrinsic system. As mentioned above the initial event in
this pathway is the activation of Hageman Factor. Recent experi-

ments suggest that this is a nonprotelytic activation and probably
involves a conformational change in the molecule which either
exposes its catalytic center or its binding sites (1, 2). It is
generally thought that the major activator of Hageman Factor in
vivo is collagen although elastin has also been implicated. Activated Hageman Factor then proteolytically attacks another zymogen Factor XI or PTA (3). This reaction has not been studied in
detail, but by analogy with other events in coagulation it appears
to involve proteolysis of Factor XI. It is of interest that neither
of these reactions is calcium dependent. Therefore, when plasma
anticoagulated with calcium chelators is used to study blood coagulation these reactions may still go to completion and large
amounts of activated Factor XI may be formed. Activated Factor
XI then apparently proteolytically attacks another zymogen Factor
IX or Christmas factor (4). This is a calcium requiring reaction
and appears to involve the release of an activation peptide from
Factor IX. Activated Factor IX in an extremely complex reaction
then proteolytically attacks Factor X leading to the formation of
activated Factor X. This reaction exhibits a requirement for
calcium ions and phospholipids as well as a protein co-factor,
anti-hemophiliac factor or Factor VIII (5). Although the enzyme-
activated Factor IX apparently can attack its substrate, Factor
X, in the absence of these co-factors, the rates are barely dis-
cernable and a stimulation of many thousand-fold is obtained in
the complete system. During the activation of Factor X, it is
likely that a complex is formed between activated Factor IX
calcium ions, phospholipids, and Factor VIII (6). At the present
time it is impossible to describe in detail the basis for this complex formation and for its enormous acceleratory effect.

The tissue factor pathway also involves the formation of a complex which proteolytically attacks Factor X. Here however only a
single reaction is involved in which tissue factor, a membrane-
bound lipoprotein, forms a proteolytically active complex with
Factor VII (7). This complex then attacks Factor X. In the case
of both the intrinsic and the tissue factor pathways of blood coagulation, the attack on Factor X appears to be the same and the
resultant enzyme, activated Factor X, is also the same (8) The
next reaction, common to both pathways, is highly reminiscent of
the activation of Factor X by the intrinsic system. Here the enzyme, activated Factor X, forms a complex with calcium ions,
phospholipids and another plasma co-factor, Factor V (9). This
complex then proteolytically attacks prothrombin yielding the

active procoagulant enzyme, thrombin.   Again, the enzyme can, in and of itself, catalyze this reaction.   However, in the presence of the co-factors, calcium ions, phospholipids and Factor V, the rate of attack is increased at least 1,000 fold.   Again details of this complex and interesting reaction are yet to be elucidated.

The final steps of blood coagulation involve the formation of fibrin from fibrinogen and the cross-linking of the resultant fibrin to form an insolubile and stable clot.   Fibrinogen is a complex molecule consisting of three pairs of polypeptide chains labeled A (α), B (β) and γ.   Thrombin catalyzes a proteolytic attack on the A (α) and B (β) chains removing small peptides from each (10)   The resulting molecule, fibrin monomer, is insoluble and readily self-associates forming a visible gel, the fibrin clot The final stabilization of the clot is accomplished by yet another enzyme, fibrin stabilizing factor of Factor XIII, which covalently links the fibrin monomers by catalyzing a transpeptidation reaction in which a glutamine on one molecule is covalently linked to a lysine on another, with the release of free ammonia (11).

As mentioned above, tissue factor is a membrane bound lipoprotein, and its function in blood coagulation is to form a proteolytically active complex with Factor VII.   It should be emphasized that tissue factor itself is a co-factor and that the catalytic center of this active complex resides in the Factor VII molecule (12).   It should also be emphasized that the co-factors in blood coagulation although lacking enzymatic activity appear to have the same rigid requirements for specificity as do the enzymes involved in this system.   Thus, tissue factor consists of a specific protein and, as will be discussed, phospholipids which also exhibit specificity.   Neither component of tissue factor alone is biologically active.   The first clear demonstration of the lipid requirement of tissue factor was accomplished in 1946 by Studer (13)   He extracted a crude tissue factor preparation with ether-alcohol and demonstrated a loss of activity.   He also demonstrated complete restitution of activity when the ether-alcohol soluble material was added to the insoluble residue.   Subsequently, Kuhn and Klesse (14) essentially confirmed this observation and added that only certain phospholipids could substitute for the naturally occurring lipids.   More recently Deutsch, Irsigler, and Lomoschitz (15) refined and extended these observations by extracting a semi-purified particulate brain tissue factor preparation with pyridine, separating the components and showing essentially an absolute requirement for the pyridine soluble material. Subsequently our laboratory (16) and that of Prydz (17) have investigated the lipid requirements of tissue factor.

In our early experiments, we started with a particulate preparation of brain tissue factor which contains 38-40% phospholipids by weight. When the phospholipids were removed by repeated extraction with organic solvents, essentially all the biological activity of tissue factor was lost. The residual particles contained only about 2% phospholipid by weight. When a brain phospholipid preparation was added back to this delipidated material, full biological activity was restored. The recombination was affected by dissolving the phospholipids in mixtures of heptane and butanol, adding the protein and flash evaporating the solvent. In parallel experiments it was shown that neutral lipids had no effect on this system. Accordingly the effect of purified phospholipids was studied, and it was found that phosphatidyl ethanolamine restored the entire biological activity of tissue factor. On a weight basis phosphatidyl ethanolamine was approximately twice as active as mixed brain phospholipids. Phosphatidyl choline was somewhat less active than the mixed brain lipids, but restored significant activity. On the other hand neither phosphatidyl inositol nor phosphatidyl serine restored activity.

In order to determine whether the head group alone was responsible for the activity of the lipids or whether there was a contribution from the fatty acid components, phosphatidyl choline was modified and tested for biological activity. Catalytic hydrogenation totally eliminated the ability of phosphatidyl choline to restore the biological activity of tissue factor. Similarly, digestion with phospholipase A also yielded an inert product as did digestion with phospholipase D. On the other hand, sphingomyelin, which also contains choline as its polar component, had essentially no activity. On the basis of these observations, then, it was concluded that the appropriate polar group is an absolute requirement for the activity of phospholipids, but that unsaturation of the fatty acids as well as their presence is also required for full activity.

Inasmuch as the protein component of tissue factor could not be further investigated due to the particulate nature of these preparations, a major effort of our laboratory was directed to the solubilization and purification of the protein component of tissue

factor. The former was accomplished by extracting the delipidated powders described above with sodium deoxycholate which
totally solubilized and preserved the activity of tissue factor (18).
The latter, however, could only be demonstrated if phospholipids
were added back to the solubilized tissue factor protein   This
was accomplished by emulsifying the lipids in solutions of deoxycholate, recombining the lipids with these solutions of the apoprotein and removing excess deoxycholate by dialysis. The
resultant product was then fully active in blood coagulation. The
apoprotein was purified by conventional techniques involving
ammonium sulfate fractionation, DEAE chromatography and gel
filtration. The final product has been purified several thousand-
fold and has been used for studying the physical interaction of the
apoprotein of tissue factor with various phospholipids.

The approach used in our laboratory was to study the binding
of purified phospholipids to tissue factor apoprotein by determining
the behavior of relipidated preparations of the apoprotein during
sucrose density gradient ultracentrifugation (19). We found that
tissue factor binds not only phospholipids which restore coagulant
activity, i. e. , phosphatidyl ethanolamine and phosphatidyl choline,
but also those which are ineffective. Therefore, binding alone is
not sufficient for restoration of activity. However, qualitative
differences were detected and phospholipids which failed to restore
activity were bound poorly. For example, complexes formed with
lysophosphatidyl choline broke up in the centrifugal field and were
thus different from those containing active lipids. The experimental
approach was to recombine the apoprotein with the appropriate
phospholipid in deoxycholate as described above. The mixture was
then applied to a sucrose gradient and centrifuged at 36, 000 rpm
for 18 hours. At this time the lipids alone would have floated to
the top of the tube while the protein alone would have pelleted at the
bottom. Complexes which formed with densities intermediate to
those of either the protein or the lipid would have reached equilibrium
and stabilized somewhere in the body of the gradient. Using this
isopycnic technique, stable complexes of phosphatidyl ethanolamine and phosphotidyl choline were detected. The density of the
complex was a function of the ratio of the lipid concentration to
that of the protein. No limiting stoichiometry was observed,
suggesting that the protein was interacting with lipid but that
lipid-lipid interactions were also of major significance. Of note
is that if the detergent, sodium deoxycholate, were omitted from
the initial step, that is the recombination of the protein and the

lipid, there was no restitution of biological activity to the apoprotein, nor did any detectable complexes form.

The results of these experiments indicate that binding of tissue factor to phospholipid is an absolute requirement for activity. As noted above, when the protein was simply added to an active lipid in the absence of deoxycholate there was no restriction of activity nor did binding occur. It is also clear, however, that binding to lipids per se is not sufficient to restore activity to the system: reduced phosphatidyl choline and lysophosphatidyl choline bound to tissue factor but restored no activity. The data do suggest, however, that lipids which stimulate biological activity form more stable complexes with tissue factor than do inert lipids. For example, phosphatidyl ethanolamine, the most active lipid, forms complexes which quickly reached equilibrium and which remained intact in the centrifugal field for at least 63 hours. The complexes formed with lysophosphatidyl choline behave quite differently during centrifugation. Whereas in the experiments using phosphatidyl ethanolamine tubes at equilibrium showed coincidence of the peaks of biological activity, protein and lipid, no such coincidence was noted when lysophophatidyl choline was substituted. There is strong evidence for complex formation with the inert lipid, however. Under the conditions used the lipid alone floated at the top of the tube and the protein pelleted at the bottom. The mixture however was distributed throughout the tube suggesting that complexes did form but were dissociable and broke up the centrifugal field. A different situation, however, was detected using reduced phosphatidyl choline. Here a stable, but biologically inert complex with tissue factor protein was formed. It appeared however that the affinity of this lipid for the protein is less than that of the active lipids. That is, far more reduced phosphatidyl choline was required to form a complex than when the native lipid was used.

It should be noted that the lipid-lipid interactions vary considerably from one phospholipid to another as manifested by different micellar properties. It is clear that the number of fatty acid chains as well as their degree of saturation play an important role in the binding to tissue factor and to the restoration of biological activity. These parameters are also reflected in the micellar properties of these lipids. In water solution, egg and brain phosphatidyl choline form micelle with estimated molecular weights of 2×10^6 daltons (20) whereas lysophosphatidyl choline forms a smaller globular structure with an estimated molecular weight of approximately 10^5 (21). Reduced phosphatidyl choline on the other hand may not even form micelle at room temperature (22). It appears that brain phosphatidyl ethanolamine micelle are similar to those formed by phosphatidyl choline. Further complications in the interpretation of these data arise from the fact that although the micellar size of phosphatidyl ethanolamine and phosphatidyl choline have the same micellar size, the fatty acids of phosphatidyl ethanolamine are less saturated, thus having a greater cross-sectional area.

The considerations of the different physical states of the various phospholipids preclude a formal analysis of the structure-function relationships in this system. What is clear, however, is that there is an absolute requirement for phospholipids for the biological activity of tissue factor and that some structural specificity is evidenced by the efficacy of phosphatidyl ethanolamine in restoring activity and the total inability of phosphatidyl serine or phosphatidyl inositol to function in this system.

As mentioned earlier, active tissue factor forms a complex with a plasma protein, Factor VII, which then proteolytically attacks factor X. In this reaction it appears that Factor VII is "directed" by tissue factor to attack its substrate, Factor X. In the absence of tissue factor, Factor VII is inert in this reaction whereas in the presence of its co-factor it explosively initiates blood coagulation. The molecular events have not yet been elucidated, although it is known from studies of the incorporation of DFP, an active site directed irreversible inhibitor of serine proteases, that the catalytic center of Factor VII is intact and functional prior to complex formation with tissue factor. It should be noted that both components of tissue factor are required for this complex formation.

As noted earlier activated Factor X requires calcium ions, phospholipids and a plasma co-factor, Factor V, to attack its substrate, prothrombin. In the intrinsic system the phospholipid requirement of this reaction is thought to be fulfilled by the plasma membranes of blood platelets. When coagulation is initiated by tissue factor, however, no additional phospholipid need be added to accelerate the conversion of prothrombin. This is because the phospholipids normally associated with the tissue factor molecule can satisfy the phospholipid requirement of prothrombin conversion. Hence in this pathway explosive thrombin formation can occur in the total absence of blood platelets or any other source of phospholipids.

Thus, in the tissue factor pathway of blood coagulation the mere addition of tissue factor and calcium ions to the plasma proteins of the coagulation system leads to rapid fibrin formation. The role of phospholipids in this reaction has been extensively studied and significant data have emerged. The fundamental question, however, of the mechanism by which various non-enzymatic molecules such as the proteins, Factor VIII and Factor V, and the lipoprotein, tissue factor, so markedly accelerate and control blood coagulation has yet to be approached.

ACKNOWLEDGEMENT

This work was supported by NIH Grant HL 16126 from the National Heart and Lung Institute.

REFERENCES

1. Ratnoff, O. D. , and Rosenblum, J. M. J. Lab. Clin. Med. 50: 941, 1957

2. Cochrane, C. G. and Weupper, K. D. J. Exp. Med. 134: 986, 1971

3. Ratnoff, O. D. and Davie, E. W. Biochemistry 1: 967, 1962

4. Fujikawa, K. , Thompson, A. R. , Legaz, M. E. , Meyer, R. G. and Davie, E. W. Biochemistry 12: 4938, 1973

5. Macfarlane, R. G. , Biggs, R. , Ash, B. J. , and Denson, K. W. E. Brit. J. Haematol. 10: 530, 1964

6. Hoagle, L. , Denson, K. W. E. and Biggs, R. Thromb. Diath. Hoemuruh. 18: 211, 1967

7. Nemerson, Y. Biochemistry 5: 601, 1966

8. Radcliffe, R. and Barton, P. G. J. Biol. Chem. 248: 6788, 1973

9. Hemker, H. C. , Esnouf, M. P. , Hemker, P. W. , Swart,
    A. C. W. and Macfarlane, R. G. Nature 215: 248, 1967

10. Bettelheim, F. R. and Baily, K. Biochem. Biophys. Acta
    9: 578, 1952

11. Lorand, L. , Konishi, K. and Jacobsen, A. Nature 194:
    1148, 1962

12. Nemerson, Y. and Esnouf, M. P. Proc. Nat. Acad. Sci.
    (USA) 70: 310, 1973

13. Studer, A. 1946. In: Jubilee Volume dedicated to Emile
    Christophe Barell. The Roche Companies, Basel.

14. Kuhn, R. and Klesse, P. C. Naturwissenschaften 44: 352,
    1957

15. Deutsch, E. , Irsigler, K. and Lomoschitz, H. Thromb.
    Diath. Haemorrh 12: 12, 1964

16. Nemerson, Y. J. Clin. Invest. 47: 72, 1968

17. Huatum, M. and Prydz, H. Thromb. Diath. Haemorrh 21:
    217, 1969

18. Nemerson, Y. J. Clin. Invest. 47:72, 1968; 48:322, 1969.

19. Pitlick, F. A. and Nemerson, Y. Biochemistry 9: 5105,
    1970

20. Gammack, D. B. , Perrin, J. H. and Saunders, L. Biochim.
    Biophys. Acta 84: 576, 1964

21. Perrin, J. H. and Saunders, L. Biochim. Biophys. Acta
    84: 216, 1964

22. Fleischer, S. , Klouwen, H. and Carpenter, E. Biochem.
    Biophys. Res. Commun. 5: 378, 1961

USE OF FIBRINOPEPTIDE A MEASUREMENTS IN THE

DIAGNOSIS AND MANAGEMENT OF THROMBOSIS

H. L. Nossel

Department of Medicine, College of Physicians and
Surgeons of Columbia University, New York, New York

CLINICAL PROBLEMS WITH REGARD TO THROMBOSIS

From the clinical and laboratory point of view, it would be
extremely useful to have laboratory tests which could help with
the diagnosis of thrombosis. These tests could be divided into
those which would diagnose the established lesion and those which
would tell the physician that the patient was at a high risk of developing thrombosis -- that is, assist in the prediction of thrombosis.
From the treatment point of view, it would be most useful to have
laboratory tests which would serve as an index of whether the
treatment was being effective or not. The most important problem
with regard to thrombosis and embolism is of course prevention.
The ability to prevent the occurrence of thrombosis and embolism
requires the availability of tests which would permit prediction of
a high risk of clinical disorder.

METHOD OF APPROACH

In its simplest terms, the thrombus is composed of two principal elements. These elements are aggregated platelets and
fibrin. The initial approach of my group has been based on the
development of assays which would permit one to follow the formation of fibrin intravascularly. It was decided to commence with
assays which would monitor the actions of identified enzymes on

fibrinogen in vivo. Three enzymes are known to affect fibrin
formation in vitro, and there is considerable circumstantial evidence that all three may be involved in vivo. We decided to develop tests which would reflect the action of each of these enzymes
in vivo separately. The first tests were based on an attempt to
quantitate the action of thrombin on fibrinogen in vivo. When
thrombin acts on fibrinogen, it proteolyzes 4 peptide bonds in the
fibrinogen molecule. These are arginylglycine bonds near the
amino terminal ends of the Aα chain and Bβ chain of fibrinogen.
The result of these proteolytic cleavages is the production of two
molecules of fibrinopeptide A and two molecules of fibrinopeptide
B and 1 molecule of fibrin from the fibrinogen molecule (1). A
number of attempts have been made to develop tests for the
presence of fibrin in solution in the blood (2, 3, 4). The approach
of my group was to develop assays for fibrinopeptides A and B.
These assays have been based on the radioimmunoassay principle.
Since in thrombin action on fibrinogen, fibrinopeptide A cleavage
precedes that of fibrinopeptide B, our initial studies were based
on the assays of fibrinopeptide A (FPA) (5, 6).

FIBRINOPEPTIDE A ASSAY

Two special reagents are required for the assay of fibrinopeptide A. These reagents are radiolabelled fibrinopeptide A and
specific antibody to peptide. The fibrinopeptide A molecule consists of 16 amino acids, but tyrosine is not present in the molecule.
In order to radiolabel the peptide with radioactive iodine, it was
necessary to couple tyrosine to the fibrinopeptide molecule. Tyrosine was accordingly coupled to the amino terminal alanine in the
fibrinopeptide A molecule. Tyrosinated peptide was labelled with
125I with the chloramine T technique of Hunter and Greenwood
(7). Specific antibodies to fibrinopeptide A were developed in
New Zealand white rabbits by immunization with native or synthetic
fibrinopeptide A coupled to serum albumin. The assay technique
involves the incubation of antiserum, test solution and radiolabelled
tyrosinated fibrinopeptide A, followed by separation of bound from
free tracer with the use of charcoal. Figure 1 shows a typical
inhibition of binding curve produced by different quantities of fibrinopeptide A. The results indicate that 50% inhibition of binding was
achieved with about 0.2 ng of fibrinopeptide A. This signifies that
0.2 ng of fibrinopeptide A can be measured accurately with the
assay.

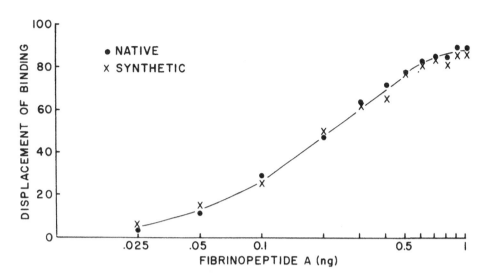

Figure 1: Inhibition of binding of ^{125}I-labeled tyrosinated peptide A by native and synthetic fibrinopeptide. 500 μl volumes that contained various concentrations of native FPA (●) or synthetic FPA (X) were tested. (Amounts shown on abscissa.)

When the assay had been developed for in vitro use, it was then necessary to apply it to the measurement of FPA in clinical blood samples. We have developed a reproducible technique for collecting blood and extracting the fibrinopeptide A from it, as well as preventing the generation of fibrinopeptide A in vitro. The technique involves the use of heparin and Traylol as an anti-coagulant solution, precipitation of fibrinogen from the plasma with ethanol and dialysis of the supernatant solution. Using this technique, we obtain between 95 and 105% recovery of fibrinopeptide A added to plasma.

Very strong immunochemical evidence is available, that the 16 amino acid fibrinopeptide A is being measured in the clinical samples without the presence of larger fragments of the fibrinogen molecule which contain the A peptide, and which could be produced by plasmin action.

CLINICAL RESULTS

Clinical measurements of fibrinopeptide A levels in 50 normal

TABLE I

FPA Levels in the Blood of Patients with Reduced Fibrinogen Levels and/or Reduced Platelet Counts

Patient	Diagnosis	Fibrinogen	Thrombin clotting time	Fibrinogen degradation products	Platelets	FPA levels		
						R2 antiserum		R.33 antiserum
						Antiserum with hirudin	Dialysate treated with thrombin	
		mg/100 ml	s	μg/ml	ml⁻¹	ng/ml		
Normal range		200–400	14–17	<2	150,000–400,000	<2	<2	<2
P. H.	Acute immunological disorder, probable drug sensitivity	0	>180	<2	50,000	80		
J. J.	Acute gram-negative sepsis	50	>180	3	62,000	4		
Y. S.	Acute sepsis with E. coli	305	19	165	125,000	41	41	52
S. B.	Dissecting aneurysm	140	23	5	32,000	17		16
C. T.	Acute myeloid leukemia	70	>120	12	19,000	11.5		11.7
C. H.	Lung carcinoma with metastases	50	>180		100,000	290		289
P. N.	Pancreatic carcinoma, femoral artery thrombosis, myocardial infarction	276	26	330	90,000	140	135	140
P. M.	Cirrhosis	90	44	21	23,000	18.5		
I. T.	Liver failure	125	37	10	80,000	6.6		
L. B.	Liver failure	85	24	0	27,000	16.5		15
G. G.	Liver failure	95	>180	0	70,000	21	25	20
V. B.	Liver failure, lymphosarcoma	85	65	20	50,000	10.8		12.4

Measurement of Fibrinopeptide A in Human Blood

individuals show a range of levels from .1 to 2 ng per ml with a
mean of 0.7 ng per ml. Clinical studies have been principally
devoted to two groups of patients. The first group includes patients
with laboratory evidence of vascular coagulation. Table I shows
the results of studies in 12 such patients. Fibrinopeptide A levels
ranged between 4 and 290 ng per ml. In a patient with a congenital
hemangioma of the leg and a state of chronic intravascular coagulation in the hemangioma, fibrinopeptide A levels have varied between 4.5 and 9.6 ng per ml over a three year period. On two
occasions, following heparin infusion in the patient, no fibrinopeptide A could be measured with the assay (Table II). A second
group of patients have normal fibrinogen levels and platelet counts.
Table III shows the results of FPA measurements in 13 such
patients. Results on 5 patients with venous thrombosis and/or
pulmonary embolism are shown. The FPA levels ranged between
6 and 23 ng per ml. One of these patients with renal transplant
rejection is of particular interest, since all conventional coagulation studies, including the fibrinogen degradation product level,
were consistently normal, yet there was evidence from a rising
blood urea of renal failure, and biopsy of the transplanted kidney

TABLE II

FPA Immunoreactivity in Plasma of Patient C. N.

Date		Concentration	
		R2	R33
		ng/ml	
6/8/71		4.8	4.6
11/22/71	right arm	5.5	5.2
	right leg	8.6	
	left leg	6.7	
11/23/71		9.6	
11/25/71	postheparin	0	
11/26/71		5.4	
	postheparin	0	
12/10/71		4.8	
12/28/71		6.1	
1/15/72		6.3	
5/4/72		4.7	
6/20/72		6.1	

The results of coagulation tests on the patient's blood were
as follows: partial thromboplastin time, 88 s (control 54 s);

TABLE III

FPA Levels in the Blood of Patients with Normal or Elevated Fibrinogen Levels and Platelet Counts

Patient	Diagnosis	Fibrinogen	Thrombin clotting time	Fibrinogen degradation products	Platelets	FPA levels R2 antiserum		R33 antiserum
						Antiserum with hirudin	Dialysate treated with thrombin	
		$mg/100\ ml$	s	$\mu g/ml$	ml^{-1}	ng/ml	ng/ml	
Normal range		200–400	14–17	<2	150,000–400,000	<2	<2	<2
G. A.	Aortic aneurysm	320	13.7	82	228,000	12.4		10.8
M. B.	Renal transplant rejection	340	14.1	0	190,000	21.3		25.0
E. C.	Renal transplant	590	11.7	10	150,000	12.4		8.4
I. M.	Pulmonary embolism	280	17.7		230,000	19.4		15
M. F.	Pulmonary embolism	330	12.2	1.3	adequate	6.0		5
C. F.	Venous thrombosis and pulmonary embolism	640	10.3	10	275,000	23	31	19.8
A. A.	Venous thrombosis	970	14.3	10	375,000	11		9.2
F. T.	Venous thrombosis	285	15	10		6.8		9.4
E. O.	Venous thrombosis	610	17	5	340,000	10	10.2	9.4
M. F.	Myocardial infarction	390	18.7	2.6		10.3		10.6
N. R.	Severe arteriosclerotic vascular disease	520	18.5	0	350,000	5.6	7.2	6.2
G. N.	Probable thrombotic thrombocytopenic purpura	920	15.4	5.2	196,000*	22		
E. C.	Meningitis	1,080	10.8		200,000	15.6	13.9	

* 78,000/µl on admission.

showed fibrin deposits in the glomeruli.   This patient has consistently had elevated FPA levels, ranging between 5 and 35 ng/ml.

In order to determine the significance of different levels of
FPA in the blood, infusions of native FPA were made into four
normal individuals.   Figure 2 shows that immediately following
infusion, approximately 75% of the infused FPA was found in the
circulating blood.   Thereafter, FPA levels declined at a rate of
equivalent to a 4 minute t 1/2.   No FPA could be found in the urine
of any of these individuals.   Studies of FPA levels were also made
immediately after infusion of heparin in six patients with evidence
of venous thrombosis and/or pulmonary embolism and in the patient
with fibrin thrombin in the glomeruli of a transplanted kidney.
Figure 3 shows that following heparin infusion, FPA levels declined rapidly at a rate equivalent to a four minute t 1/2.   From
these data, it is possible to make estimations of the rate of

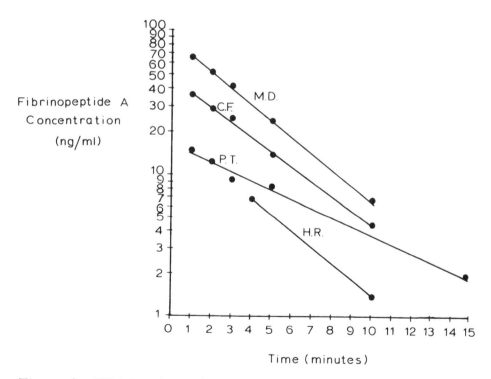

Figure 2: FPA levels in the plasma of four normal subjects
infused with fibrin clot supernate containing native FPA.

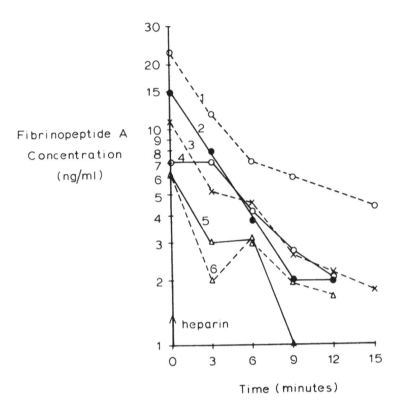

Figure 3: Plasma FPA concentrations in six patients with elevated
A peptide levels before and after infusion of heparin.

1.	O --- O	C. F.	thrombophlebitis and pulmonary embolism
2.	●———●	I. M.	pulmonary embolism
3.	X ----X	A. A.	thrombophlebitis
4.	O———O	F. T.	thrombophlebitis
5.	△———△	M. F.	pulmonary embolism
6.	△ --- △	M. B.	renal transplant and renal thrombosis.

10,000 U of heparin were given at 0 time as indicated in the figure.
The pre-heparin sample was collected 30 s before infusion of the
heparin and the assumption was made that the level had not
changed in the 30 s before the heparin infusion was made.

proteolytic change of the fibrinogen which could be responsible for the FPA levels measured. Based on the four minute t 1/2, we may estimate that a 2 ng per ml FPA level could be produced by thrombin proteolysis of 200 mg of fibrinogen per 24 hours, which would represent about 10% of the normal total fibrinogen catabolism of 2.2 g per 24 hours in a 70 kg individual. This figure is consistent with previously held views that in normal individuals, thrombin proteolysis is not a major determinant of fibrinogen catabolism (8). In patients with elevated fibrinopeptide A levels, a 10 ng per ml level could be produced by proteolysis of 1 g of fibrinogen per 24 hours. Thus far, this technique appears to be a sensitive and specific indicator of fibrinogen proteolysis, probably by thrombin, in vivo. Since levels can be measured in normal individuals, it is possible that small increases in steady state intravascular clotting may be detected with this technique. Thus far, significantly elevated levels have been observed in a number of patients with clearly evident venous thrombosis and/or pulmonary embolism. Following heparin infusion, a rapid decline of FPA level was obtained. This finding indicates that the technique may be useful to monitor the results of therapy of in vivo clotting.

ACKNOWLEDGEMENTS

This work was supported by research grants from the National Institutes of Health (Program Project Grants HL-15486 and HL-15596 and SCOR grant HL-14236 and the New York Heart Association. Dr. Nossel is the recipient of Career Development Award HL-46355.

Figures 1-3 and Tables I-III are reproduced from the Journal of Clinical Investigation 54: 43, 1974.

REFERENCES

1. Blomback, B. In: Blood Clotting Enzymology. Walter H. Seegers, editor. Academic, New York, 1967, pp. 143-215.
2. Kisker, C. T. and R. Rush. J. Clin. Invest. 50: 2235-2251, 1971.
3. Niewiarowski, S. and V. Gurewich. J. Lab. Clin. Med. 77: 665-676, 1971.

4. Fletcher, A. P. , N. Alkjaersig, J. O'Brien, and V. G.
    Tulevski. Trans. Assoc. Am. Physicians Phila. 83: 159-167,
    1970.

5. Nossel, H. L. , L. R. Younger, G. D. Wilner, T. Procupez,
    R. E. Canfield, and V. P. Butler, Jr. Proc. Nat. Sci. U. S. A.
    68: 2350-2353, 1971.

6. Nossel, H. L. , I. Yudelman, R. E. Canfield, V. P. Butler, Jr. ,
    K. Spanondis, G. D. Wilner, and G. D. Quershi. J. Clin.
    Invest. 54: 43-53, 1974.

7. Hunter, W. M. In: Handbook of Experimental Immunology.
    D. M. Weir, editor. F. A. Davis Co. , Phila. , 1971, pp. 608-
    654.

8. Hjort, P. F. and R. Hasselback. Throm. Diath. Haemorrh.
    6: 580-612, 1961.

MODIFICATIONS OF PLATELET FUNCTIONS BY DIETARY FATS

S. Renaud

INSERM, Unite 63, Lyon-Bron, France

Several epidemiologic studies have shown that coronary heart disease (CHD) was closely related to the saturated fat intake (1, 2). The dietary fats might exert their effect by changing the vessel wall morphology, i. e. , by inducing atherosclerosis but also by predisposing for arterial thrombosis, which is most of the time the final occluding event. In addition, mural thrombi can contribute to the formation of atherosclerotic plaques (3, 4).

In venous thrombosis, epidemiologic studies have also suggested that dietary fats might be a predisposing factor since this condition appears to occur only in the populations susceptible to CHD (5, 6).

In addition to Norway (7) as well as in Germany (8) a marked decrease in the incidence of pulmonary embolism as well as CHD (9) has been reported during World War II. This decrease in thrombotic episodes was related to the consumption of dietary fats (7, 8, 9). Finally, experimental studies have shown that the long chain saturated fatty acids might be the responsible factors in the dietary fats (10).

It is therefore feasible that saturated dietary fats might predispose to thrombosis through a direct effect on certain blood components. In the present report we will examine mostly the influence of dietary fats on blood platelets which in thrombosis appear to have a key role chiefly by forming aggregates, the earliest event in thrombus formation, and promoting coagulation through the so-called platelet factor 3 (PF_3 for lack of a more precise term). In addition, the study of PF_3 in connection with dietary fats appear to have a special interest since it is the only clotting factors of which the active part is a lipid.

PLATELET FACTOR 3 ACTIVITY

Whether the clot promoting activity of platelets is released as indicated by some studies (11) or is a property of the membrane surface (12), is still a matter of controversy. However what appears to be well documented is that the active moiety of this PF_3 is a phospholipid or a mixture of phospholipids of which the most active is phosphatidyl serine (PS) (13, 14, 15) followed by phosphatidyl inositol (PI) (16, 41) or phosphatidyl ethanolamine (PE) (17) depending on the experimental conditions. Of interest is that PS does not appear to be present in carefully prepared platelet-poor plasma, and that such plasma has a markedly prolonged clotting time. Intact platelets, resuspended in this plasma, will bring back the clotting time to normal (17). Therefore intact platelets present a clot promoting activity, but this activity can be markedly increased by damaging them in various ways (contact with glass, kaolin, sonication). As an example, the clotting activity of 50×10^3 totally disrupted platelets by 30 seconds sonication, has been observed (18) (Figure 1) to be more powerful than this of 1000×10^3 intact platelets.

We have also noted (18) that the total clotting activity of platelets obtained by sonication can be entirely reproduced by the total phospholipids contained in these platelets (Figure 1), provided these phospholipids are uniformly resuspended in plasma, also by sonication. Finally it seems that the activity of these total phospholipids cannot be reproduced by the fractions PS or PS + PI alone. The five main phospholipid fractions PS, PI, PE, PC and SPH have to be added to plasma to duplicate the clotting activity of the total phospholipids.

However this does not necessarily mean that ordinarily, the clot promoting activity of platelets (PF_3) is the result of the activity of the above mentioned five phospholipid fractions.

Another interesting feature of PF_3 is that it might be the

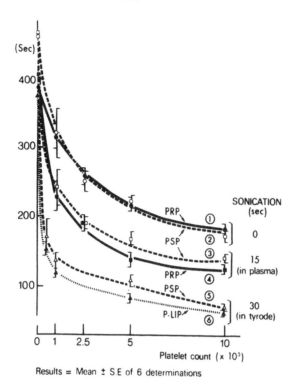

Results = Mean ± S E of 6 determinations

<u>Figure 1:</u> Recalcification clotting time in rats, showing compari-
son between the clotting activity of platelet-rich plasm (PRP) and
of washed platelets (PSP) resuspended in their platelet-poor plasm
without (O) or after having damaged platelets by sonication.

Comparison is also made between the clotting activity of
washed platelets, totally disrupted by sonication (30 sec) and the
total phospholipids (P - Lip) extracted from the same platelets
and separated by TLC.   The phospholipids were resuspended in
the platelet-poor plasma by 30 seconds sonication (Courtesy of
Thrombosis Diathesis Haemorrhagica 30: 557, 1973).

limiting factor of coagulation under normal conditions.   Although
further studies have to be conducted to clearly determine this, in
various conditions such as hyperlipemia (19) pregnancy or contraceptive treatment (20), the platelet-rich plasma clotting time
which is markedly correlated with the whole blood clotting time
(Figure 2), is also correlated with the PF_3 as determined in

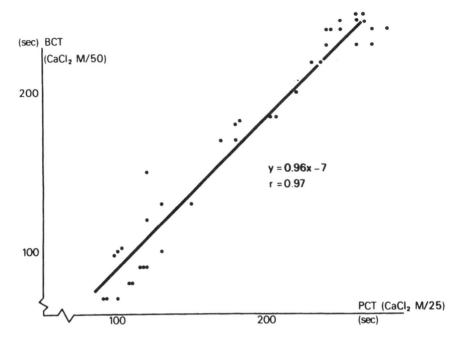

Figure 2: Correlation in normo- and hyperlipemic rats between
the whole blood (ECT) and the platelet-rich plasma (PCT) recalcification clotting time, prepared in siliconized glassware, the final
determination being performed in duplicate in plastic, as in previous studies (16, 17).

For both tests the blood was collected in siliconized syringes
containing sodium citrate (3. 8%, 1 volume for 9 volumes of blood)
and stored at 25°C. The BCT was determined as soon as possible
after the blood removal since it was not stable as is the PCT.
These determinations were performed on blood of rats fed for 10
weeks either laboratory chow or a butter rich hyperlipemic diet
as previously reported (19).

washed platelets, resuspended in a standard platelet-poor plasma.
In other terms, it seems that under these conditions, the whole
blood clotting activity is mostly dependent upon the activity of PF_3.
Since the plasmatic clotting factors are largely in excess for a
normal clotting, an increase in their activity as occuring in hyperlipemia or in contraceptive treatment, does not seem to result in

a shortening of the clotting time. By contrast, the consequence of an increase in PF_3 activity appears to be a clotting acceleration, in other terms as <u>in vitro</u> hypercoagulability.

DIETARY FATS AND PF_3 ACTIVITY

Feeding to rats for 9 to 11 weeks certain purified diets rich in fat, predispose these animals to large thrombosis. Depending on the initiating agent (endotoxin, epinephrine, ellagic acid), the thrombi are located either in hepatic veins (21), in the cardiac cavities (22) or even in the coronary arteries. This predisposition depends on the type of fat included in the diet (22). In the hours following the injection of the initiating agent, the animals fed butter or long chain saturated fatty acids, present an incidence of thrombosis close to 100% while the animals fed corn oil have no thrombosis or a very low incidence. In the butter-fed animals the platelet-rich plasma clotting time (PCT) is markedly shortened as compared to the animals fed corn oil or laboratory chow (19, 23).

By contrast, the cephalin time (CEP-CT) in which most of the platelets have been removed by slow speed centrifugation and the PF_3 activity replaced by cephalin, do not show any significant difference between the butter or the corn oil fed animals (19, 23). This indicates that even if certain plasmatic clotting factors presented an increased clotting activity, they could not be responsible for the shortened PCT. Finally when the platelets from the butter or corn oil fed animals were washed and resuspended in a standard platelet-poor plasma, a test we called platelet factor 3 clotting time (PF_3-CT), those platelets from the butter fed rats could induce a similar shortening in the clotting time to this observed with the PCT. This therefore demonstrated that the hypercoagulability observed in the butter fed rats was due to platelets. Since the lipid extract of these platelets could also reproduce the same shortening in theclotting time, we concluded that the hypercoagulability noted in butter fed animals was due to PF_3 the only clotting factor contained in the lipid extract.

In rats fed for 10 weeks a more physiological diet containing solely 29% butter or 25% corn oil and 0. 1% cholesterol, we obtained also a significant shortening of the PCT which could be also reproduced by the platelets resuspended in a standard platelet-poor plasma (16) (Figure 3).

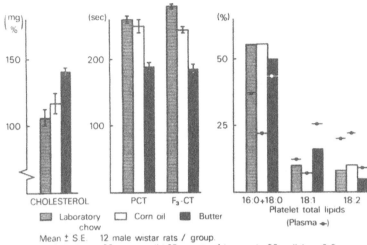

Figure 3: Influence on serum cholesterol, the recalcification
platelet-rich plasma clotting time (PCT), the platelet factor 3
clotting time (F_3-CT) and the fatty acid composition of platelet
or plasma total lipids, of various diets in rats. As shown above,
the diet was either laboratory chow (Ralston Purina Co. of Canada)
or a purified diet containing either butter 29% or corn oil (25%) +
water (4%). The serum cholesterol, PCT, F_3-CT and fatty acid
composition of platelet and plasma lipids were performed as in
our previous studies (19, 28).

In rabbits fed laboratory chow to which was simply added 0.1%
cholesterol and 10% butter alone or butter + corn oil, identical results to those noted in the rat were obtained, indicating that also in
this animal, butter could induce a hypercoagulability entirely due to
PF_3 (19).

In coronary patients who presumably have been eating a diet
rich in saturated fats, a hypercoagulability was also observed, apparently due, as in animals, to an increase in the acitivity of PF_3
(24), determined in washed platelets. As a confirmation of the
role of PF_3 in these coronary patients, the clotting time shortening
obtained with the whole platelets, could be reproduced by the total
phospholipids from these platelets, separated from the other lipids

by thin-layer chromatography (24).   Other investigators, utilizing
a different technique to evaluate PF_3, have also found an increase
in its activity, in patients with ischemic heart disease (25).

DIETARY FATS AND PLATELET LIPID CHANGES

Andreoli and Coll (26) have shown that rapid changes in the
platelet fatty acid pattern can be induced by incubating various
fatty acids with platelets in vitro.   In human subjects Nordoy and
Rodset (27) have reported that a dietary change with more unsaturated fatty acids, will be subsequently reflected in the platelets.
These investigators did not observe any change in the platelet
cholesterol or phospholipids level, but an increase in the linoleic
acid content of various platelet phospholipids at the expense of
palmitic and oleic acids (27).   The change in the platelet fatty acid
composition was also associated with a decrease in the PF_3 activity.

Under our conditions, in rats fed butter as compared to corn
oil, we have observed drastic changes in the fatty acid composition
of plasma and platelets total lipids (28).   The most striking result
in the butter fed animals, was an increase in oleic acid in both
plasma and platelets, at the expense of the polyunsaturated fatty
acids (28).

Even in rats fed diets not containing cholic acid, it is chiefly
an increase in oleic acid at the expense of linoleic acid, which we
obtained in the group fed butter (Figure 3).

As already mentioned, the butter fed animals presented a
hypercoagulability apparently due to an increase in PF_3 activity
(Figure 3).

In subsequent studies rats (29) and rabbits (30) were fed 5
different fats (cocao butter, butter, coconut oil, olive oil and corn
oil), the platelet phospholipids separated by thin-layer chromatography in two dimensions and the clotting activity of the PS + PI
fractions compared to the PCT and to the quantitative and qualitative changes observed in these fractions.   In both rats and rabbits,
there was no significant quantitative difference in the PS + PI
fractions, between the groups fed the various fats.

By contrast, we noted an increase, mostly in oleic acid but also in stearic acid at the expense of the polyunsaturated fatty acids in the PS + PI fractions of the animals fed the most thrombogenic fats. This change in the fatty acid composition of the phospholipids studied was correlated with their clotting activity and the platelet-rich plasma clotting time (PCT). In rat, it was also correlated with the severity of thrombosis initiated by an endotoxin injection (29).

In the platelet PS of human subjects from Cincinnati, eating the typical American food, rich in saturated fats, Iacono and Coll (31) found a higher level of stearic and oleic acids than in the platelets of subjects from Milan or Sicily, of which the diet contains more unsaturated fatty acids. In patients with a recent myocardial infarction, we found (28) that the total platelet lipids, as compared to normal men having no risk factor for CHD, presented an increase in palmitic, stearic and oleic acid at the expense of the polyunsaturated fatty acids.

In addition, it has been shown, at least in the plasma phospholipids, that by increasing the polyunsaturated fatty acids in the diet for six months, this change resulted in a decrease in the content mostly, of oleic acid, and an increase in this of linoleic acid (32).

As far as the PF_3 activity is concerned, it seems that in the phospholipids, an increase in the content of oleic acid at the expense of the polyunsaturated, might be the change able to induce the most drastic increase in this PF_3 activity. These results are also concordant with in vitro work on synthetic phospholipids in which only dioleyl phospholipids presented clotting activity (33, 34). Utilizing phosphatidyl choline commercially available, we found that the most active was the dioleyl followed by the distearoleyl, with the least active being the dipalmitoyl (16).

DIETARY FATS AND PLATELET AGGREGATION

In our studies with rats fed hyperlipemia diets, we found a highly significant increase in the susceptibility of platelet to thrombin-induced aggregation, in the animals fed the most thrombogenic fats (22, 35). In rabbits fed butter, as compared to corn oil, a similar result was obtained (19).

In rats fed a more physiologic diet, Hornstra did not find any significant difference in the susceptibility of platelets to aggregation as evaluated by the turbidimetric method. However, with the filter-loop technique, this investigator found an association between thrombotic tendency induced by the fats fed and the susceptibility to aggregation (36).

In man, numerous studies (37, 38, for citing only a few) indicate that in occlusive arterial disease, therefore presumably in subjects having eaten saturated fats, there is an increase in the susceptibility of platelets to aggregation by ADP. We have found that it was mostly to thrombin (24) as in hyperlipemic animals, that the platelets were the most susceptible, particularly in patients with severe stenotic lesions (24).

The mechanisms by which dietary fats affect the susceptibility of platelets to aggregation appear largely unknown. Changes in the fatty acid composition of platelet phospholipids might be involved in this susceptibility, since these phospholipids play a prominent structural role in platelet membranes. However prostaglandin synthesis in the platelet as well as the influence of plasma lysolecithin which have been shown recently to affect markedly platelet aggregation (39, 40), might be involved in the effect of dietary fats on platelet behaviour.

CONCLUSIONS

From the studies reported here, it could be concluded that:

- Dietary saturated fats appear to predispose man to thrombosis, a result which can be reproduced in experimental animals.

- The dietary fats might predispose to thrombosis at least in part through blood platelets by increasing
  a) their susceptibility to platelet aggregation,
  b) their clot promoting activity, so-called platelet factor 3 (PF_3).

- The lipid moiety of PF_3 (the only clotting factor of which the active part is a lipid) is probably a mixture of phospholipids of which the most active is the phosphatidyl serine.

- The saturated dietary fats might induce an <u>in vitro</u> hyper-coagulability mostly through an increase in PF_3 activity.

- The increase in the activity of PF_3 does not result from a change in the concentration but rather in the fatty acid pattern, of the platelet phospholipids, namely, an increase in stearic and mostly oleic acid, at the expense of the polyunsaturated fatty acids.

- Human subjects presenting coronary heart disease (CHD) as well as populations prone to CHD, eating saturated fats, exhibit an increase in stearic and oleic acid in the platelet lipids or phospholipids.

ACKNOWLEDGEMENTS

The author would like to gratefully acknowledge the financial support of the INSERM organization and the "Fondation pour la Recherche Medicale."

REFERENCES

1. Stamler, J. : Med. Clin. 57: 5, 1973.
2. Stormorken, H. : In "Dietary Fats and Thrombosis". Haemostasis 2: 1, 1973/74.
3. Duguid, J. B. : J. Path. Bact. 60: 57, 1948.
4. Haust, M. D. , More, R. H. and Movat, H. Z. : Amer. J. Path. 35: 265, 1969.
5. Thomas, W. A. , Davies, J. N. P. , O'Neal, R. M. and Dimakulangan, A. A. : Amer. J. Cardiol. 5: 41, 1960.
6. Gore, I. , Hirst, A. E. and Tanaka, K. : Arch. Int. Med. 113: 323, 1964.
7. Jensen, R. A. : Acta Med. Scand. 103: 263, 1952.
8. Hamperl, H. : Klin. Wschr. 247, 1965.
9. Strom, A. and Jensen, R. A. Lancet 1: 126, 1951.
10. Renaud, S. : Thromb. Res. 4 (suppl. 1): 25, 1974.
11. Webber, A. J. and Johnson, S. A. : Amer. J. Pathol. 60: 19, 1970.
12. Marcus, A. J. and Zucker-Franklin, D. J. : Amer. Oil. Chem. Soc. 42: 500, 1965.

13. Troup, S. B. , Reed, C. F. , Marinetti, G. V. , and Swisher, S. N. : J. Clin. Invest. 39: 342, 1960.
14. Marcus, A. J. , Ullman, H. L. , Safier, L. B. and Ballard, H. S. : J. Clin. Invest. 41: 2198, 1962.
15. Woodside, E. E. , Therriault, D. G. and Kocholaty, W. : Blood 24: 76, 1964.
16. Renaud, S. and Gautheron, P. : Haemostasis 2: 53, 1973/74.
17. Gautheron, P. , Dumont, E. and Renaud, S.: Thromb. Diath. Haemorrh. , in press.
18. Renaud, S. , Gautheron, P. and Rosenstein, H. : Thromb. Diath. Haemorrh. 30: 557, 1973.
19. Renaud, S. and Lecompte, F. Circulation Res. 27: 1003, 1970.
20. Lecompte, F. and Renaud, S. : Thromb. Diath. Haemorrh. 29:510, 1973.
21. Renaud, S. : Lab. Invest. 14:424, 1965.
22. Renaud, S. and Godu, J. : Lab. Invest. 21: 512, 1969.
23. Renaud, S.: Thromb. Diath. Haemorrh. 30 (Suppl. 56): 11, 1973.
24. Renaud, S. , Gautheron, P. , Arbogast, R. and Dumont, E. : Scand. J. Haematol. 12: 85, 1973.
25. Nordoy, A. and Rodset, J. M. : Acta. Med. Scand. 188: 133, 1970.
26. Andreoli, V. M. , Maffei, F. and Thonon, G. C.: Haemostasis 2: 118, 1973/74.
27. Nordoy, A. and Rodset, J. M. : Acta Med. Scand. 190: 27, 1971.
28. Renaud, S. , Kuba, K. , Goulet, C. , Lemire, Y. and Allard, C.: Circulat. Res. 26: 552, 1970.
29. Gautheron, P. and Renaud, S. : Thromb. Res. 1: 353, 1972.
30. Renaud, S. and Gautheron, P.: Atherosclerosis, in press.
31. Iacono, J. M. , Zellner, D. C. , Paoletti, R. , Ishikawa, T. , Frigeni, V. and Fumagalli, R. : Haemostasis 2: 141, 1973/74.
32. Wilson, W. S. , Hulley, S. B. , Burrows, M. I. and Nichaman, M. Z. : Amer. J. Med. 51: 491, 1971.
33. Hecht, E. R.: In "Lipids in Blood Clotting", Thomas, Springfield, p. 81, 1965.
34. O'Brien, J. R. : Brit. J. Exper. Path. 38: 529, 1957.
35. Renaud, S. , Kinlough, R. L. , and Mustard, J. F. : Lab. Invest. 22: 339, 1970.
36. Hornstra, G. : Haemostasis 2: 21, 1973/74.
37. Dreyfus, F. and Zahavi, J. : Atherosclerosis 17: 107, 1973.

38. O'Brien, J. R., Heywood, J. B. and Heady, J. A. : Thromb. Diath. Haemorrh. 16: 752, 1966.

39. Smith, B. J., Ingerman, C., Kocsis, Y. J. and Silver, M. J. : Thromb. Res. 4 (Suppl. 1): 49, 1974.

40. Gillet, M. P. T. and Besterman, E. M. M. : Thromb. Res. 4 (Suppl. 1): 85, 1974.

41. Zolton, R. P. and Seegers, W. H. : Thromb. Res. 4: 437, 1974.

Risk Factors Other Than Diet

DIABETES AS A RISK FACTOR FOR ARTERIOSCLEROTIC VASCULAR DISEASE

Margaret J. Albrink, M. D.

West Virginia University School of Medicine, Department of Medicine, Morgantown, West Virginia

The well known association between diabetes and arteriosclerotic cardiovascular disease (ASHD) suggests that impaired glucose tolerance is a major risk factor for ASHD. The association can be seen from the point of view of the diabetic, who has increased vascular disease when compared to non-diabetics, or from the point of view of the patient with ASHD, who has increased frequency of diabetes when compared with persons without vascular disease.

ASHD is the commonest cause of death of diabetics in the U.S., accoutning for more than half of all deaths in diabetics.

At the Joslin Clinic, which has the largest experience of any one center with diabetes, the death rate from ASHD for diabetics has been increasing over the past decades, just as it has for non-diabetics (1, 2). In 1960-66, 53% of their diabetics died of ASHD, about twice that of the average population.

A number of autopsy studies have also shown that diabetics suffer about twice as much ASHD as non-diabetics. A possible bias exists in these clinical and autopsy studies since they were drawn from selected populations. However, the same trend of increased death from ASHD is seen in unbiased population studies. The Framingham study has followed a defined population sample of over 5000 men and women between ages of 30 and 62 at entry. Persons identified as diabetic at the time of entry or during the

study have suffered nearly three times as many cardiovascular
deaths as expected in non-diabetics of the same age and sex (3).
Coronary artery disease was the most common manifestation of
the vascular disease but peripheral vascular disease was also
prominent.

Another population study, that of Tecumseh, Michigan, found
a high prevalence of coronary artery disease, about 50 per cent,
in diabetics (4). In this study the interrelation between diabetes
and ASHD was also examined from the point of view of the patient
with coronary heart disease. Of persons in the population identified as having coronary heart disease nearly half had hyperglycemia, significantly more than age and sex-matched persons (4).
A number of other studies have reported similar findings, about
50 per cent of patients with ASHD having impaired glucose tolerance.

Age is a factor in susceptibility of diabetics to ASHD. According to the Joslin Clinic, nearly half (42%) of diabetics under
age 20 die of the renal complications. Over age 20, however,
ASHD becomes more prominent. In the UGDP study of mild adult
onset diabetics of less than one year's duration 85% of the deaths
were from cardiovascular disease (5). The immunity of women
from ASHD does not appear to be enjoyed by diabetic women.
The Framingham study if any thing suggested increased risk to
women with diabetes, particularly women taking insulin (3).

The duration of diabetes appears to increase the risk of ASHD.
The Joslin Clinic charted the mortality experience of a cohort
aged 0 to 20 years at onset. The relative mortality increased
with each decade of duration of diabetes, a reflection chiefly of
ASHD death (2).

A correlation between severity of diabetes, or blood sugar
level, and susceptibility to ASHD, has been difficult to demonstrate. In the population of patients with coronary artery disease
the diabetes is often of mild degree. The Framingham study
showed increasing rate of ASHD with increasing blood sugar within the normal range. Table I shows for example the cumulative
experience for Framingham males aged 55-64 (6). The incidence
of coronary heart disease increased with increase in casual blood
sugar concentration. Similar information for the diabetic range
of blood sugars is not available.

Table I

Average annual incidence rate for coronary heart
disease per 10,000 persons at risk. Adapted from
Framingham Study, 18 year follow-up. (6)
Men, aged 55-64

Casual blood glucose	man-years	smoothed rate/10,000
29-69	1752	196
70-89	5154	199
90-109	1614	209
110-129	390	218
130-524	322	229
All	9232	203

The association between diabetes and ASHD is thus well established. The question must be asked whether the impaired glucose
tolerance is the risk factor or whether the risk is incurred from
some factor associated with diabetes. The Framingham Study
showed that diabetes was a risk factor independent of blood pressure, smoking, relative weight, age and sex (3). A number of
studies, however, suggest that related factors may also be of
importance. The absence of ASHD in diabetics in less industrialized parts of the world suggests that environmental factors such
as diet rather than diabetes per se are responsible for the increased
ASHD in affluent diabetics.

A cluster of related metabolic abnormalities is associated
with coronary artery disease. Mild diabetes, hypertriglyceridemia,
usually of Fredrickson's type IV, insulin resistance and hyperinsulinism are common in patients with ASHD. The obesity is
usually of the adult onset type (7) associated with large adipose
cells which are insensitive to insulin. Because of the occurence
together of these abnormalities it is difficult to assign an individual role to impaired glucose tolerance.

The association between impaired glucose tolerance and serum
triglycerides has been shown in a number of studies. Fasting blood
sugar rises slightly but definitely with increasing plasma triglyceride concentration (7), and indeed hypertriglyceridemia may signify
some degree of impaired glucose tolerance. The association
between impaired glucose tolerance and elevation of plasma triglyceride concentration was also shown in the Tecumseh Study (8).

Persons with coronary heart disease and impaired glucose tolerance showed significantly higher triglycerides than persons with
coronary heart disease and normal glucose tolerance or without
coronary disease regardless of glucose tolerance.

The Framingham Study showed that for the diabetic, hypertriglyceridemia (as very low density lipoproteins, VLDL) was
higher in diabetics than non-diabetics, perhaps accounting for
the greater incidence of ASHD in the diabetics (3). Hypertriglyceridemia, not cholesterol, is thus the hyperlipidemia most
characteristic of the diabetic and many contribute substantially
to the risk of ASHD.

Diabetics as a rule have lower insulin levels than normal
persons, particularly after a glucose meal. A subgroup of diabetics, particularly obese diabetics, has increased rather than
decreased insulin concentrations. In these instances the impairment of glucose tolerance is manifest as insulin resistance with
only slightly impaired glucose tolerance. Such insulin resistance
and hyperinsulinism is commonly associated with hypertriglyceridemia. Hyperinsulinism has also been associated with ASHD in
several studies. In our laboratory a group of middle aged persons
with ASHD were compared with a group without known vascular
disease. Both plasma insulin and glucose were higher in the group
with vascular disease (Figure 1). The impaired glucose tolerance
in the ASHD group is thus of the hyperinsulinemic type.

Hypertension is another risk factor associated with diabetes
and some authors think that the hypertension accounts for the
greater death rate from ASHD. Pell, studying an industrial
group, showed that the increased ASHD of diabetics could be attributed to associated hypertension. The rate of ASHD of non-
hypertensive diabetics was lower than that of hypertensive diabetics and was not significantly greater than for non-diabetics (9).

The relationship between diabetes and ASHD suggests that
treatment of diabetes might be an important part of the treatment
and prevention of ASHD, and that treatment of hyperlipidemia
might improve the outlook of diabetics. There are a few data to
support or refute this supposition. Diabetics have almost universally been excluded from studies of the effect of dietary or
pharmacologic treatment of hyperlipidemia on ASHD.

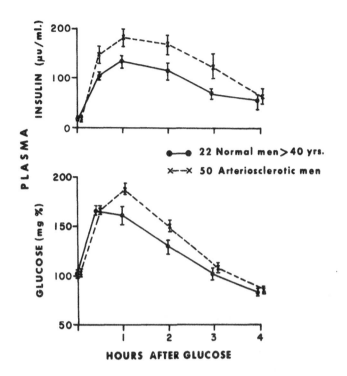

Figure 1: Plasma glucose and insulin concentrations of normal
men and persons with ASHD before and after ingestion of a solution of 100 grams glucose.   (Albrink, M. J. , unpublished observations.)

The effect of treatment of diabetes on the large vessel complications is also unclear.   The UGDP study showed no beneficial
effect of lowering of blood sugar on the vascular complications
of mild maturity diabetics (5).   Thus, patients receiving optimal
treatment with insulin (IVAR) did indeed show lower blood sugars
than patients treated by diet alone (placebo group) over a six year
period.   However, the mortality of the IVAR group was similar
to that of the placebo group.   The maintenance of lower blood sugar
in the IVAR group was thus not associated with decreased mortality
from cardiovascular causes during the time this particular group
of patients was under way.

The association between diabetes and ASHD is thus unexplained.
Hypertriglyceridemia, hyperinsulinemia and hypertension may
play a role.   Clinical trials aimed at investigating the effect of diet
and drugs on hyperlipidemia in diabetes are badly needed and should

yield information of importance not only for diabetics but for the coronary-prone western world.

SUMMARY

Clinical and population studies have uniformly shown a greater incidence of arteriosclerotic vascular disease (ASCVD) in diabetics than in non-diabetics, and increased incidence of impaired glucose tolerance in patients with ASCVD than without it. Of persons with existing ASCVD nearly half have impaired glucose tolerance. Amongst diabetics, ASCVD is the commonest cause of death. The relationship of ASCVD to duration and severity of diabetics is not clear.

The diabetes associated with ASCVD is associated with a cluster of metabolic abnormalities including mild obesity of the adult onset type with insulin resistance of the peripheral tissues, with hyperinsulinemia and hypertriglyceridemia. Diabetes is also associated with hypertension. The increased ASCVD could be caused in part by one or more of these associated factors, all of which carry risk of ASCVD. In addition, the impaired glucose tolerance itself may contribute in some unknown way.

ACKNOWLEDGEMENT

This work was supported, in part, by NIH grant 5 RO1 AM 09252 and a Research Career Award 5 KO6 HL00486.

REFERENCES

1. Bradley, R. F. : Cardiovascular disease. In Joslin's Diabetes Mellitus, Eleventh Edition, Editors Marble, A. , White, P. , Bradley, R. F. , and Krall, L. P. Lea and Febiger, Philadelphia, 1971, pp. 417-477.
2. Kessler, I. I. : Mortality experience in diabetic persons. A twenty-six year follow-up study. Amer. J. Med. 51: 715-24, 1971.
3. Garcia, M. J. , McNamara, P. M. , Gordon, T. , and Kannel, W. B. : Morbidity and mortality in diabetics in the Framingham population. Sixteen-year follow-up study. Diabetes 23: 105-111, 1974.
4. Ostrander, L. D. , Jr. , Francis, T. , Jr. , Hayner, N. S. , Kjelsberg, M. O. , and Epstein, F. H. : The relationship of

cardiovascular disease to hyperglycemia.   Annals Int. Med.
62: 1188-98, 1965.

5.   The University Groups Diabetes Program.   A study of the
     effects of hyperglycemic agents on vascular complications
     in patients with adult-onset diabetes.   Part II.   Mortality
     results.   Diabetes 19: supp. 2. , 787-830, 1970.

6.   The Framingham Study.   An epidemiological investigation
     of cardiovascular disease.   Section 30.   Some characteristics
     related to the incidence of cardiovascular disease and death;
     Framingham Study, 18-year follow-up.   Editors, Kannel,
     W. B. , and Gordon, T.   DHEW Publication No. (NIH) 74-599.

7.   Albrink, M. J. and Meigs, J. W. :   Interrelationship between
     skinfold thickness, serum lipids and blood sugar in normal
     men.   Amer. J. Clin. Nutr. 15: 255-261, 1964.

8.   Ostrander, L. D. , Jr. , Neff, B. J. , Block, W. D. , Francis,
     T. , Jr. , and Epstein, F. H. : Hyperglycemia and hypertri-
     glyceridemia among persons with coronary heart disease.
     Annals Int. Med. 67: 34-41, 1967.

9.   Pell, S. : The identification of risk factors in employed
     populations.   Trans. N. Y. Acad. Sci. 36: 341-56, 1964.

HYPERTENSION AND OTHER RISK FACTORS

Quentin B. Deming

Albert Einstein College of Medicine of Yeshiva
University, Bronx, New York

My assignment is to discuss factors which increase the rate
of atherogenesis and which, thereby, increase the frequency of
infarctions in heart, brain or elsewhere.

The correlation between blood pressure and the rate of occurrence of these morbid events is so well established by many beautiful studies that it cannot usefully be questioned.

The Build and Blood Pressure Study reported in 1959 by Lew
(1) for the Society of Acturies analyzed data on 4 million lives and
102,000 deaths. It established that life expectancy in both sexes,
at all ages varies inversely with arterial blood pressure.

Similar data from Framingham, Albany, Chicago and other
places have established that this relationship is continuous at all
blood pressure levels. It is extremely close for cardiac infarction
but it is even closer for cerebral infarction.

Gubner showed from the Build and Blood Pressure data that a
very modes elevation of blood pressure to 148-177/93-102 increased
the probability of a man sustaining a cardiac infarct before the age
of 40, 3.6 x. But it increased his probability of having a stroke
15 x. These analyses did not include consideration of cholesterol.

Kannel, in his analysis of 14 years of follow-up of the Framingham population considered that "serum cholesterol plays an

important role under age 50 in discriminating coronary heart disease for women and up to age 62 for men. "

But he stressed "The dominant feature is the role of systolic blood pressure in all the various cardiovascular outcomes. "

And he added that for brain infarction or for CHD in older women "one would generally do nearly as well in discrimination, relying on systolic blood pressure alone, as one can when all three measurements are used" meaning cholesterol and weight as well.

As early as 1941, Clawson had shown that 77% of all deaths classified at autopsy as due to coronary sclerosis were associated with hypertension (25). The correlation was better with women than with men.

Similar series are now legion.

The evidence is absolute. The frequency of cardiac infarction correlates with blood pressure. The frequency of stroke correlates with blood pressure and in both instances the correlation is closer than with any other "risk factor" except one - age.

It is necessary to correct for the effect of blood pressure when evaluating the role of any other "risk factor".

For instance, the Framingham study at 14 years (2) showed that a 55 year old man with a cholesterol of 280 had no more risk of coronary heart disease than one with a cholesterol of 190 if the first had a systolic of 110 and the second had a systolic of 160 (a blood pressure many doctors would still call normal at 50).

Despite the absolute nature of the data relating blood pressure to these events, the theoretical and the clinical problems remain complex.

The Veteran's Administration study, reported by Freis (3), has established that pharmacologic control of diastolic blood pressures above 90 in males does result in decreased frequency of some morbid events. It has not established that the incidence of cardiac infarction is affected and of course it has established nothing about women. Easy extrapolation of the results to these groups is made

unacceptable by available experimental work. I will deal with the
sex difference later. Here I will only recall that a number of experimental studies, like those of Pick and Katz (26) have demonstrated that the response of coronary arteries need not be identical to that of cerebrals or aorta. I like to think this difference
may be explicable by the differences in hemodynamic stresses to
which the vessels are exposed. The coronary arteries are unique
in having no flow during systole and in being supported from the
outside by the myocardium for much of their lengths. Whether
this adequately explains the difference in response to estrogens
is not clear. But it does amount to a difference in degree of exposure of the two vessels to the stress of increased blood pressure.

The complexity of the relationship between blood pressure and
the various other risk factors: age, sex, cholesterol, smoking,
diabetes; is very great. In addition to correlating with atherosclerosis, many of them correlate with each other.

The correlated events we were referring to are infarctions.
Infarction is not dependent exclusively on atherosclerosis. The
precipitating events of infarction, hemorrhage and thrombosis,
may be influenced or triggered by factors distinct from atherogenesis. However, the distinction can also be overstressed. The
events do not occur without a damaged vessel wall.

1. Thrombosis. There may or may not be such a thing as
a hyperthrombotic state, in man. It has been shown in rats and
indeed it correlates with serum cholesterol concentration and so
perhaps with blood pressure, but in man it is still an inference-
perhaps affected by smoking, perhaps affected by estrogens, but
probably unimportant unless there is pre-existing vascular damage
on which it can localize.

2. Hemmorrhage, is of course made more likely at a time
when arterial pressure is particularly high, but even so, it always
occurs where a vessel is damaged.

Pickering has emphasized the importance of Charcot-Bouchard
aneurisms in the small vessels of the brain as a source of hemorrhagic stroke. They result from hypertension. He considers
them distinct from atherosclerosis. It is conventional to think of
the changes in small vessels, like this, as different in kind from
the changes in large vessels, which we call atherosclerosis. The

small vessel starts with a different anatomy, characterized by more muscle and less collagen and elastin. The fact that the final appearance of the damaged vessel is different does not prove that the initiating pathogenesis was not the same.

Both hemorrhage and thrombosis occur where the vessel is damaged. Our principal concern therefore must still be the process of modification and degeneration of the vascular wall itself.

Whether we consider morbid events or atherosclerosis, the best of all ocrrelates is age. This correlation is so good that only 30 years ago atherosclerosis was considered by many to be part of the aging process. A graph (4) from the U.S. National Health Survey shows the very steep rise in incidence of cardiac infarction with age. It also shows the familar and dramatic difference in incidence between the sexes and the break in the female curve near the edge of menopause.

One problem in interpreting the effect of age is that one could show a fair degree of correlation between age and most of the discreet "risk factors".

Average blood pressure of a population rises with age.

Average cholesterol of a population rises with age.

The incidence of diabetes, even the incidence of smoking, rise with age.

My own preference is to look at age as no more than the cumulative sum of a group of time dependent variables. However, as I will show, some of these variables are dependent on each other.

Could, for instance, some of the apparent correlation between serum cholesterol and atherosclerosis result from separate dependencies of both atherosclerosis and serum cholesterol on blood pressure?

Both dependencies do exist.

In rats, raising the blood pressure by any means (hormonal, renal, vascular, or simply salt feeding, raises the serum cholesterol and even increases the amount of cholesterol in the liver and in the whole animal (5).

A colony of inbred caged rats on a fixed regimen is ideal for demonstration of an effect of one variable on another. A demonstration in man of dependence of serum cholesterol on blood pressure - though often suggested - has never been clearly made.

It has however been shown (6) that lowering blood pressure of hypertensives with a variety of agents does result in a fall in their serum cholesterols. An interdependence probably does exist.

An interesting relationship can be observed in rats between blood pressure, diet and serum cholesterol. Rat strains vary in the lability of their serum cholesterol concentration. In the most responsive ones - cholesterol rises with systolic blood pressure while the animal is on a normal diet and has a low serum cholesterol concentration but a high cholesterol intake results in very high serum cholesterols regardless of blood pressure and the relation to blood pressure is obscured. In the least responsive strains neither blood pressure nor diet alone has much effect but if the animal is on a high cholesterol intake the serum concentration rises fast with rising blood pressure.

For each strain there is some combination of diet and blood pressure that reveals the dependence of serum cholesterol on both factors and some conditions that make the animal appear unresponsive to one or the other.

Other effects of blood pressure on cholesterol metabolism have been shown. At least to the extent that incorporation of labelled acetate is a measure of synthesis, hypertensive rats synthesize cholesterol more rapidly than do normotensive rats (7). This is true in vivo, in both the liver and the aorta. But what I find most intriguing about this is that this is true in vitro. That is, aortas or livers removed from rats which were hypertensive, synthesize cholesterol more rapidly than do livers or aortas removed from normotensive rats. The difference in cholesterol metabolism then in not a direct result of pressure but is a result of a change in the tissue which had been previously brought about by pressure. These changes are not small, they are big, 10-100 fold.

One interpretation of these facts might be that the same factors which affect arterial wall also affect serum cholesterol independently. While we may eventually find a causal sequence, present data suggest that: blood pressure affects arterial wall and appears to affect serum cholesterol independently; age affects arterial wall and appears to affect serum cholesterol independently.

At any rate - despite the clear demonstration that hypertension can increase serum cholesterol there are multiple reasons for believing this is not the principal mechanism for its effects on arterial wall or atherogenesis.

While we know that abnormal elevation of serum cholesterol in many species does facilitate atherogenesis, in both rat and man it has been clearly shown that the amount of cholesterol in arterial wall is rather independent of serum cholesterol and is correlated with blood pressure.

Marie Daly has compared the concentration of cholesterol in the aortic walls of normotensive and hypertensive rats on low cholesterol and high cholesterol diets (8).

Within the 14 weeks of this experiment, the atherogenic diet increased the serum cholesterol of normotensive animals from 82 to 1257 mg% but the aortic cholesterol did not change (35 μg/mg N_2 in the first group and 31 in the second). Hypertension did increase the aortic cholesterol to 46 though it raised the serum cholesterol only slightly (to 135). However, in the presence of the changes in the aorta wall induced by hypertension, diet and its attendant hypercholesterolemia (1206 mg%) had a profound effect on aortic cholesterol, raising it to 67 μg/mg N_2.

These data seem quite consistent with the extraordinary studies of Paterson and colleagues (9). In 1960, they reported measurements of the lipid extractable from the cerebral and coronary arteries of patients on whom measurements of blood pressure and of serum cholesterol had been available during life.

Except when serum cholesterol was above 300 mg% they found no suggestion of a correlated increase in atherosclerosis. In fact they found no more lipid in the arteries of patients with serum cholesterol between 250 and 299 than they did in the arteries of those with serum levels between 150 and 199.

On the other hand, there was a clear correlation between arterial wall lipid at autopsy and blood pressure during life.

These observations certainly suggest that the effect of blood pressure on atherogenesis is not dependent on any effect blood pressure may have on serum cholesterol.

Even more obvious evidence is derived from the local nature of lesions. The concentration of cholesterol in the serum (whether induced by blood pressure, diet or genes) is identical at all sites in the vascular system but the lesions are localized where pressure and turbulence are maximal and where external support to the vessel is minimal. And they are in the high pressure greater circuit, not in the low pressure lesser circuit.

One could argue that these are structurally vulnerable sites for some reason other than exposure to mechanical stress but this argument is negated by: appearance of lesions in large or small vessels distal to a renal artery stenosis, though they are present on the non-stenosed side; and particularly the argument is made untenable by experiments with parabiotically twinned rats.

It is possible to establish pairs, the members of which differ in blood pressure but in which the cross circulation keeps the serum cholesterol equal. A clip on its left renal artery has established hypertension in one animal. The cross circulation kept cholesterol equal in the two, but an infarct occurs in the myocardium of the hypertensive animal.

Extensive aneurism formation is seen in the mesentery of a hypertensive (this is common in severe hypertension in rats) but not in the mesentery of his equally hypercholesterolemic but normotensive mate. Yellow cholesterol deposits accumulate in the damaged vessels, not in the undamaged vessels of the mate. In these twin pairs, although the concentration of cholesterol in the serum is the same, the concentration of cholesterol in aorta wall is grossly different. When atherosclerosis develops, that too is asymmetrical.

On analysis of data from 13 such pairs, it was found that the hypertensive animal showed more extensive atherosclerosis than the normotensive animal in 12 or 13 instances. The probability that this would occur by chance is less than 1%. Therefore the effect of blood pressure on atherogenesis is not dependent on the effect of blood pressure on serum cholesterol.

Brunner and Laragh (10) have interpreted their clinical data to suggest that renin, or angiotensin, may be vasculotoxic and may account for damage to the vessel wall directly, while incidentally being pressor and so producing an apparent correlation. They suggest that hypertension with high renin is accompanied by atherosclerosis and its sequellae and hypertension with low renin is not.

The parabiotic twin pairs exchange blood volumes one or two times per hour. The half life of renin in the rat is about 30 minutes, so the renin concentration of these animals should have been at least partly equallized, yet the lesions were unequal, which of course they should be if the atherosclerosis is pressure invoked rather than renin invoked.

A more certain way of investigating this would be to produce hypertension by methods having different effects on renin and aldosterone. We have done this.

    1. Hypertension by renal artery stenosis = renin ↑ angiotensin ↑ mineralocorticoid ↑
    2. Hypertension produced by DCA and NaCl = renin ↓ angiotensin ↓ mineralocorticoid ↑
    3. Hypertension produced by NaCl alone = renin ↓ angiotensin ↓ mineralocorticoid ↓
    4. Hypertension by renal artery stenosis and nephrectomy = renin ↓ angiotensin ↓ mineralocorticoid ↓

All of these forms of hypertension produce an increase in the rate of dietary atherogenesis.

The evidence then suggests that there is some direct effect of pressure on the vessel wall which produces an alteration in its anatomy or physiology which can persist in the absence of the pressure.

This takes us back to the effects of aging on the vessel wall.

In 1938 Karsner (12) pointed out the dramatic effect of elevation of blood pressure on the thickness of aortic media. We presented a graph showing that the thickness of aortic media of normotensives increases with age but that the media of hypertensives in the second decade has already achieved dimensions that the normotensive would not reach until the 5th or the 6th decade.

Karsner concluded, "The changes in the younger hypertensives represent precocious senile alterations."

I think he had it backwards. It is not an explanation of hypertension to call it accelerated again and then ask what aging is. Rather I think he has shown us that the changes we have associated with aging are no such thing. They are the effects of response to tangential tension (to muscle stretching). They are the product of stretch and time. The less the stretch stimulus the slower the response. It is probable that the range of atherosclerotic involvement is elderly "normotensives" may in fact parallel the range of blood pressures within what we accept as normal.

Wolinsky has extended this parallel between hypertension and aging and compared the effects of each on a number of attributes of arterial wall.

In addition to an increase in diameter (with concomittant increase in tangential stress and decrease in distensibility) both are accompanied by increases in collagen, elastin, mucopolysaccharides, oxygen consumption and oxydative enzymes, atheroma of course, and - most important for our discussion today - smooth muscle. (In fact, I will indicate that the increase in smooth muscle accounts for all the others.)

Injury and degeneration of arterial wall from any cause may initiate atherosclerosis. We are looking for reasons why a normal stimulus (pressure) should initiate degeneration. A number of years ago, Dr. Marie Daly, having been struck by the medial hypertrophy produced by hypertension and having demonstrated a marked increase in oxygen consumption by these thickened vessels, suggested that simultaneously increasing the demand for oxygen and the distance oxygen had to diffuse might lead to hypoxia and necrosis in the deeper areas.

Damaged or necrotic muscle cells are characteristic of hypotensive damage of small vessels and Wolinsky (13) and Curreri (14) have shown increased lysosome concentrations in hypertensive and atherosclerotic artery walls.

Daly's suggestion then was very simple - it was that smooth muscle hypertrophy itself might be the crucial factor in vascular degeneration and atherosclerosis.

To test this hypothesis we sought a way to stimulate hyper-trophy of medial smooth muscle without raising intralaminal blood pressure. We reasoned that if the collagen and elastin structure of the arteries was weakened the smooth muscle cells would carry a larger proportion of the normal blood pressure load and should hypertrophy.

Our rats treated from weaning with the lathyrogen, β amino propionitrile showed fractured elastic lamellae in the aorta. The severe manifestation of such treatment is development of actual aneurisms of aortic arch.

When such animals and control animals are maintained on an atherogenic diet the animals with weakened elastin and, therefore, presumably hypertrophied medial smooth muscle show markedly accelerated atherogenesis.

With one exception - the least severely involved lathyritic animal showed more atheroma than did the most severely involved control.

The distribution of lesions is also consistent with the hypo-thesis that muscle hypertrophy is primary. The atherosclerosis in hypertensive animals is most severe peripherally, where there is a higher proportion of muscle and less fibrous protein to share the load. The atherosclerosis in the lathyritic rats is most severe proximally where the usually large amount of fibrous protein is now weakened and the normal pressure must be sustained by originally scanty muscle.

In the last few years a great deal has been learned about the smooth muscle cells of artery wall. Wolinsky (15) has reviewed this beautifully. This cell is the principal cell of the artery and serves multiple functions. It is capable of contraction. It secretes the extracellular proteins - collagen, elastin and mucopolysaccha-rides as well as cholesterol. It is present in the subendothelium as well as the media and "it is the major, if not the only cellular ele-ment in the atherosclerotic plaque."

This cell responds to a large variety of stimuli. "Virtually any perturbation of the vessel wall results in damage to or pro-liferation of medical and subendothelial muscle cells."

Hypertension, in direct proportion to blood pressure, pro-
vokes proliferation of these cells, and exuberant accumulation of
elastin, collagen and mucopolysaccharides as well as lysosomes.

A variety of substances, including lipids may also stimulate
these cells.

Let us review the experimental results with hypertension.
Elevation of blood pressure, regardless of the stimulus used to
raise the pressure, has been shown to produce vessel hypertrophy
and increased atherogenesis in many species - rats, chickens,
dogs, rabbits, monkeys, man.

Pharmacologic control of this previously elevated blood pressure has been shown to decrease the accelerated rate of atherogenesis (15).

Wolinsky (18) has shown that elevation of blood pressure produces increases in thickness of media, in diameter, tangential
tension and an increase in the absolute amounts first of smooth
muscle later of collagen, elastin and mucopolysaccharide. "The
degree of proliferation of smooth muscle cells and accumulation
of extracellular fibrous proteins is predictably and linearly related to the level of calculated wall tension. "

Further, he has shown that if the blood pressure is restored
to normal, the hypertrophied muscle mass was capable of reversal, though not as completely in males as in females. However,
the collagen and elastin increased by hypertension do not reverse
(16).

Perhaps the most striking and intriguing of Wolinsky's findings in rats relates to the difference between males and females.
In the male, reversal of hypertension does not reverse medial
thickness to normal; in the female it does (16).

In rats, estrogen treatment has a distinctly inhibitory effect
on the aortic wall response to hypertension (17). The increase
in weight of arterial wall is prevented. The increase in muscle
is prevented. The increase in collagen, elastin and polysaccharide
(products of the muscle) is prevented. The degradation of collagen and elastin is accelerated. The increase in oxygen consumption is prevented. The increase in DNA is prevented. The

increase in lysosomes and their enzymes is prevented.

Conversely - oophorectomy of the female rat (like hypertension and aging) increases oxygen consumption by the aorta and increases accumulation of connective tissue in the aorta. Androgen in large doses can also stimulate accumulation of fibrous proteins even in the absence of elevated blood pressure.

It was pointed out earlier that medial hypertrophy is proportional to wall stress and it was suggested that this represents a response of the muscle cells to stretching and that all the other changes follow from the increase in muscle. The effect of estrogen modifies this first response. In its presence, hypertension fails to produce the muscle hypertrophy which it produces in its absence. Therefore, Wolinsky pointed out the coexistence of a high pressure and a thin wall means a peculiarly high calculated wall stress. If stress acted directly to produce damage, atherosclerosis should be greater with estrogen but it is less. If filtration pressure at the intima were the key, atherosclerosis should be unaffected by estrogen but it is less.

Some of these effects have been seen with other compounds (14).

Cortisone can suppress aortic lysosomal enzymes and can prevent development of lesions in hyperlipidemic rabbits even while making the lipid levels in serum still higher.

Colchicine has been reported to inhibit cell proliferation and plaque formation in lipid fed rabbits.

In some hands, pyridinolcarbamate suppresses dietary atheroma in rabbits.

Therefore a number of agents may be found eventually to modify the mesenchymal response of arterial wall to blood pressure and diet. However, for today, we will look only at estrogen because the striking effects listed above are consistent with clinical data and there seems so obvious and immediate clinical indication.

Gertler and White in 1954 (27) analyzed 1000 consecutive patients with clinical coronary disease and found it 19 times more common in men than women under 35 and 15 times more common

in men than women under 40.   James, in 1955, pointed out the
sharp rise in incidence of infarction in women after the 5th decade,
(usually about 16 years after menopause).

As Wolinsky has shown in the hypertensive rat, so many have
shown in women, that bilateral oophorectomy is followed by more
rapid atherosclerosis. Wuerst in 1953 (19) examined the coronaries of 49 women who had died more than two years after oophorectomy and compared the degree of coronary sclerosis to that found
in 600 hearts from woemn and 600 hearts from men of comparable
ages. On the average, the degree of coronay sclerosis was
greater than that in control women but was still less than that of
control men (who had lacked estrogen not for two years but all
their lives).

Robinson in 1959 (20) reported increased coronary heart
disease and peripheral vascular disease in women who had bilateral oophorectomy prior to natural menopause as compared
to a similar group of women who had hysterectomy without castration.

Oliver and Boyd in 1959 (21) compared 31 patients followed
20 years after unilateral oophorectomy to 36 patients followed 20
years after bilateral oophorectomy. They reported that 9/36 of
the latter as compared to 1/31 of the former developed CHD. The
β value of this difference is less than 0.01. Incidentally, the serum cholesterol and C/P ratio were also higher in the bilaterally
oophorectomized group.

Davis, in a 1961 study (22) of long term estrogen substitution,
concluded, "the incidence of abnormal electrocardiograms was
lower in the hormonally treated castrates than in untreated women
both naturally menopausal and oophorectomized."

The conclusion that castration of the premenopausal woman
increases atherosclerotic disease and that it is malpractice not to
give hormone replacement after this procedure is inescapable.

The numerically much more important question of whether the
natural menopause should be allowed in women with hypertension
or indeed in any women, is more difficult to answer.

The attention of doctors interested in atherosclerosis was

directed first to coronary artery disease, the number one killer,
and first to men, because its incidence is 10-20 times higher in
young men than in young women. But there is a sharp break in
the curve of CHD in women in the 5th decade and the hypertensives who are spared CHD show a terrible incidence of a worse
infarction, stroke.

Boyd, in his beautiful presentation in Utrecht in 1973 (28)
stressed the effects of estrogen on lipid metabolism in general
and cholesterol metabolism in particular and the possible relevance of these to atherosclerosis. He described the cyclical
variation of plasma cholesterol in young women (lowest at mid-
cycle when estrogen is maximal) the rise in plasma cholesterol
following ovariectomy. He showed that estrogens lower cholesterol in a dose dependent manner but he pointed out that the dose
required to lower cholesterol is higher than the "estrogenic" dose.

When Oliver and Boyd treated 100 male survivors of cardiac
infarction with ethanyl estradiol, they caused a uniform depression
of plasma cholesterol and C/P ratio and a rise in alpha/beta ratio,
but they showed no change in morbidity. Marmorsten reported
similar results with estradiol but different results with Premarin.

Rivin, in 1954 (29), described a group of men (aged 46-91)
who had received high doses of estrogen (75 mg stilbestrol) over
3 months to 7 years for management of cancer of the prostate.
He found less sclerosis in the coronaries, aorta and cerebrals
than in untreated men. Considering the ages and the inevitability
of atherosclerosis in such patients, one has to ask whether this is
evidence of reversal, of diminishment of previously established
atherosclerosis. It is an interesting report and perhaps consistent with Wolinsky's work, but the doses make it clinically irrele-
vant for the moment.

The work of Oliver and Boyd (23) and of Marmorsten (24),
testing estrogen in men, is suggestive but conflicting. They have
lowered serum cholesterol. They do not agree about effects on
morbidity. They both have focussed their attention on men and
therefore have incurred the problem of testing the effects of estrogen in the presence of androgen and in the presence of atherosclerosis already established in the androgen stimulated arteries
of older men. There is a much more promising group to test.
Wolinsky's studies in the ovariectomized and estrogen replaced

rat, even in the presence of hypertension suggest that the changes
in artery wall which we believe underly atherogenesis may be prevented from occurring in the first place.

The terribly important question is: whether if physiologic not
pharmacologic estrogen levels were maintained in women throughout life, the effects of blood pressure and diet might be muted
throughout life as they are in the premenopausal woman. All the
experimental evidence suggests that this would be so. The time
is overdue for a large controlled comparison of the incidence of
stroke and heart disease in populations of women with and without
estrogen replacement. The population at risk is more than 50%
of those over 45. The other side effects rather than being unde-
sirable are desirable. The probability of achieving more than we
can with dietary and blood pressure manipulation (each of which
carry difficult social problems and side effects) is high.

SUMMARY

The effects of diet and serum cholesterol while important,
are much more important under some circumstances (high blood
pressure, low estrogen) then under other circumstances (low blood
pressure, high estrogen).

The value of modification of serum lipids, if any, can not be
determined by simply measuring the lipids and the value of modifying the blood pressure and maintaining youthful estrogen levels
(in older women) seems more probable.

REFERENCES

1. Lew, E. A., Build and Blood Pressure Study, Vols. 1 and 2.
    Chicago, Society of Actuaries, 1959.
2. The Framingham Study. An Epidemiological Investigation of
    Cardiovascular Disease. Serum Cholesterol, Systolic Blood
    Pressure and Framingham Relative Weight as Discriminators
    of Cardiovascular Disease, Section 23. Editors: William B.
    Kannel, M. D. and Tavia Gordon.
3. Veterans Administration Cooperative Study Group on Anti-
    hypertensive Agents. J. A. M. A. 213: 1143-52, 1970.

4. Coronary Heart Disease in Adults - Data from the National Health Survey 1960-62. U.S. Public Health Service No. 1000, Series 11, No. 10.

5. Deming, Q.B., Mosbach, E.H., Bevans, M., Abell, L., Daly, M.M., Martin, E., Brun, L., Halpern, E. and Kaplan, R. J. Exper. Med. 24: 882, 1958.

6. Deming, Q.B., Hodes, M.E., Baltazar, A., Edreira, J.G., Torosdag, S. Amer. J. of Med. 24: 882, 1958.

7. Adel, H.N., Deming, Q.B., Daly, M.M., Raeff, V., Brun, L. J. Lab. and Clin. Med. 66: 4, 1965.

8. Gross, Franz, Editor, <u>Antihypertensive Therapy (Principles and Practice)</u>, An International Symposium, Springer-Verlag, 1966.

9. Paterson, J.C., Mills, J. and Lockwood, C.H. Canad. Med. Assoc. J. 82: 6-11, 1960.

10. Paterson, J.C., Dyer, L. and Armstrong, E.C. Canad. Med. Assoc. J. 82: 6-11, 1960.

11. Brunner, H.R., Laragh, J.H., Baen, L., et al New England J. Med. 286: 441-449, 1972.

12. Karsner, H.T. Trans. A. Assoc. Physicians 53: 54-59, 1938.

13. Wolinsky, H., Goldfischer, S., Schiller, B. and Kasak, L. Circulation Research 34: 233, 1974.

14. Curreri, P.W., Kothari, H.V., Bonner, M.J. and Miller, B.F. Proc. Soc. Exptl. Biol. Med. 130: 1253-1256, 1969.

15. Wolinsky, H. Circulation Research 32: 543, 1973.

16. Deming, Q.B., Daly, M.M., Brun, L., Kaplan, R., Schechter, M. and Bloom, J. <u>Hypertension Recent Advances</u>, Lea and Febiger, pp. 160-163, 1961.

17. Deming, Q.B., Daly, M.M. and Wolinsky, H. Hypertension: A Precursor of Arteriosclerosis in Hypertension: Mechanisms and Management, Onesti, G., Kim, K.E. and Moyer, J.M., Editors. Grune and Stratton, Inc., 1973.

18. Wolinsky, H. Circulation Research 30: 341, 1972.

19. Wuerst, J.H., Jr., Dry, T.J. and Edwards, J.E. Circulation 7: 801-809, 1953.

20. Robinson, R.W., Higano, N. and Cohen, W.D. A.M.A. Arch. Int. Med. 104: 908-920, 1959.

21. Oliver, M.F. and Boyd, G.S. Lancet 2: 690-694, 1959.

22. Davis, M.E., Jones, R. and Jarolim, C. Amer. J. Obst. and Gyn. 82: 1003-1018, 1961.

23. Oliver, M.F. and Boyd, G.S. Circulation 13: 82-91, 1956.

24. Marmorsten, J., Moore, F., Hopkins, C.E., Kuzmaot and Weiner, J. Proc. Soc. Exptl. Biol. Med. 111: 400-408, 1962.

25. Clawson, B.J. Amer. Heart J. 22: 607-624, 1941.

26. Pick, R., Clark, G.B. and Katz, L. Progr. Biochem. Pharmacol. 4: 354-362, 1968.

27. Gertler, M.M. Coronary Heart Disease in Young Adults. Harvard University Press, Cambridge, 1954.

28. Boyd, G.S. Frontiers of Hormone Research, Vol. 2. Karger, Basel, 1973.

29. Rivin, A.R. and Sim, P.D. Circulation 9: 533-539, 1954.

THE HERITABLE HYPERLIPOPROTEINEMIAS AND ATHEROSCLEROSIS

Charles J. Glueck, M. D. , and Ronald W. Fallat, M. D.

University of Cincinnati, College of Medicine,
Lipoprotein Research Laboratory and General Clinical
Research Center, Cincinnati, Ohio

INTRODUCTION

Hyperlipidemia can be caused by occasional or constant environmental factors, by genetic factors, by other primary diseases, or by various combinations (11-14, 16, 17, 28, 36, 37, 46, 48, 54, 57). Probably less than 10% of individuals from free living populations whose plasma cholesterol and triglyceride concentrations are above the upper 95th percentile are carriers of genes for familial hyperlipoproteinemia (6, 46). A large numerical majority of individuals with hyperlipidemia have acquired the disorder primarily through diet, excessive alcohol intake, drugs, or other primary disease states (most frequently diabetes, hypothyroidism, nephrotic syndrome, liver disease). Hypercholesterolemia and hypertriglyceridemia acquired secondary to dietary habits are highly sensitive to minor changes in habitual life style. For the most part, the familial hyperlipoproteinemias require major changes in dietary habits and often the conjunction of diet and drug therapy is required to normalize blood lipids.

The familial hyperlipoproteinemias, particularly familial hypercholesterolemia, familial combined hyperlipidemia, and familial hyperglyceridemia are closely associated with accelerated and severe atherosclerosis (1, 6, 7, 12-14, 16, 21-23, 29, 33, 46, 49, 57-60). Early identification of the familial hyperlipoproteinemias, preferably in childhood, offers the opportunity for primary prevention of atherosclerosis at a stage where it may be reversible (2, 9, 16-22, 24, 27, 35, 37, 39, 42, 56, 60, 62, 64).

My discussion will attempt to review the relationship between premature atherosclerosis and familial hyperlipidemias and the genetics of the common familial hyperlipoproteinemias, with the caveat that development of discrete biochemical markers for the familial hyperlipoproteinemias will provide the most definitive approach to these disorders (4, 5).

FAMILIAL HYPERLIPIDEMIAS AND ATHEROSCLEROSIS RISK

Although the hyperlipidemias are only one of multiple risk factors for ischemic heart disease, they are particularly important factors (33). As suggested by the studies of Carlson (6) and others (45, 59), the event rate for ischemic heart disease probably increases linearly with increasing fasting concentrations of plasma cholesterol and triglycerides. Plasma triglycerides and cholesterol are risk factors for ischemic heart disease independent of each other. A combined elevation of plasma cholesterol and triglyceride may be associated with the highest risk for ischemic heart disease (6).

The close association of familial hypercholesterolemia and ischemic heart disease has been particularly well documented (1, 6, 7, 16, 23, 46, 50, 52, 54, 57). Stone, Levy et al, studied 547 first degree relatives of patients with well documented familial type II hyperlipoproteinemia (57). Coronary artery disease was present in 29. 2% of hypercholesterolemic relatives, more than twice the event rate (12. 5%) in normal relatives. Angina pectoris and death or infarction from coronary artery disease were 3-4 times more common in the relatives with hypercholesterolemia than in the normocholesterolemic relatives. The cumulative probability of coronary events by age 40 was 19% for hypercholesterolemic male relatives and less than 1% for normal relatives. By age 60, 65% of the male type II relatives had had a coronary event as compared to only 15. 6% of normal relatives. The coronary event rate was somewhat lower in women. By age 50, 25% of type II relatives, and by age 60, 36% of the women were affected as opposed to 14. 3% of the normal kindred members.

The studies of Stone, Levy et al (57) were in agreement with earlier similar results from Slack and co-workers (58, 59). In kindred members from families with familial hypercholesterolemia, ischemic heart disease events had occurred in 5.4% of men and no women by age 30, 51.4% of the men and 12.2% of the women by age 50 and 85.4% and 57.5% respectively by age 60. These two studies clearly document then, that both men and women with familial hypercholesterolemia have an extraordinary excess of morbidity and mortality from ischemic heart disease at relatively early ages. A similar but quantitatively less accelerated event rate was reported by Slack et al (59) in patients from families with various hypertriglyceridemias, primarily type IV hyperlipoproteinemia. Thirty percent of kindred members were affected by age 50, and 53% by age 60.

Other family studies with the propositus being an individual with a premature ischemic event revealed familial aggregation of premature ischemic heart disease. Nikkila and Aro (46) have studied 412 first degree relatives of 101 survivors of myocardial infarction. The index patients were 101 consecutively admitted patients under age 50 with unequivocal electrocardiographic evidence for myocardial infarction. When their families were studied, roughly a third of the families were completely normal. In 33 families there was one other hyperlipoproteinemic member with type II-A and IV lipoprotein phenotypes predominant. There was a significant clustering of familial hyperlipoproteinemia in 33 of the 101 families examined. Of these, only 9 families had a pure "or single type" familial disease with types II-A, II-B and IV represented. Twenty-four of the 33 familial hyperlipoproteinemic families had combined hyperlipidemia characterized by mixtures of the II-A, II-B and IV phenotype. These findings were extremely similar to a comparable study by the Seattle group (23) in families of young myocardial infarction survivors.

The Cincinnati group also approaches the problem by studies in kindreds where the propositus had an early myocardial event (21). Seventy kindreds were referred where one parent had a documented myocardial infarction before age 50. The average age of infarction was age 40 and there were 64 men and 6 women. In this very young study group, some form of familial hyperlipoproteinemia appeared to be present in 60 of the 70 kindreds. Familial hypercholesterolemia, combined hyperlipidemia and hypertriglyceridemia were particularly common. As in other lipid clinics, referral

of the families was probably biased to the more severe premature
atherosclerosis and the more quantitatively marked severe hyperlipidemia. In the 223 children born to these 70 kindreds, elevations of cholesterol and triglyceride or both were quite common.
A third of these healthy, normal children had some form of hyperlipoproteinemia, and two-thirds were normal. In the 69 children
with hyperlipoproteinemias, roughly 50% had elevations of cholesterol and LDL cholesterol with normal triglycerides, the type
II-A phenotype. Roughly, 15% had combined elevations of cholesterol and triglyceride, the type II-B phenotype. A considerable
number of the children had elevations of triglyceride alone.
Similar data has previously been reported by Tamir et al (60).

Elevations of cholesterol and triglyceride, or triglyceride
alone are intimately associated with the development of premature
heart disease. Hence, an awareness of the close association of
the familial hyperlipidemias with atherosclerosis should prompt
the practicing physician to carefully mine a valuable resource in
terms of preventive medicine, that is, families with known hyperlipidemias or families with known histories of premature atherosclerosis.

HERITABLE HYPERLIPOPROTEINEMIAS

Using quantitative lipid and lipoprotein measurements and extensive family screening much has been learned about the apparent
inheritance of the hyperlipidemias.

Low density lipoprotein cholesterol or LDL is under well
characterized genetic control over a wide concentration range.

Abetalipoproteinemia, a rare genetic disorder of the LDL
metabolism (3, 8, 15, 26, 30, 36, 51), is inherited as an autosomal
recessive. Two exceptional cases of abetalipoproteinemia have
been reported which were the result of homozygous inheritance
of hypobetalipoproteinemia (8).

Hypobetalipoproteinemia is characterized by reduction of
cholesterol levels to about 40% of normal (8, 15, 38, 43, 47, 63).
Its prevalence is unknown but it is considerably more common
than abetalipoproteinemia with a minimal prevalence of 1/400
kindreds in a pilot study by the Cincinnati group (8). Hypobetalipoproteinemia is transmitted as an autosomal dominant trait.

Hyperbetalipoproteinemia is transmitted as an autosomal
dominant with an estimate of the heterozygote frequency of about
1 in 200 (62) to 1 in 600 (23). Homozygotes with hyperbetalipoproteinemia are relatively rare, and usually have lethal atherosclerosis by age 25. Familial hypercholesterolemia (hyperbetalipoproteinemia) is probably the best studied of the inherited
hyperlipoproteinemias and is closely associated with a remarkable increase in cardiovascular event rate (1, 2, 4, 5, 7, 11-17, 23-25,
27, 28, 31, 32, 40, 45, 46, 54, 57-60). Kwiterovich et al (37) have
recently summarized their experience with a large number of
kindreds with well characterized familial hypercholesterolemia.
The distribution of LDL cholesterol in the offspring of affected
kindreds represented a biomodal pattern with only minimal over-
lap. Approximately 50% of children born to normal X hyperbeta
matings had elevated LDL cholesterol. These data were comparable to those by Schrott et al (54), and were entirely consistent
with transmission of familial hypercholesterolemia as an autosomal dominant trait. Low density lipoprotein cholesterol, in
contrast to total cholesterol, was shown to be the best conventional
clinical marker of the disorder.

Perhaps the most common familial hyperlipidemia associated
with premature cardio-, peripheral, or cerebral vascular disease
is familial combined hyperlipidemia. This disorder was recognized in variable forms by Nikkila and Aro (46), Goldstein et al
(23, 24), Rose (50) and others (19, 41, 62). As summarized by
Goldstein et al (23), combined hyperlipidemia was very common
in kindreds where the propositus had sustained a premature myocardial infarction. In those individuals in whom "monogenic"
hyperlipoproteinemia could be fully identified, 30% of the kindreds
could be classified as having familial combined hyperlipidemia
and 14% had familial hypertriglyceridemia. Affected kindred members with familial combined hyperlipidemia may have elevations of
cholesterol or triglyceride or both. Familial combined appears
to be transmitted as a simple Mendelian autosomal trait with the
presence of three different lipoprotein phenotypes, types II-A,
II-B, and IV, felt to represent variability in expression of a single
abnormal gene. The frequency distribution of plasma triglyceride
in adult first degree relatives appears to be bimodal. Cholesterol
levels were found to be unimodal, but shifted to the right of controls. Familial combined hyperlipidemia is currently felt to be
determined by a single gene with primary action on triglyceride
metabolism and secondary effects on cholesterol metabolism (23).

High density lipoprotein cholesterol is also characterized by complex genetic control. An-alphalipoproteinemia is a very rare disorder transmitted as an autosomal recessive (10-16). Hypo-alphalipoproteinemia has never been described. Recently our group has studied 12 kindreds with apparent hyperalphalipoproteinemia inherited as an autosomal dominant trait (Glueck et al, Circulation Supplements, in press, 1974). In the 62 offspring from these 12 kindreds alphalipoprotein cholesterol was 70 or more in 32/62, 52%. The ratio of offspring with elevated alphalipoprotein cholesterol to those with normal alpha was 32:30 (1.07), not significantly different from 1.0 ($X^2 = 0.063$), the ratio predicted for a dominant trait. There was no female:male difference in alpha in the 32 offspring with familial hyperalpha. Alpha in 21 females was 82 ± 10, similar to alpha in 11 men, 86 ± 16 mg/100 ml. Patients with familial hyperalphalipoproteinemia had no unique physical or neurologic features, no xanthomas. Familial hyperalphalipoproteinemia was transmitted vertically through three generations in 4 kindreds.

Chylomicrons and Very Low Density Lipoproteins (VLDL) are also under a complex and less well understood set of genetic controls. Type I hyperlipoproteinemia (familial hyperchylomicronemia) is transmitted as an autosomal recessive (11-16) and is not associated with any increase in cardiac event rate. The extremely common Type IV hyperlipoproteinemia (familial hypertriglyceridemia) is probably inherited as an autosomal dominant (11-16, 20, 23, 61). The genetics of types III and V hyperlipoproteinemias are considerably less well defined, but type III appears to be inherited as an autosomal recessive (10-16), and type V as an autosomal dominant (10-16).

Of the heritable hypertriglyceridemias, type IV (familial hypertriglyceridemia) is probably the most common, has the closest association with premature atherosclerosis, and is genetically distinct from both familial hypercholesterolemia and familial combined hyperlipidemia (11-14, 16, 20). Affected kindred members have elevations of triglyceride and VLDL cholesterol. The disorder is transmitted as a simple Mendelial autosomal dominant trait (16, 20). The frequency distribution of triglyceride in adult first degree relatives of hypertriglyceridemic propositi is bimodal. In contrast to familial hypercholesterolemia, this familial hypertriglyceridemia cannot be diagnosed in cord blood (62), and only 20% of children less than age 21 (at genetic risk), manifest hypertriglyceridemia (20).

DISCRETE BIOCHEMICAL MARKERS OF HERITABLE
HYPERLIPOPROTEINEMIAS

Until recently analysis of the genetics of the hyperlipoproteinemias was severely limited by the lack of a specific and unique
genetic marker, forcing reliance on measures of lipids and lipoproteins and extensive kindred analysis. Goldstein and Brown
have now provided an imaginative and elegant method for quantitative analysis of the expression of the heterozygous and homozygous
trait of familial hypercholesterolemia by tissue culture methods
(4, 5, 25). They studied low density lipoprotein binding, degradation,
and LDL mediated suppression of HMG-CoA reductase activity in
cultured fibroblasts from normals, heterozygotes and homozygotes
with familial hypercholesterolemia. Normal fibroblasts bound
approximately twice as much I-125 LDL as fibroblasts from subjects
heterozygous for type II, whereas fibroblasts from homozygotes
essentially has very little binding of LDL.

The degradation of the bound LDL was approximately twice as
high in fibroblasts from normals as compared to those from heterozygotes, whereas cells from homozygotes degraded very little of
the small amount of LDL that was bound. Introduction of LDL into
the culture medium repressed the activity of HMG-CoA reductase
to only 10% of its previous level in lipoprotein-poor medium in
normals. In heterozygotes, however, there is considerably less
suppression by introduced LDL whereas homozygotes cells were
essentially non-repressed. Brown and Goldstein have identified
the apparent biochemical defect in familial hypercholesterolemia
as a genetic deficiency in a cell surface receptor for LDL. In
heterozygotes, a 60% reduction in LDL receptors leads to a concentration dependent defect in regulation. Attainment of equal
rates of cholesterol synthesis and LDL degradation in normal and
heterozygous cells requires a two to three-fold higher concentration of LDL in the heterozygote.

In normal cells binding of LDL to the receptor regulates
cholesterol metabolism by suppressing cholesterol synthesis and
increasing LDL degradation. In the heterozygote, the number of
functional receptor sites is reduced to 40% of normal, and at
levels of LDL below saturation approximately a 2.5-fold higher
concentration of LDL must be present to produce the same absolute number of occupied receptor sites and hence the same sup-
pressive effect as in normal cells. Thus this brilliant work now
allows us a more discriminate indicator of familial hypercholesterolemia, an indicator useful on a molecular biochemical level.

HERITABLE HYPERLIPOPROTEINEMIAS IN CHILDREN, PRIMARY PREVENTION OF ATHEROSCLEROSIS

In the past the diagnoses of the genetic hyperlipidemias have been primarily made in adults. Recently it has become clear that the genesis of atherosclerosis is in childhood (17, 21, 22, 39, 48). Hence, in conclusion, I would like to briefly review the data from our group (18-22, 61, 62), and many other research groups (2, 9, 17, 27, 35, 37, 42, 53, 56, 60, 64) suggesting that many of the heritable hyperlipidemias can be diagnosed in childhood.

In two separate studies done in our laboratory we are able to make the diagnosis of neonatal and familial hypercholesterolemia, characterized by three generation vertical transmission, in 0.4% or approximately 1 in 200 live births (22, 62). If two generation horizontal and vertical transmission were counted as familial disease, the prevalence would increase to about 0.8%. Neonatal hypercholesterolemia and combined hyperlipidemia together have been diagnosed by Goldstein in 0.45% of consecutive unselected live births (24). With a familial type II parent as propositus, 50% of infants born to parents with known type II have elevations of cord blood LDL (35).

The diagnosis of type IV cannot be made in neonates because cord blood triglyceride reflects pre- and intra-partum stress (61). Pediatric familial type IV in screening studies in school children in the Cincinnati area is relatively common and probably present in approximately one-half of 1% of unselected school children. Where the parent is a known propositus with familial hypertrigly-ceridemia, 20% of children under age 21 with parents with known type IV are also found to have elevations of triglycerides (20).

CONCLUSIONS

1. The genetic hyperlipoproteinemias are common, are easily diagnosed and are often expressed in children or in infants.

2. Familial combined hyperlipidemia, hypercholesterolemia and hypertriglyceridemia are all associated with a markedly aug-mented atherosclerotic cardiovascular event rate.

3. The clinical importance of early diagnosis, family screening, and lipid sampling in high risk or free living populations must be emphasized.

4. Exciting progress at a biochemical molecular level (in tissue culture, for example) provides better understanding of the genetic hyperlipoproteinemias and possible avenues for its better therapy.

REFERENCES

1. Adlersberg, D. , Parets, A. D. , and Boas, E. P. : J. A. M. A. 141: 246, 1949
2. Andersen, G. E. , and Clausen, J. : Z. Ernaehrungswiss 11: 120, 1972
3. Bassen, F. A. , and Kornzweig, A. L. : Blood 5: 381, 1950
4. Brown, M. S. , Dana, S. E. , and Goldstein, J. L. : J. Biol. Chem. 249: 789, 1974a
5. Brown, M. S. and Goldstein, J. L. : Science 185: 61, 1974b
6. Carlson, L. A. , and Bottiger, L. E. : Lancet 1: 865, 1972
7. Carter, C. O. , Slack, J. , Myant, N. B. : Lancet 1: 400, 1971
8. Cottrill, C. , Glueck, C. J. , Leuba, V. , Millett, F. , Puppione, D. , and Brown, W. V. : Metabolism 23: 779, 1974
9. Darmady, J. M. , Fosbrooke, A. S. , and Lloyd, J. K. : British Medical Journal 2: 685, 1972
10. Fredrickson, D. S. : J. Clin. Investigation 43: 228, 1964
11. Fredrickson, D. S. , Lees, R. S. , and Levy, R. I. : In Progress in Biochemical Pharmacology. Vol. 2, edited by R. Paoletti, D. Kritchevsky and D. Steinberg. Basel, Karger, p. 343, 1966.
12. Fredrickson, D. S. , Levy, R. I. , Lees, R. S. : New Eng. J. Med. 276: 32-44, 94-103, 148-156, 215-224, 273-281 (Jan. 5, 12, 19, 26 and Feb. 2), 1967
13. Fredrickson, D. S. : Proc. Nat. Acad. Sci. U. S. A. 1138: 46, Nov. , 1969
14. Fredrickson, D. S. : British Med. J. 2: 187, 1971
15. Fredrickson, D. S. , Gotto, A. M. , and Levy, R. I. : In the Metabolic Basis of Inherited Disease, edited by Stanbury, J. B. , Wyngaarden, J. B. , and Fredrickson, D. S. McGraw-Hill, N. Y. , 3rd ed. , 1972, pp. 499-513.
16. Fredrickson, D. S. and Levy, R. I. : In Metabolic Basis of Inherited Disease, edited by Stanbury, J. D. , Wyngaarden, J. B. ,

and Fredrickson, D. S. McGraw-Hill, N. Y., 3rd ed., 1972, pp. 545-614

17. Fredrickson, D. S. and Breslow, J. L.: Ann. Rev. Med. 24: 315, 1973

18. Glueck, C. J., Heckman, F., Schonfeld, M., Steiner, P., and Pearce, W.: Met. 20: 597, 1971

19. Glueck, C. J., Fallat, R., Buncher, R., Tsang, R., and Steiner, P.: Met. 22: 1403, 1973a

20. Glueck, C. J., Tsang, R., Fallat, R., Buncher, C. R., Evans, G., and Steiner, P.: Met. 22: 1287, 1973b

21. Glueck, C. J., Fallat, R., Tsang, R., and Buncher, C. R.: Amer. J. Dis. Child. 127: 70, 1974a

22. Glueck, C. J., Fallat, R. W., and Tsang, R. C.: Amer. J. Dis. Child., in press, 1974b

23. Goldstein, J. L., Schrott, H. R., Hazzard, W. R., Bierman, E. L., Motulsky, A. G.: J. Clin. Invest. 52: 1544, 1973a

24. Goldstein, J. L., Albers, J. J., Hazzard, W. R., Schott, H. R., Bierman, E. L., and Motulsky, A. G.: J. Clin. Invest. 52: abstract 127, p. 35A, 1973b

25. Goldstein, J. L. and Brown, M. S.: Proc. Nat. Acad. Sci.: 70: 2804, 1973c

26. Gotto, A. M., Levy, R. I., John, K., and Fredrickson, D. S.: N. E. J. M. 284: 813, 1971

27. Greten, H., Wengeler, H., and Wagner, H.: Nutr. Metabol. 15: 128, 1973

28. Harlan, W. R., Jr., Graham, J. B., and Estes, E. H.: Medicine 45: 77, 1966

29. Heinle, R. A., Levy, R. I., Fredrickson, D. S., and Gorlin, R.: Amer. J. Cardiol. 24: 178, 1969

30. Isselbacher, K. H., Scheig, R., Plotkin, G. R. and Caulfield, J. B.: Medicine 43: 347, 1964

31. Jensen, J., Blankenhorn, D. H., and Konerup, V.: Circulation 36: 77, 1967

32. Jensen, J., and Blankenhorn, D. H.: The Am. J. Med. 52: 499, 1972

33. Kannel, W. B., Castelli, W. P., Gordon, T. and McNamara, P. A.: Annals of Internal Medicine 74: 1, 1971

34. Khachadurian, A. K.: Am. J. Med. 37: 402, 1964

35. Kwiterovich, P. O., Levy, R. I. and Fredrickson, D. S.: Lancet 1: 118, 1973

36. Lees, R. S., Wilson, D. E., Schonfeld, G., and Fleet, S.: Prog. in Med. Genetics 9: 237, 1973

37. Kwiterovich, P. O., Jr., Fredrickson, D. S., and Levy, R. I.: J. Clin. Invest. 53: 1237, 1974

38. Levy, R. I. , Langer, T. , Gotto, A. M. , and Fredrickson, D. S. : Clin. Res. 18: 539, 1970

39. Levy, R. I. and Rifkind, B. M. : Amer. J. Cardiol. 31: 547, 1973

40. Lewis, B. and Myant, N. B. : Clinical Science 32: 201, 1967

41. Loeper, J. , Rouffy, J. , Loeper, J. : Arch. Mal. Coeur. 12: Suppl. 1: 3-15, 1970-71

42. Lloyd, J. K. and Wolff, O. H. : In, Endocrine and Genetic Diseases of Childhood. Edited by L. I. Gardner. W. B. Saunders, Philadelphia, 1969, p. 937.

43. Mars, H. , Lewis, L. A. , Robertson, A. L. , Jr. , Butkus, A. , and Williams, G. H. , Jr. : Am. J. Med. 46: 886, 1969

44. Miettinen, T. A. , Penttila, I. M. , and Lampainen, E. : Clinical Genetics 3: 271, 1972

45. Nevin, N. C. and Slack, J. : Journal of Medical Genetics 5: 9, 1968

46. Nikkila, E. A. , and Aro, A. : Lancet 1: 954, 1973

47. Richet, G. , Durepaire, H. , Hartmann, L. , Ollier, M. P. , Polonovaki, J. , and Maitrot, B. : Presse Med. 77: 2045, 1969

48. Rifkind, B. M. : Clinics in Endocrinology and Metabolism, Volume 2, B. M. Rifkind, editor. W. B. Saunders, Philadelphia, 1973, pp. 1-151.

49. Roberts, W. C. , Levy, R. I. and Fredrickson, D. S. : Arch. Pathol. 90: 45, 1970

50. Rose, H. G. , Kranz, P. , Weinstock, M. , Guliano, J. , and Haft, J. I. : Am. J. Med. 54: 148, 1973

51. Salt, H. B. , Wolff, O. H. , Lloyd, J. K. , Fosbrooke, A. S. , Cameron, A. H. , and Hubble, D. V. : Lancet 2: 325, 1960

52. Schaefer, L. E. , Adlersberg, D. , and Steinberg, A. G. : Circulation 17: 537, 1958

53. Schreibman, P. H. , Wilson, D. E. , and Arky, R. A. : New Eng. J. Med. 281: 981, 1969

54. Schrott, H. G. , Goldstein, J. L. , Hazzard, W. R. , McGoodwin, M. C. and Motulsky, A. G. : Annals of Int. Med. 76: 711, 1972

55. Schwartz, J. F. , Rowland, L. P. , Eder, H. , Marks, P. A. , Osserman, E. F. , Hirschberg, E. , and Anderson, H. : Arch. Neurol. 8: 438, 1963

56. Segal, M. M. , Fosbrooke, A. S. , Lloyd, J. K. , and Wolf O. H. : Arch. Dis. Child. 45: 73, 1970

57. Stone, N. J. , Levy, R. I. , Fredrickson, D. S. , and Verter, J. : Circulation, supplement IV, XLVIII, II-14, 1973

58. Slack, J. and Nevin, N. C. : J. Med. Genet. 5: 4, 1968

59. Slack, J. : Lancet 2: 1380, 1969

60. Tamir, I., Bojamower, Y., Levtow, O., Heldenberg, D., Dickerman, Z., and Werbin, B.: Archives of Disease in Childhood 47: 808, 1972

61. Tsang, R. and Glueck, C.J. Amer. J. Dis. Children 127: 78, 1974

62. Tsang, R., Fallat, R.W., and Glueck, C.J.: Pediatrics 53: 458, 1974

63. Van Buchem, F.S.P., Pol. G., de Gier, J., Bottcher, C.J.F., and Pries, C.: Amer. J. Med. 40: 794, 1966

64. Wolff, O.H.: Proc. Roy. Soc. Med. 60: 1147, 1967

SMOKING AND CARBON MONOXIDE UPTAKE AS A RISK FACTOR IN ATHEROSCLEROTIC CARDIOVASCULAR DISEASE

Knud Kjeldsen, M. D.

Department of Clinical Chemistry A, Rigshospitalet, University Hospital, DK-2100 Copenhagen, Denmark

For many years nicotine has been considered responsible for the association between tobacco smoking and the development of atherosclerotic cardiovascular disease, due to its pronounced pharmacological effects on the cardiovascular system. In animal experiments, however, nicotine has no atherogenic effect when administered in amounts relatively much higher than the nicotine uptake by a smoker, but may cause necrosis and calcifications of the medial arterial layers (1), which suggests probable importance in the development of the Monckeberg type of arteriosclerosis in man.

Intimal-subintimal injuries of arterial walls indistinguishable from early atherosclerosis are, however, produced in experimental animals by another compound in tobacco smoke: carbon monoxide. Rabbits exposed to carbon monoxide for 13 weeks, leading to carboxyhemoglobin concentrations of 10-11 per cent, develop focal intimal-subintimal changes in a significantly higher degree than nonexposed control animals. These are characterized by a pronounced subintimal edema accompanied by various degenerative and reparative processes (2). Significant intimal changes have also been demonstrated in the coronary arteries of primates after a short low-level carbon monoxide exposure (3). When feeding carbon monoxide exposed rabbits (16-18 per cent carboxyhemoglobin) cholesterol for 8-10 weeks, the aortic content of cholesterol increases from 2.5 to 5 times (4). This effect of carbon monoxide

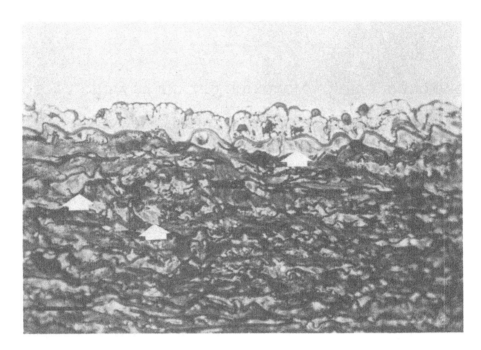

Figure 1: Light micrograph (phase contrast) of 1 μm thick section
from luminal part of aorta of experimental rabbit. Note the considerable widening of the edematous subendothelial space containing smooth muscle cells. Note also the protruding endothelial
cells and subendothelial "blister"-formation. In the luminal media
scattered edematous areas are seen (arrows).
Toluidine blue.
Bar represents 10 μm.

Figure 2: Myocardium from experimental rabbit. Photomontage
showing different grades of myofibrillar injury. A: Z bands are
widened and have a washed out appearance. To the left the myofibrils are intact, but to the right they are breaking up between the
Z bands. Note also the accumulation of ribosomes close to the
mitochondria. B: Most of the filaments between the Z bands have
disappeared. The mitochondria are circular with a homogeneous
matrix. C: Myofibrils are broken into small pieces and the
normal structure is disorganized. Bars indicate 1 μm.

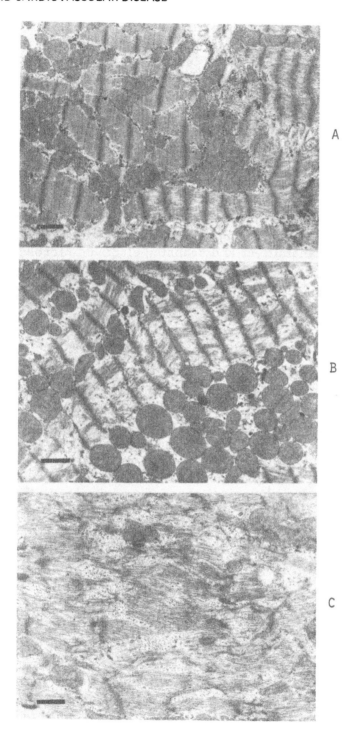

has been confirmed by other laboratories (5). Experiments in primates have also shown an increase in the number and size of lipid containing lesions in the intramural coronary arteries with carbon monoxide exposure and cholesterol feeding (6). Exposure to hypoxia (16 per cent oxygen in the inspired air) for 8-10 weeks has a similar effect on the cholesterol uptake of the arterial walls as exposure to carbon monoxide (7), while hyperoxia (26-28 per cent oxygen) has an opposite effect (8).

The primary effect of carbon monoxide on the cardiovascular system is an increased endothelial permeability, leading to sub-endothelial edema, which is easily demonstrable by ordinary light by ordinary light microscopy (Fig. 1) and also has been described in detail by transmittent and scanning electron microscopy (9). The edema is probably caused by an increased flux of plasma components through insufficient endothelial junctions. Secondary the edema will lead to proliferation of the vascular smooth muscle cells and increased formation of fibrils and extracellular matrix (10).

Severe ultrastructural changes are also found in the rabbit myocardium after a low-level carbon monoxide exposure for 2 weeks, the most impressive findings being local areas of partial or total necrosis of the myofibrils and degenerative changes of the mitochondria (Fig. 2). Other observations in this study include extra- and intracellular edema, capillary wall edema, increase in the number of ribosomes, and reparative fibrotic changes. The morphological changes are similar to those found in arterial hypoxia (11).

Both the arterial and myocardial changes can occur after only 4-5 hours exposure to carbon monoxide (16-18 per cent carboxyhemoglobin) (12).

Since the arterial and myocardial damage caused by carbon monoxide exposure in experimental animals is achieved by carboxyhemoglobin concentrations comparable to those found in some heavy smokers, these experimental results strongly indicate that the carbon monoxide content of tobacco smoke is a toxic compound of major importance. In population studies on association between carboxyhemoglobin levels in smokers and the occurrence of atherosclerosis has been demonstrated (13), and it has later been calculated that smokers with carboxyhemoglobin levels of 5 per cent or higher have a 21 times higher incidence of athero-sclerotic disease than smokers with values of 3 per cent or lower (15).

REFERENCES

1. Schievelbein, H. , Longdon, V. , Longdon, W. , Grumbach, H. , Remplik, V. , Schauer, A. and Immich, H. Z. Klin. Chem. 8: 190, 1970.
2. Wanstrup, J. , Kjeldsen, K. and Astrup, P. Acta Path. Microbiol. Scand. 75: 353, 1969.
3. Thomsen, H. K. Atherosclerosis 20: 233, 1974.
4. Astrup, P. , Kjeldsen, K. and Wanstrup, J. J. Atheroscler. Res. 7: 343, 1967.
5. Birnstingl, M. , Hawkins, L. and McEwen, T. Eur. Surg. Res. 2: 92, 1970.
6. Webster, W. S. , Clarkson, T. B. and Lofland, H. B. Exptl. Mol. Pathol. 13: 36, 1970.
7. Kjeldsen, K. , Wanstrup, J. and Astrup, P. J. Atheroscler. Res. 8: 835, 1968.
8. Kjeldsen, K. , Astrup, P. and Wanstrup, J. J. Atheroscler. Res. 10: 173, 1969.
9. Kjeldsen, K. , Astrup, P. and Wanstrup, J. Atherosclerosis 16: 67, 1972.
10. Ross, R. and Glomset, J. A. Science 180: 1332, 1973.
11. Kjeldsen, K. , Thomsen, H. K. and Astrup, P. Circulation Res. 34: 339, 1974.
12. Thomsen, H. K. and Kjeldsen, K. Arch. Environ. Health 29: 73, 1974.
13. Kjeldsen, K. Smoking and Atherosclerosis (Thesis) Copen-hagen, Munksgaard, 1969.
14. Wald, N. , Howard, S. , Smith, P. G. and Kjeldsen, K. Brit. Med. J. I: 761, 1973.

RISK OF CORONARY DISEASE AND CORONARY COMPLICATIONS BY NEURAL AND PSYCHOLOGICAL FACTORS

Alberto Zanchetti and Alberto Malliani

Istuti di Ricerche Cardiovascolari e di Semejotica Medica I, Universita di Milano, and Centro per le Ricerche Cardiovascolari del CNR, Milano, Italy

The problem of the involvement of neuropsychological factors in coronary disease can be usefully seen to consist of three separate, though obviously interrelated questions.

1. The first question is whether psychological factors, or behaviour, can influence development of chronic coronary disease. And, subordinately, whether this hypothetical influence is mediated through, or is independent of, the standard risk factors of vascular disease (blood lipids, arterial pressure, and so on). And, finally, through what neural, hormonal or metabolic pathways is this influence exerted.

2. The second question is whether psychological factors, or perhaps neural non-psychic factors, can precipitate an acute coronary event, in presence or even in absence of chronic coronary disease. Here again we can ask ourselves through what pathways can the mind or behaviour exert this precipitating influence.

3. The third question is about neural or neuro-hormonal reflex mechanisms which can be elicited while coronary disease is developing, and most often, when acute events occur. These neural mechanisms may consist in an alteration of normally protective reflexes or in an activation of noxious ones, and re-

sult in a dangerous complication such as arrhythmia or hypertension, which can transform an otherwise remediable illness in
a killing disease.

The difference between the three sets of questions need not
be emphasized. The available evidence about each topic is also
quite different; it is less and less by inference and more and
more factual as we progress from the first to the second problem,
and from the second to the third.

It will be no surprise, therefore, if in this review the order
of the problems to be discussed is going to be turned upside down,
and we will start from the third question, the one about cardiac
reflexes in the ischaemic heart. It is hoped in fact that there will
be some advantage by proceeding from sounder knowledge toward
knowledge by analogy or by inference to end up with mere hypotheses to be tested.

NEURAL REFLEX MECHANISMS DURING ACUTE
CORONARY EVENTS

We will concentrate on reflexes arising from the diseased
myocardium and capable of detrimental effects on the myocardium
itself.

Our group has extensively investigated these reflexes, their
pathways, their effects and the nature of the activating stimulus.
The stimulus is unlikely to be ischaemia itself, or chemical
substances released by ischaemia. Rather than chemoreceptors,
the receptors involved appear to be mechanoreceptors (1) probably sensitive to changes in ventricular stiffness or volume
caused by ischaemia. Afferent and efferent discharges course
through the cardiac sympathetic nerves, through what can be
defined as sympatho-sympathetic reflex (2, 3, 4), the effect of
which consists of an increase in myocardial contractility (5) and
in heart rate (6). Beside sympatho-sympathetic reflexes, also
vago-vagal reflexes occur (7, 8) and more complex interrelationships between the two, as it has been shown that stimulation of
sympathetic afferents can reduce the discharge of vagal efferents,
and vice-versa, with a sort of reciprocal organization (9). And
finally, it should also be recalled that especially sympathetic
afferent fibres, by mediating cardiac pain, can also elicit more

widespread cardiac, vascular and hormonal changes, as observed during emotional behaviour.

It is time now to ask ourselves what may be the role of these cardiac reflexes. The dangers inherent in the so-called Bezold-Jarisch effect (10, 11) of vago-vagal reflexes are well-known: bradycardia, atrioventricular block, systemic hypotension too often occur complicating the course of acute myocardial infarction. The role of a reflex increase in cardiac sympathetic activity is at a first sight less clear. A reflex increase in myocardial contractility might be an important mechanism to oppose ventricular dilation and cardiogenic shock. On the other hand, this potentially protective reflex might easily turn out to become a detrimental one, by imposing an additional oxygen consumption to the myocardium and by facilitating arrhythmias. Extracardiac responses, such as peripheral vasoconstriction and catecholamine release, might further contribute to load the heart and to the risk of arrhythmias.

Indeed, there is both experimental and clinical evidence that cardiac reflexes may add further detrimental action to the direct one of coronary occlusion. Almost forty years ago it was shown that the mortality of dogs after coronary occlusion was reduced by previous denervation of the heart (12, 13), and the role of cardiac nerves in facilitating arrhythmias has recently been re-emphasizing (14). On the clinical side, there is plenty of evidence for increased catecholamine release during acute myocardial infarction (15, 16), and the protective role of the beta-blocking drugs toward arrhythmias of the early stage is well established (17). Recently, Webb et al. (18) have suggested that as many as 36% of 74 patients seen within 30 min of the onset of acute myocardial infarction show clinical signs of sympathetic over-activity, and that 55% have signs of parasympathetic overactivity. There is also evidence that incidence of sympathetic and para-sympathetic overactivity is different according to the location of the myocardial infarction: sympathetic overactivity predominates in cases of anterior infarction, while parasympathetic disturbances largely predominate in patients with diaphragmatic lesions. Atropine and practolol could effectively abolish these signs of autonomic disturbance: the overall hospital mortality in these patients was 9.7% only, a figure quite lower than expected. Of course these data have to be considered very cautiously, particularly because of the difficulty of measuring sympathetic activity in man,

nonetheless they stress a problem worth being more actively
investigated in the future.

NEURAL AND PSYCHOLOGICAL MECHANISMS PRECIPITATING ACUTE CORONARY DISTURBANCES

It is common clinical experience than an acute coronary
event, be it anginal attack or myocardial infarction or a cardiac
sudden death, can be precipitated by an emotional disturbance.
More difficult it is to establish how often this does occur and to
translate delightful fireside anecdotal reports into more stringent
quantitatively controlled data.

Dreyfuss and his co-workers (19, 20) point out that stressful
life experiences of a crescendo type often precede myocardial
infarction, and similar data are reported by Pearson and Joseph
(21). In their experience more than half of the infarct episodes
in men as well as in women in a controlled study have followed
periods of such tension usually extending over a few weeks.

There are of course several ways through which emotional
stimuli can precipitate an acute coronary disturbance. Emotional-
ly-induced sympathetic activation can directly, or indirectly,
through catecholamine release, elicit tachycardia, increase
cardiac output, and augment arterial pressure, so increasing
volume and pressure loads to the myocardium. A mechanism
for a more enduring rise of blood pressure after emotion can be
surmised from recent work of our group, who has shown a con-
spicuous increase in renin release from the kidney during electrical stimulation of the so-called "defense area" in the hypothalamus
of the cat. Renin release may be thought to cause a lasting increase
in arterial pressure as well as salt and water retention, both effects being obviously detrimental to a failing myocardium.

Another mechanism by which emotional stimuli may precipitate an acute coronary disturbance, is a catecholamine-mediated
influence on blood coagulation. Emotional conditions, such as an
examination or leaving the hospital for home, have been found to
increase blood viscosity (23) and clotting time (24), to influence
fibrinolysis (25, 26), and to facilitate platelet aggregation (27).
Also electrical stimulation of the hypothalamus can increase
factor VIII in animals (28). Finally catecholamines are known to

release free fatty acids (29, 30), and these in turn have been found to increase the incidence of dangerous and sometimes fatal, cardiac arrhythmias (31). We only mention the possibility of neurally induced coronary vasomotor changes because this seems at the moment a rather remote possibility (see 32).

We have been left with the hypothesis that neural mechanisms, not necessarily tied with emotions, might be involved in precipitating the so-called spontaneous anginal attacks. A few years ago Guazzi et al (33, 34) performed a penetrating study of patients with Prinzmetal's variant angina pectoris, and described haemodynamic changes, such as bradycardia, decrease of cardiac output, and rise in right atrial pressure. However, in no anginal attack these haemodynamic modifications preceded the typical electrocardiographic alterations, and Guazzi et al, could rightly rule out that this form of angina is triggered by circulatory modifications which acutely increase cardiac work or oxygen requirements. What is the primary cause of both the electrocardiographic and haemodynamic changes remains unknown. The possibility that this cause consists in an altered neural discharge to the heart is attractive, of course, but is only very indirectly supported by the excellent therapeutic results obtained by admini- of a beta-adrenergic receptor blocking drug, propranolol (35). Quite recently, Maeri et al, have confirmed Guazzi's observations (36).

To sum up, neural involvement in causing the unknown sudden change responsible for Prinzmetal's angina, especially in those cases with an apparently intact coronary tree, is a very attractive hypothesis, but so far a totally undemonstrated assumption. Similar considerations can be made about the possibility of neural or catecholamine involvement in precipitation of those cases of myocardial infarction in which there is no anatomical evidence of acute thrombotic occlusion and whose immediate mechanism is unknown. It is now clear that these cases are far more frequent than previously deemed (37).

NEURAL AND PSYCHOLOGICAL FACTORS RESPONSIBLE FOR DEVELOPMENT OF CHRONIC CORONARY DISEASE

There are three fundamental approaches to this problem: epidemiological, psychological and physiological.

A first way of using epidemiology for assessing the respective
role of neural and non-neural factors in coronary disease, would
be an attempt to estimate what proportion of coronary disease
can be explained in terms of the currently recognized major risk
factors and how much remains to be accounted for by other factors
which might be mediated by the nervous system.   Among coronary
patients studied by Epstein (38), 85% did harbour at least one of
three major risk factors considered (elevation of blood lipids, of
blood pressure or excessive smoking).   However, it was also
found that 80% of the entire male population studied, and preva-
lently without coronary disease, showed evidence of at least one
risk factor.   It seems evident that the three risk factors considered cannot entirely explain the cases of coronary disease: something more is needed to turn a healthy person into a patient.   This
critical attitude does not indicate, of course, whether this "something more" is psychosocial stress, and whether it acts through
or independently of the other risk factors.

Some further insight comes from psychosociological and
psychoepidemiological studies.   The values of this approach are
self-evident.   The present limitations, however, are at least as
equally important, and mostly concern difficulties of methodology.
These not only consist of the difficulty of grasping the human mind
in a scientifically quantitative way, though more and more precise
methods are being suggested and used.   Difficulties also consist in
the need of very sophisticated, multi-layer designs of analytical
rather than descriptive epidemiology.   This brings up to current
trends of research.   Recent times have certainly seen a great
progress from anecdotal reports of controlled studies, with more
objective evaluation of behaviour, from consideration of an omni-
comprehensive "stress" to definition of selective behavioural
patterns or psychological traits, and finally and most importantly,
from retrospective to prospective studies (see 39).

Certainly, the most significant piece of work is the prospective study carried out by Friedman and Rosenman (40, 41) for more
than a decade on the coronary risk for patients displaying what
they defined the "coronary-prone behaviour pattern", or "type A
behaviour", that is a behavioural syndrome characterized by
extremes of competitiveness, striving for achievement, repressed
aggressiveness, haste, hyperalertness, explosiveness of speech,
tenseness of facial musculature, and feeling of being pressed by
time and challenged by responsibility.   In their Western Collabora-

tive Group Study they followed 3500 employees of eleven corpora-
tions for 8-1/2 years: men aged 39-49 years at intake, who had
the type A pattern, incurred 2. 7 times more coronary disease than
did men the same age without the coronary prone behaviour pattern
(type B). In the elder age decase, 50-59 years, type A men sustained 1. 7 times the coronary incidence of type B's. Epidemiological evidence in favour of type A as a risk factor is really impressive, although its correct definition in precise psychological
terms is open to some question (42).

How can physiological work help in clarifying the role of
neural mechanisms in the development of coronary disease? A
first way is the demonstration, both in animals and man, that
neural factors and emotions can influence some of the standard
risk factors of coronary disease. As far as lipids are concerned,
which are the main interest of this meeting, situations such as
examinations or other stressful experiences have been shown to
raise blood cholesterol (43-46) and triglycerides (47-49), and
Gunn et al. (50) have succeeded in producing experimental atherosclerosis in the rabbit by combining a high cholesterol diet with
chronic electrical stimulation of the hypothalamus. We have
already mentioned that catecholamines can release free fatty
acids (29, 30), and these can in turn lead to atheroma. I have
also summarized evidence about neural effects on blood clotting.
Finally, neural influences on arterial pressure, another risk
factor for atherosclerosis, are too well known (51).

Some recent physiological studies also provide evidence in
support of the claim that not just every kind of stress but specific
behaviours might be related to cardiovascular disease. A claim
like that of Rosenman and Friedman, must necessarily assume
that different types of behaviour are associated to neural and
hormonal manifestations at least differing in part.

Recent work from our group has shown that this was the case
for haemodynamics. Cardiovascular changes during the immobile
confrontation of a cat with another threatening cat are different
and even opposite in several respects to those occurring when
confrontation gives way to actual fighting (52-53). Immobile
confrontation is associated with bradycardia, decreased cardiac
output, decreased total peripheral resistance and marked con-
striction of muscle blood vessels, while all these variables change
to the opposite direction during fighting. Moreover, confrontation
with an aggressive dog or hunting a mouse can produce in the cat

opposite vasomotor effects on the limb circulation, as compared
with the effect of confrontation with another cat (54). Therefore,
different emotional behaviours possibly subserved by different
brain circuits can be accompanied by partly different haemodynamic manifestations.

On the hormonal side, some current work by Henry et al.
seems extremely promising. By extending their studies on
chronic psychosocial stimulation in colonies of mice (55), Henry
et al, (56) have observed that the chronic emotional arousal of
dominant males who had been aggressively striving for weeks to
establish their territory, was accompanied by a rise of blood
pressure and by a four-fold increase of medullary tyrosine hydroxylase (whose induction is determined by sympathetic activity),
while their plasma corticosterone and adrenal weights remained
near normal; therefore dominant mice showed a cardiovascular-
hormonal responses such as in Folkow's defence pattern (57),
and no signs of Seyle's stress reaction. By contrast, subordinate
males had unchanged blood pressure and tyrosine hydroxylase
levels, but there was approximately 50% increase of their plasma
corticosterone and their adrenal weights doubled; therefore they
showed evidence of a stress instead of a defence reaction. It is
also extremely interesting that in Henry's experiments socially
stimulated mice, besides developing high blood pressure, showed
elevated incidence of atherosclerosis (55).

There is some preliminary evidence that different hormonal
patterns may also occur during different types of emotional behaviour in man. Aggressive emotional situations seem to be
associated with predominant noradrenaline release, while a higher
adrenaline release seems to occur during passive emotions, like
fear (47, 57, 58). As noradrenaline seems to be a more effective
releaser of free fatty acids, these observations might have some
bearing on development of atheroma in Rosenman and Friedman's
coronary-prone aggressive type of behaviour.

CONCLUSIONS

By dissecting the problem of the relationships of neural and
psychological factors in coronary disease into a series of questions, we are now in a condition to provide some answers, a few
suggestions and a lot of further hypotheses.

To the question whether neural reflexes, some of which involving the emotional experience of cardiac pain, can occur upon coronary occlusion, we can answer a very definite yes; and we can also define most of the pathways and interrelationships involved, and suggest therapeutic measures to avoid dangerous complications.

To the question whether an acute coronary disturbance can be precipitated by emotional or neural factors, we can answer that there are single instances in which such a psychoneural cause of a myocardial infarction or of an anginal attack and even of sudden death seems very likely. But how often this does occur, this we cannot say at the moment.

To the final question about the primary cause of chronic coronary disease, we have only hints to offer and suggestions to develop, but hints are no longer so vague, and some of the suggestions are such as to lend themselves to experimental testing in the future. Furthermore, there is some experimental evidence as to how behavioural risk factors may interrelate with other risk factors, particularly hyperlipidemia and hypertension, in the development of atheroma and coronary disease.

REFERENCES

1. Malliani, A., Recordata, G., and Schwartz, P. J. J. Physiol. 212: 457, 1973

2. Brown, A. M. J. Physiol. 190: 35, 1967

3. Malliani, A., Schwartz, P. J. and Zanchetti, A. Am. J. Physiol. 217: 703, 1969

4. Brown, A. M. and Malliani, A. J. Physiol. 212: 685, 1971

5. Malliani, A., Peterson, D. F., Bishop, V. S. and Brown, A. M. Circulation Res. 30: 158, 1972

6. Malliani, A., Parks, M., Tuckett, R. P. and Brown, A. M. Circulation Res. 32: 9, 1973

7. Costantin, L. L. Am. J. Cardiol. 11: 205, 1963

8. Dokukin, A. V. Fed. Proc. Transl. Suppl. 23: T296, 1964

9. Schwartz, P. J. , Pagani, M. , Lombardi, F. , Malliani, A.
    and Brown, A. M. Circulation Res. 32: 215, 1973

10. Bezold, A. , Von, and Hirt, L. Untersuch. Physiol. Lab.
    Wurzburg 1: 73, 1967

11. Jarisch, A. and Zotterman, Y. Acta Physiol. Scand. 16:
    31, 1948

12. Cox, W V and Robertson, H F. Am. Heart J. 12: 285,
    1936

13. Schauer, G. , Gross, L. and Blum, L. Am. Heart J. 14:
    669, 1937

14. Gillis, R A   Am. Heart J. 81: 677, 1971

15. Valori, C. , Thomas, M and Shillingford, J. P. Am. J.
    Cardiol. 20: 605, 1967

16. Jewitt, D. E. , Mercer, C. J., Reid, D , Valori, C. , Thomas,
    M. , and Shillingford, J P. Lancet 1: 635, 1969

17. Jewitt, D. E. , Mercer, C. J. and Shillingford, J. P. Lancet
    2: 227, 1969

18. Webb, S. W. , Adgey, A A. J and Pantridge, J. F   Brit.
    Med. J. 3: 89, 1969

19. Dreyfuss, F. and Abramov, A. Cardiovascular Regulation,
    C. Bartorelli and A Zanchetti (Eds.), Milan, Cardiovascu-
    lar Research Institute, 1971, pp. 209-211

20. Dreyfuss, F. Neural and Psychological Mechanisms in
    Cardiovascular Disease, A. Zanchetti (Ed.), Il Ponte, Milan,
    1972, pp 109-117

21. Pearson, E. H. and Joseph, J. Lancet 1: 415, 1963

22. Zanchetti, A. and Stella, A. 80. Tagung. Dtsch. Ges. inn.
    Med , Wiesbaden, 1974, Bergmann, in press

23. Schneider, R. A. Life Stress and Bodily Disease. Baltimore, Williams and Wilkins, 1950, vol. 29, pp. 818-831

24. Dreyfuss, F. J. Psychosom. Res. 1: 252, 1956

25. Ogston, D., McDonald, G. A. and Fullerton, H. W. Lancet 2: 521, 1962

26. Cash, J. D and Allan, A. G. E. Brit. Med. J. 2: 545, 1967

27. Zahavi, J. and Dreyfuss, F. II Congr. Int. Soc. Thrombosis Hemostasis, Oslo, 1971

28. Gunn, C. G. and Hampton, J. W. Am. J. Physiol. 212: 124, 1967

29. Himms-Hagen, J. Pharmacol. Rev. 19: 367, 1967

30. Ostman, J. and Effendic, S. Acta med. scand. 187: 471, 1970

31. Oliver, M. F., Kurien, V. A. and Greenwood, T. W. Lancet 1: 710, 1968

32. Zanchetti, A. and Malliani, A. Causes and Prevention of Coronary Disease, in press

33. Guazzi, M., Polese, A., Fiorentini, C., Magrini, F. and Bartorelli, C. Brit. Heart J. 33: 84, 1971

34. Guazzi, M., Polese, A., Fiorentini, C., Magrini, F. and Bartorelli, C. Cardiovascular Regulation, C. Bartorelli and A. Zanchetti (Eds.), Cardiovascular Research Institute, Milan, 1971, pp. 245-255

35. Guazzi, M., Magrini, F., Fiorentini, C. and Polese, A. Brit. Heart J. 33: 889, 1971

36. Maseri, A., Pesola, A., Contini, C., Chierchia, S., Marchesi, C., Mimmo, R. and Parodi, O. Europ. J. Clin. Invest. 4: 1974, in press

37. Baroldi, G., Radice, F., Schmid, G. and Leone, A. Am. Heart J. 87: 65, 1974

38. Epstein, F. H. Neural and Psychological Mechanisms in
    Cardiovascular Disease. A. Zanchetti (Ed.), Il Ponte,
    Milan, 1972, pp. 85-92

39. Neural and Psychological Mechanisms in Cardiovascular
    Disease. A. Zanchetti (Ed.), Il Ponte, Milan, 1972, pp.
    1-137

40. Rosenman, R. H. , Friedman, M. and Straus, A. J. A. M. A
    189: 15, 1964

41. Rosenman, R. H. , Friedman, M. Straus, R. , Jenkins, C. D. ,
    Zyzanski, S. and Wurm, M. J. Chron. Dis. 23: 173, 1970

42. Mertens, C. and Segers, M. -J. Neural and Psychological
    Mechanisms in Cardiovascular Disease. A. Zanchetti (Ed.),
    Il Ponte, Milan, 1972, pp. 285-296

43. Thomas, C. B. and Paasikivi, J. J. Psychosom. Res. 15:
    25, 1971

44. Grundy, S. M. and Griffin, C. A. J. A. M. A. 171: 1794, 1959

45. Dreyfuss, F. and Czaczkes, J. W. Arch. Int. Med. 103:
    708, 1959

46. Wolf, S , McCabe, W. R. , Yamamoto, J. , Adsett, C. A. and
    Schottstaedt, W. W. Circulation 26: 379, 1962

47 Taggart, P. and Carruthers, M. Lancet 1: 363, 1971

48. Taggart, P. , Carruthers, M. and Sommerville, W. Lancet
    2: 341, 1973

49. Schwartz, D. and Patois, E. J. Atheroscler. Res. 7: 537,
    1967

50. Gunn, C. G. , Friedman, M. and Byers, S. O. J. Clin.
    Invest. 39, 1963, 1960

51. Zanchetti, A. Neural and Psychological Mechanisms in
    Cardiovascular Disease. A. Zanchetti (Ed.), Il Ponte,
    Milan, 1972, pp. 15-31

52. Adams, D. B. , Baccelli, G. , Mancia, G. , and Zanchetti, A
     Nature 220: 1239, 1968

53. Adams, D. B. , Baccelli, G, , Mancia, G, , and Zanchetti, A.
     J. Physiol. 212: 321, 1971

54. Zanchetti, A. , Baccelli, G. , Mancia, G. , and Ellison, G. D.
     Physiology, Emotion and Psychosomatic Illness. Ciba
     Foundation Symp. 8, Associated Scientific Publishers,
     Amsterdam, 1972, pp. 201-223

55. Henry, J. P. , Ely, D. L. , and Stephens, P. M. Neural and
     Psychological Mechanisms in Cardiovascular Disease.
     A. Zanchetti (Ed.), Il Ponte, Milan, 1972, pp. 211-223

56. Henry, J. P. , Ely, D. L. and Stephens, P. M. 80, Tagung
     Dtsch. Ges. inn. Med. , Wiesbaden, 1974, in press

57. Taggart, P. , Carruthers, M. and Somerville, W. Symposium
     on Beta-Blockers, in press

58. Levi, L. Society, Stress and Disease. Oxford University
     Press, 1971

Animal Models for
Atherosclerosis Research

NEW ANIMAL MODEL FOR ATHEROSCLEROSIS RESEARCH

Charles E. Day and Walter W. Stafford

Diabetes and Atherosclerosis Research, The Upjohn
Company, Kalamazoo, Michigan

SUMMARY

Japanese quail were investigated for their utility as a model
for the discovery and evaluation of anti-atherosclerosis compounds.
Although they possessed suitable characteristics for a screening
animal, their development of atherosclerosis was too variable
to make them a practical model. A search was conducted to find
a means to make quail uniformly atherosclerotic. To this end a
line of quail susceptible to experimental atherosclerosis (SEA)
were selectively bred. Thus, the SEA Japanese quail is a new
animal model for atherosclerosis research.

INTRODUCTION

Animal models suitable for use in pharmaceutical discovery
and evaluation must meet more stringent requirements than models
used for basic research. Most drug discoveries result from random screening of organic compounds in a suitable test system.
Generally the success rate is quite low, so large numbers (thousands)
of compounds must be screened. If a whole animal is used for
screening, then several immediate considerations are apparent.
The animal must be readily available, inexpensive, and small. In
addition, it should be easy to maintain, dose, and handle routinely.
Rats and especially mice fit these requirements almost ideally.
This is in no small part why mice and rats are the number one and
two animals used in biomedical research in the pharmaceutical
industry.

Mice can be mass produced quite inexpensively. For example,
The Upjohn Company alone produces over one half million per year.
If 10 mice, 30g each are placed on a test compound for 1 week at
a screening dose of 50 mg/kg/day, then approximately 100 mg of
compound is needed for the test. Housing space and labor for
mouse maintenance are minimal. This example serves to illustrate
the good economic sense that an animal with the characteristics
of a mouse makes for drug screening operations.

Unfortunately, both rats and mice are very poor models for
atherosclerosis. They generally have low serum cholesterol and
extremely diminuitive low density lipoprotein (LDL). They also
are quite resistant to the development of atherosclerotic lesions.
Animals that do develop atherosclerosis, such as rabbits, chickens,
monkeys, and pigeons are too big and/or too expensive to use for
screening of anti-atherosclerotic agents.

About 2 years ago atherosclerosis development in Japanese
quail was reported (1), and subsequently confirmed by other investigators (2, 3). Japanese quail (Coturnix coturnix japonica)
are small (approximately 100g), hardy animals that can be rapidly
and inexpensively mass produced. In addition they can be easily
handled, dosed, bled, and maintained. For these reasons we
turned our attention to the utility of these animals for a screening
model for anti-atherosclerotic agents over 2 years ago. This
report deals largely with our experience with development of
coturnix as an atherosclerosis screening model.

MATERIALS AND METHODS

Japanese quail were obtained from a closed stock colony maintained at The Upjohn Company. This colony was derived from stock
obtained from 4 separate university colonies maintained in the
U. S. A. We originally fed a standard chicken mash diet (4). The
standard maintenance is now Purina Game Bird Startena[R] or Game
Bird Layena[R]. Data in this report are from animals fed the chicken
mash diet. For cholesterol feeding experiments crystalline
cholesterol is normally fed at a level of 2% in the ground diet. To
induce atherosclerosis birds are commonly placed on cholesterol
diet for 15 weeks. At the end of each experimental period birds are
bled via the right jugular vein. Up to 2 ml can be drawn without
apparent injury to the animal. The maximum amount that can be

obtained is 4 to 5 ml from each bird.   At this level the mortality
rate is fairly high.   The animal is decapitated, and the thoracic
aorta and brachiocephalic and subclavian arteries (just after the
first branch point) are removed as one piece.   The arteries are
placed in physiological saline, cleaned, opened longitudinally, and
scored for gross atherosclerotic lesions by three independent
observers on a scale of 0 to 100.   After blotting, the arteries are
weighed and then homogenized in a combination tissue grinder and
screw cap test tube with 0. 5 ml redistilled isopropanol.   After
grinding, 5. 0 ml isopropanol is added.   Tubes are capped, shaken,
and allowed to extract overnight at room temperature.   Cholesterol
concentration is then determined in the isopropanol extract by an
automated $FeCl_3$ method (5).

Male British Range, English White, Tuxedo, Manchurian
Golden, and Pharaoh D1 strains of Japanese quail were purchased
from Marsh Farms, Garden Grove, California 92643.   All quail
rearing and breeding equipment was purchased from either Marsh
Farms or C. Q. F. Manufacturing Company, Savannah, Georgia
31402.   Both cockerel and porcine aortic elastins were prepared
according to the method of Kramsch, Franzblau, and Hollander
(6).   Elastin was suspended in complete Freund's adjuvant and
injected subcutaneously at 5 separate sites (nape of neck, under
each wing, and on both sides of cloaca) with a total of 3 injections
given over a period of 6 weeks.

RESULTS AND DISCUSSION

From our initial studies with coturnix one fact was quite
apparent.   Fewer than half of a given population from our stock
colony developed atherosclerotic lesions in response to dietary
cholesterol (For example see F_0 data in Table V).   In birds in
which gross atherosclerosis was detectable, the extent of lesions
was highly variable, ranging from <1% surface area involvement
to virtually 100%.   A few male quail (approximately 10%) developed
severe atherosclerosis with almost total occlusion of major arteries
exiting from the heart.   Because of the high variance of lesions
quail from our stock colony were not suitable for evaluating anti-
atherosclerosis agents.   It was necessary then to develop a method
to make the animals uniformly atherosclerotic.

Table I

EFFECT OF SEVERAL ATHEROSCLEROTIC COMPOUNDS IN JAPANESE QUAIL

TREATMENT	INCIDENCE OF ATHEROSCLEROSIS	AORTIC ATHEROSCLEROSIS SCORE	AORTIC CHOLESTEROL (mg/g)	SERUM CHOLESTEROL (mg/dl)	WEIGHT CHANGE (g)
CONTROL	0/8	1.0	1.85	706	0.6
NEGATIVE CONTROL (NO CHOLESTEROL)	0/9	1.0	1.22	230*	1.0
10% COCONUT OIL	1/8	1.2	2.04·	450	5.4
0.05% THIOURACIL	2/8	2.1	2.09	1221	3.2
0.5% CHOLIC ACID	5/7	13.2*	4.31	1528*	-0.3
0.05% THIOURACIL + 0.5 % CHOLIC ACID	4/7	3.7	2.40	2163*	3.0
0.05% DESOXYPYRIDOXINE	0/7	1.0	1.59	665	-4.4
0.2% SUDAN IV	7/9	11.3*	2.28	964	0.4
1% CHOLESTANOL	2/9	2.4	1.84	513	-1.3
1% CHOLESTANOL (NO CHOLESTEROL)	0/9	1.0	1.28	282*	-1.3
POOLED % STANDARD DEVIATION		122	62	53	

*SIGNIFICANTLY DIFFERENT FROM CONTROL (P ≤ 0.05)

To accomplish the desired objective, we initiated a three-pronged approach to the problem. One possible solution was enhancement of atherosclerosis by chemical induction. Ideally this method would be one by which the diet could be modified in such a way as to produce extensive and uniform lesions. Time consuming methodologies, such as surgical procedures, were ruled out since disease had to be produced in hundreds of animals. Results on a few of the compounds tried in cholesterol fed quail are listed in Tables I and II. Only cholic acid, at a level of 0.5-1.0% in the diet, consistently produced a significant increase in the atherosclerosis score. This increase was primarily in the brachiocephalic artery (Table II). In one experiment quail immunized with porcine aortic elastin at 4 mg/kg had a significant elevation in their brachiocephic atherosclerosis score. No attempt was made to confirm this observation since the immunization procedure was too time consuming to make it suitable as a routine technique for inducing atherosclerosis in large numbers of animals.

Table II

EFFECT OF ATHEROSCLEROTIC COMPOUNDS IN JAPANESE QUAIL

TREATMENT	INCIDENCE OF ATHEROSCLEROSIS			ATHEROSCLEROSIS SCORE			ARTERIAL CHOLESTEROL (mg/g)	SERUM CHOLESTEROL (mg/dl)
	AORTA	BRACHIO-CEPHALIC	SUB-CLAVIAN	AORTIC	BRACHIO-CEPHALIC	SUB-CLAVIAN		
CONTROL	4/13	4/13	3/13	3.1	3.3	2.7	2.46	653
0.5% CHOLIC ACID	5/14	14/14	12/14	2.6	20.0*	15.1*	2.49	907
1.0% CHOLIC ACID	9/15	14/15	13/15	7.2	27.8*	16.5*	4.15	1486*
0.5% CHOLIC ACID + 0.2% SUDAN IV	9/13	11/13	11/13	13.3	30.6*	22.7*	4.02	1204*
0.2% SUDAN IV	9/15	12/15	11/15	3.9	8.2	7.2	2.46	470
COCKEREL ELASTIN S.C.	8/15	7/15	7/15	3.4	5.0	3.7	2.08	767
PORCINE AORTIC ELASTIN S.C. (4 mg/kg)	5/6	6/6	6/6	11.4	28.2*	18.0	3.60	1825*
PORCINE AORTIC ELASTIN S.C. (40mg/kg)	1/7	4/7	0/7	1.2	2.3	1.0	3.06	628
1% PARAFFIN	7/18	12/18	7/18	2.8	6.7	4.1	2.21	548

* SIGNIFICANTLY DIFFERENT FROM CONTROL (P ≤ 0.05)

A second approach to finding uniform atherosclerosis in quail was to examine the different strains or stocks of birds that were readily available. We placed 5 different strains - British Range (black), English White, Manchurian Golden, Tuxedo (black and white) and Pharaoh D1 - on a cholesterol diet and examined birds for gross atherosclerosis, arterial cholesterol, and serum cholesterol. No strain was more susceptible to atherosclerosis than were our stock colony birds (Table III). One strain, Tuxedo, appeared to be more resistant to atherosclerosis than our stock animals. Both gross atherosclerosis and arterial cholesterol were significantly reduced when compared to controls. No atherosclerosis has been seen in any animal that has not been on a cholesterol diet (Table IV). The investigation of different quail strains was not a fruitful approach.

Table III

STRAIN DIFFERENCES IN ATHEROSCLEROSIS DATA IN CHOLESTEROL FED JAPANESE QUAIL

STRAIN	INCIDENCE OF AORTIC ATHERO-SCLEROSIS (o/o)	AORTIC ATHERO-SCLEROSIS SCORE	ARTERIAL CHOLESTEROL (mg/g)	SERUM CHOLESTEROL (mg/dl)
STOCK	48 (20/42)	5.9	3.73	967
BRITISH RANGE	56 (10/18)	4.2	2.20	874
ENGLISH WHITE	50 (9/18)	4.2	2.21	774
MANCHURIAN GOLDEN	54 (6/11)	2.8	2.08	584
TUXEDO	9 (1/11)	1.1*	1.54*	585
PHAROAH DI	30 (3/10)	1.6	2.38	716
OHIO STATE	21 (3/14)	1.9	1.78*	669

† DATA TRANSFORMED TO LOGARITHMS AND EXPRESSED AS ANTI-LOG MEANS

* SIGNIFICANTLY DIFFERENT FROM STOCK COLONY (P< .05)

Table IV

STRAIN DIFFERENCES IN CONTROL JAPANESE QUAIL

STRAIN	INCIDENCE OF ATHERO-SCLEROSIS (o/o)	ATHERO-SCLEROSIS SCORE	ARTERIAL CHOLESTEROL (mg/g)	SERUM CHOLESTEROL (mg/dl)
BRITISH RANGE	0 (0/6)	0	1.17	259
ENGLISH WHITE	0 (0/7)	0	1.10	254
MANCHURIAN GOLDEN	0 (0/8)	0	1.19	263
TUXEDO	0 (0/4)	0	1.11	296
PHAROAH DI	0 (0/7)	0	1.37	314

Table V

SUMMARY OF ATHEROSCLEROSIS DATA
ON JAPANESE QUAIL

GROUP	GENE-RATION	INCIDENCE OF AORTIC ATHERO-SCLEROSIS (%)	AORTIC ATHERO-SCLEROSIS SCORE	ARTERIAL CHOLESTEROL (mg/g)	SERUM CHOLESTEROL (mg/dl)
STOCK	F0	44 (34/77)	21	5.45	886
SEA	F1	73 (45/62)	35	6.05	785
REA	F1	16 (4/25)	3	1.92	357

Table VI

SEX DIFFERENCES IN ATHEROSCLEROSIS DATA
FROM JAPANESE QUAIL

GROUP	GENE-RATION	SEX	INCIDENCE OF AORTIC ATHEROSCLEROSIS (%)	AORTIC ATHEROSCLEROSIS SCORE	ARTERIAL CHOLESTEROL (mg/g)	SERUM CHOLESTEROL (mg/dl)
STOCK	F0	MALE	48 (20/42)	29	6.29	1205
STOCK	F0	FEMALE	40 (14/35)	12	4.43	505
SEA	F1	MALE	68 (21/31)	41	7.35	1195
SEA	F1	FEMALE	77 (24/31)	29	4.79	375
REA	F1	MALE	17 (2/12)	4	1.63	488
REA	F1	FEMALE	15 (2/13)	1	2.19	235

Our third approach to the problem of developing uniformly atherosclerotic quail was selective breeding. We randomly paired a colony of our stock animals, placed them on a cholesterol diet, and reared offspring from each pair. After 15 weeks on cholesterol the parents were sacrificed, and their aortas examined and graded for atherosclerosis. Offspring from parents with high atherosclerosis scores were selected for one line. The birds were designated as Susceptible to Experimental Atherosclerosis (SEA). One pair had no atherosclerosis and low arterial and serum cholesterol. Its offspring were selected for a second line designated Resistant to Experimental Atherosclerosis (REA). Brother-sister matings were made for each line, and the rearing procedure described above repeated. From a summary of data on the first generation of selective breeding (Table V), it can be seen that a segregation was achieved in this generation. There was a significant different between SEA and REA in atherosclerosis score, arterial cholesterol and serum cholesterol. Although the incidence of atherosclerosis for both male and female are about the same, the lesions in male animals tend to be more severe (Table VI). Serum cholesterol levels are also higher for males. It is interesting to note that the data for male REA is virtually identical to the male Tuxedo quail data (Table VII).

We measured a number of serum chemistry values on SEA and REA quail. The only consistent difference was serum alkaline phosphatase levels. Alkaline phosphatase was significantly less in SEA when compared to REA quail. However, this finding may have no physiological significance since it is quite probable that aortic atherosclerosis and alkaline phosphatase were independently co-selected.

Our breeding program with SEA and REA quail is continuing now into the fourth generation. Although there are still problems to be resolved, the SEA quail could prove to be a valuable tool for anti-atherosclerosis drug discovery.

REFERENCES

1. A. D. Ojerio, G. J. Pucak, T. B. Clarkson and B. C. Bullock. Lab. Animal Sci. 22: 33-39, 1972.

2. R. C. Bayer, R. K. Ringer and E. A. Cogger. Poultry Sci. 51: 925-929, 1972.

3. R. L. Smith and D. M. Hilker. Atherosclerosis 17: 63-70, 1973.

4. D. M. Tennent, H. Siegel, G. W. Kuron, W. H. Ott, and C. W. Mushett. Proc. Soc. Exptl. Biol. Med. 96: 679-683, 1957.

5. W. D. Block, K. J. Jarrett, and J. B. Levine. In: Automation in Analytical Chemistry, ed. by L. T. Skeggs, Mediad Incorporated, New York, 1966, pp. 345-347.

6. D. M. Kramsch, C. Franzblau and W. Hollander. J. Clin. Invest. 50: 1666-1677, 1971.

EFFECTS OF VARIOUS HYPOLIPIDEMIC DRUGS ON FATTY

ACID COMPOSITION OF LIVER AND SERUM LIPIDS

Rene Maier and Klaus Muller

Research Department, Pharmaceuticals Division,
CIBA-GEIGY Ltd., CH-4002 Basel, Switzerland

Despite the extended clinical application hypolipidemic drugs have experienced in the last years, very little hard facts have become known on their mechanism of action. At present drugs belonging to only a few chemical structures are or were in use, namely,

- the arloxy fatty acids;
- the derivatives of nicotinic acid;
- the thyronines;
- cholesterol and bile acid sequestrants;
- and, most recently, compounds with antioxidant properties.

From large scale studies on patients with and without hyperlipidemia we have learned to recognize more or less beneficial effects of these drugs.

Concerning the mode of action most attention has been attributed to changes in circulating lipids and their lipid classes, but only little attention has been given to the fatty acid composition of these fractions. More than ten years ago Jurand and Oliver (1) observed in serum lipids of patients with ischaemic heart disease after treatment with clofibrate an increase in oleic acid and a decrease in linoleic acid content in the cholesterol esters and phosphatides, but hardly any change in the triglycerides. Similar observations were reported by Berry et al (2) and some years later also by Hagopian and Robinson (3).

In order to further investigate this shift in certain fatty acids of the ester fractions we undertook a study on rats with the followin compounds: clofibrate, C 13437-Su, also known as Nafenopine, L-thyroxine and nicotinic acid. The first two drugs mentioned belong to the group of aryloxy fatty acids.

EXPERIMENTAL

In our experiments we used male albino rats of about 220 g body weight. They were treated once daily over a period of 14 days. All drugs were dispersed in polyethylene glycol or water and administered orally by stomach tube, except L-thyroxine which was injected subcutaneously. Until sacrifice the animals were kept on normal diet and under controlled lighting conditions. The rats were bled from the carotid artery under light ether anaesthesia. Serum and organs were extracted according to the procedure of Folch et al (4). The total lipid extract was subjected to column chromatography to be separated into lipid classes. Their fatty acid composition was determined by gas liquid chromatography.

The doses of the drugs were chosen in such a way that they either elicited maximal or near maximal hypolipidemic effects or to warrant good tolerance during the 14 days of treatment.

RESULTS

Table 1 shows the effect of Nafenopine (C 13437-Su), L-thyroxine (L-T_4) and nicotinic acid (NA) on liver wet-weight, total lipids and percent lipid classes after 10 days of daily treatment.

The aryloxy acids showed the well-known hepatomegalic effect, which is absent after L-thyroxine and nicotinic acid. The lipid content in increased after the aryloxy acid although not to the same extent as the livers enlarged. Thyroxine and nicotinic acid treatment had no effect on total liver lipids. None of the drugs had any effect on the cholesterol ester fraction which is anyhow only a few percent. On triglycerides, however, the aryloxy acids elicited a decrease which was made up for by the phospholipid fraction. The two remaining drugs did not change the distribution of lipid classes.

Table 1 - Liver Lipids

	N	Dose mg/kg	Route	wet-weight in g	Lipid Extract in mg	Lipid Classes in % of total lipids		
						CE	TG	PL
Controls	10	-	-	7.7 $\pm$ 0.2*	362 $\pm$ 22	2	21	74
C 13437-Su	10	100	p.o.	17.2 $\pm$ 0.6	569 $\pm$ 40	2	9	89
L-T$_4$	10	0.3	s.c.	8.4 $\pm$ 0.3	380 $\pm$ 15	2	23	74
NA	10	300	p.o.	11.4 $\pm$ 0.3	380 $\pm$ 22	2	20	79

* Standard error of the mean

In Table 2 the fatty acid composition of liver lipid classes is shown. In cholesterol esters (CE) the palmitic acid (16:0) content was reduced after clofibrate and slightly elevated after L-thyroxine. Oleic acid (18:1) concentration was substantially increased and that of linoleic acid (18:2) much reduced after both aryloxy acids. The two other drugs did not show this effect. A similar overall picture was observed in the triglyceride fraction. Palmitic acid remained uninfluenced by all drugs, except of L-thyroxine, but oleic acid content was augmented drastically after Clofibrate and Nafenopine. Linoleic acid concentration was reduced after all drugs, but most pronounced by the aryloxy acids.

The phospholipid fraction showed the same general trend, although the changes were less marked. Palmitic acid remained unchanged, but oleic acid content increased after the aryloxy acids, L-thyroxine and nicotinic acid showed no effect. Very little influence on linoleic acid concentration was seen after all drugs.

As expected the serum lipids closely followed those of liver. In Table 3 the lipid classes are shown as percent of total serum lipids and the composition of the major fatty acids thereof. Both Clofibrate and Nafenopine increased the cholesterol ester and lowered the triglyceride content. Phospholipids remained unaltered. Palmitic acid content stayed constant in all lipid classes after Clofibrate and Nafenopine. Oleic acid concentrations, however, were clearly increased in cholesterol esters and triglycerides and somewhat less pronounced in phospholipids. Linoleic

Table 2

Percent composition of major fatty acids in liver lipid classes.

	Dose mg/kg	Route	Cholesterol esters			Triglycerides			Phospholipids		
			16:0	18:1	18:2	16:0	18:1	18:2	16:0	18:1	18:2
Controls			28.6 ±3.4	26.2 ±2.5	25.7 ±2.1	33.8 ±0.9	26.7 ±0.4	34.7 ±1.3	31.8 ±1.2	7.6 ±0.7	18.5 ±0.8
Clofibrate	300	p.o.	17.6 ±1.7	48.9 ±2.3	14.4 ±0.9	31.4 ±1.7	53.1 ±2.9	15.3 ±3.2	31.2 ±1.5	13.8 ±1.4	16.4 ±0.7
C 13437-Su	100	p.o.	25.8 ±2.8	37.7 ±3.0	11.2 ±1.4	30.4 ±0.7	50.8 ±0.9	10.9 ±1.0	30.1 ±1.4	15.2 ±0.4	12.8 ±0.6
L-T$_4$	0.3	s.c.	33.1 ±0.8	18.2 ±3.4	27.1 ±3.9	44.5 ±3.5	23.4 ±1.8	23.8 ±2.3	31.9 ±3.1	6.7 ±0.4	16.3 ±2.1
NA	300	p.o.	25.1 ±0.6	27.7 ±1.5	31.7 ±1.3	36.5 ±1.0	27.2 ±0.2	27.7 ±0.1	31.8 ±3.4	7.7 ±0.3	20.2 ±0.7

Each value is composed of 4-7 determinations ± SEM.

acid concentrations weren't much reduced in cholesterol esters and phospholipids and somewhat more in the triglyceride fraction. In order to find out whether this shift in fatty acid composition is only a phenomenon elicited by fairly large doses we performed a dose-response relation with Nafenopine. In Figure 1 the concentrations of oleic and linoleic acid of liver and serum triglycerides are shown. Both fatty acids are altered in a linear relationship to the dose of the drug. A significant change occurs with a dose of 10 mg/kg and more, coinciding with the lowest effective dose in respect of its hypolipidemic effect on serum triglycerides.

In an attempt to determine how quickly the changes in fatty acid composition are achieved, rats were treated with a fixed dose of 100 mg/kg of Nafenopine for various periods of time. Table 4 shows the time-course of oleic and linoleic acid content of the liver and serum lipid classes. In cholesterol esters of both liver and serum lipids oleic acid content started to rise immediately after the beginning of treatment up to the fourth day, thereafter no further increase occurred. Similarly the linoleic acid content

Table 3 - Serum Lipids

	Dose mg/kg	Route	Lipid classes in % of total lipids			Fatty acid composition in % of								
			CE	TG	PL	CE			TG			PL		
						16:0	18:1	18:2	16:0	18:1	18:2	16:0	18:1	18:2
Controls	-		8.9	50.0	34.7	14.1	10.1	35.5	26.3	30.5	37.0	31.6	13.9	18.9
Clofibrate	100	p.o.	22.6	36.2	41.3	15.3	19.1	37.4	24.7	42.7	31.9	39.9	14.8	20.4
C 13437-Su	10	p.o.	25.3	38.1	39.2	14.0	20.0	28.5	23.0	37.8	26.9	29.9	20.7	15.4

Values are the mean of three pools from 3-4 rats.

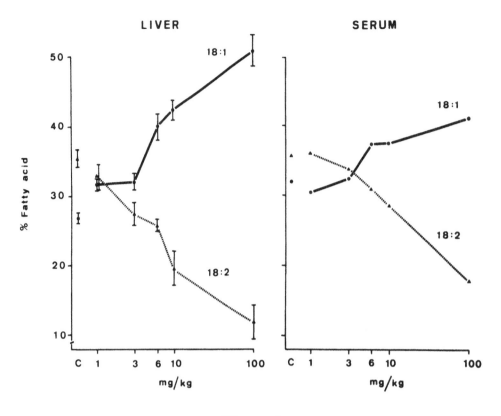

Figure 1

dropped during the first 4 days of treatment and attained thereafter a plateau at this reduced value.   Of the residual fatty acids not
shown, palmitic acid was reduced by about 20% while stearate and
arachidonate remained fairly constant.

A similar overall picture was found in the triglyceride fraction.
Oleic acid content rose up to the fourth day and that of linoleic
acid decreased within the same period of time.   No change was seen
in palmitic and palmitoleic acid concentrations.

In the phospholipid fraction oleic acid content is also increased
and that of linoleic acid decreased, although less marked as e. g. ,
in the triglycerides.   It is interesting to note that the shift in the
content of oleic and linoleic acid starts simultaneously with the
beginning of the treatment and reaches a new steady state from
the fourth day on, although enlargement and fat content of the liver
is by no means settled by this time.

Table 4 - Time-course of changes in oleic and linoleic acids
content after 100 mg/kg Nafenopine

	Days of treatment	CE		TG		PL	
		18:1	18:2	18:1	18:2	18:1	18:2
Liver	0	15.4	13.6	35.3	24.7	3.4	17.6
	2	24.4	10.6	40.3	19.3	7.0	12.8
	4	29.2	7.8	51.0	12.9	8.4	12.8
	6	23.4	8.0	42.3	10.7	9.4	10.4
	8	25.2	6.9	50.4	13.7	7.1	10.4
	10	27.4	8.1	48.3	8.9	9.0	11.3
Serum	0	10.5	35.1	35.0	31.6	9.7	27.9
	2	19.2	33.5	37.8	27.4	14.7	23.1
	4	22.7	27.0	50.4	18.5	18.4	23.9
	6	25.4	27.5	53.6	16.3	16.8	18.5
	8	18.7	27.8	52.1	17.2	15.1	24.8
	10	21.6	29.6	50.5	21.2	16.9	16.1

Each value represents the mean of 4-7 determinations.

DISCUSSION

These results show that drugs of aryloxy acid structure induce
a change in fatty acid composition, which occurs quickly and
reaches soon a new steady state. In contradiction to others we
found this shift in oleic and linoleic acid content most pronounced
in the triglycerides and cholesterol esters and somewhat less in
the phospholipids of both serum and liver lipids. In an attempt to
interpret this phenomenon the following points might be considered:

- A reduced absorption of linoleic acid from the gut;
- An enhanced catabolism of linoleic acid in liver or
  periphery;
- An increased incorporation of linoleic acid into adipose
  tissue or structural units such as membranes;
- or, since we measured only fatty acids in esterified form,
  a reduced esterification rate in liver.

In order to shed some light on these possibilities the following preliminary experiments were performed:

Table 5 - Effect of C 13437-Su on major fatty acids

		16:0	18:1	18:2
Epididymal Fat	Controls	30.2 ± 0.8	31.0 ± 0.4	29.3 ± 0.7
	C 13437-Su	27.5 ± 0.7	33.9 ± 0.4	29.6 ± 0.7
Liver Triglyceride	Controls	33.6 ± 1.3	27.4 ± 0.8	30.0 ± 2.6
	C 13437-Su	33.9 ± 2.8	44.9 ± 2.7	13.2 ± 1.9

Concerning absorption from gut the thoracic duct lymph was collected from rats treated with 100 mg/kg Nafenopine daily for 14 days and from untreated controls after a challenge of cotton seed oil. The drug elicited no change in the percent composition of either fatty acid.

Carboxyl-labelled palmitic and linoleic acid were converted to $^{14}CO_2$ to the same extent by rats treated with Nafenopine over a period of 14 days. Although these findings do not strictly preclude a greater oxidation of linoleic acid in liver, it seems rather unlikely to happen.

Preferential deposition of linoleic acid in adipose tissue does not occur as shown in Table 5.

Treatment with 100 mg/kg Nafenopine for 14 days did not change the percent composition of these three major fatty acids as compared to the controls. In the triglycerides of liver lipids of the same rats, however, the shift in oleic and linoleic acid is quite extensive.

Obviously, none of the suggested points seems to offer a clue to the mechanism by which this altered fatty acid composition comes about. Moreover, it is not known whether this shift is a bad or a beneficial effect in view of the therapeutic value of these drugs. Bearing in mind that polyunsaturated fatty acids are known to exert advantageous effects on serum lipids one could speculate that these drugs operate, at least in part, via the same unknown mechanism as polyunsaturated fatty acids.

SUMMARY

1. Treatment of rats with hypolipidemic drugs elicited an increase in oleic and a decrease in linoleic acid content in cholesterol esters, triglycerides and phospholipids of serum and liver lipids.

2. The change was most pronounced in triglycerides followed by cholesterol esters and phospholipids.

3. The shift was dose-dependent, starting with doses eliciting hypolipidemic effects.

4. The shift became obvious immediately after beginning of treatment and reached after 4 days a new steady state.

5. This effect was shared by both drugs of aryloxy fatty acid structure, but was not seen with either L-thyroxine or nicotinic acid.

6. The mechanism underlying this phenomenon is thus far unknown, but in our view it merits further attention.

REFERENCES

1. J. Jurand and M. F. Oliver. J. Atheroscler. Res. 3: 547, 1963.
2. C. Berry, A. Moxham, E. Smith, A. E. Kellie and J. D. N. Nabarro. J. Atheroscler. Res. 3: 380, 1963.
3. M. Hagopian and R. W. Robinson. J. Atheroscler. Res. 8: 21, 1968.
4. J. Folch, H. Lees and G. H. Sloane Stanley. J. Biol. Chem. 226: 497, 1957.

SOME ASPECTS OF THE CHIMPANZEE AS A MODEL FOR EXPERIMENTAL ATHEROSCLEROSIS

M. Vastesaeger[1], H. Peeters[2], V. Blaton[2],
C. Petrovas[3], and J. Mortelmans[4]

[1]- Professor of Social Cardiology, University of
Brussels, Belgium; [2]- Simon Stevin Instituut voor
Wetenschappelijk onderzoek, Brugge, Belgium;
[3]- Centre d'Etude des Maladies des Arteres Coronaires,
Brussels, Belgium; [4]- Royal Zoological Society,
Antwerpen, Belgium

The main objective of experimental atherosclerosis is to start in anima vili the atherogenic process in such a way as to be able to study its cause or causes, its development and its effects. However, such an ambitious program is nearly impossible to carry out if one wishes to extrapolate the experimental observations in spontaneous human atherosclerosis. Indeed, the latter is a multifactorial phenomenon in which metabolic elements play without a doubt a major but certainly not the only role.

Up to what point can one believe that glucid and lipid metabolism in birds such as the chicken and the pigeon, in herbivorous rodents such as the rabbit, in omnivorous rodents as the rat and in carnivorous such as the dog is superposable to that of man?

Besides considering the great facility for inducing arterial lesions in the rabbit with a cholesterol-rich diet, a simplistic reasoning often leads to forgetting the role played by hemodynamics and by the resistance of the artery to its metabolic and hemodynamic aggressors. Stehbens (1974) showed recently that one could provoke in sheep (which are only slightly vulnerable to spontaneous atherosclerosis) by a local hemodynamic disturbance without any perturbation of the animals metabolism or of its plasma biochemistry, atheromatous lesions rich in lipids and complicated by thrombosis.

Well, who can assert that the resistance of the artery to one or another aggressor, either metabolic or hemodynamic, is the same in the different species commonly used in experimental atherosclerosis, while in one same species one can prove that there could exist between races some considerable differences in vulnerability. White Carneau and Show racers are a classic example of such a racial difference in sensitivity to both spontaneous and experimental atherosclerosis (Clarkson et al, 1959; Richard, 1965; Lofland, 1965).

These are not the only difficulties which await the experimentalist in atherosclerosis. Effectively, whatever the species he may select, it is either invulnerable to spontaneous atherosclerosis or on the contrary, sensitive to this illness. This statement places experimental atherosclerosis on the horns of a dilemna:

Either: to experiment upon species, such as the rabbit which is not vulnerable to spontaneous atherosclerosis but is metabolically different from man; transposing the experimental data to spontaneous disease would then be very hazardous and lead to erroneous dogma (Mann, 1966).

Or: to use species vulnerable to spontaneous atherosclerosis and metabolically close to man; in such conditions, sorting out the natural evolution of the spontaneous lesions from the experimental atherogenesis is a knotty, or may be, an insoluble problem.

We have lived in this respect an edifying experience.

Phylogeny, anatomy, and cholesterol metabolism (Mann, 1972) bring the chimpanzee closer to man than any other sub-human primate. In their natural habitat, chimpanzees feed on an omnivorous diet, comparable in many aspects to the human diet (Goodall, 1963). Furthermore, in a colony of 63 captive chimpanzees, the mean plasma cholesterol was much higher than in any observed group of captive monkeys, and the dispersion of individual values (120-470 mg%) was as wide as in a western human population (Vastesaeger and Delcourt, 1966). It seems also highly probable that besides dietary factors, stress has a non-negligible influence on plasma cholesterol in chimpanzees as well as in man (Delcourt et al, 1964). Last but not least, one more similarity between man and the chimpanzee may be found in the precociousness of the first alterations of intimal sclerosis, which are systematically present in the coronary arteries of the newborn in both species.

In the light of these considerations, some 10 years ago, our team started experimental investigations on 16 captive chimpanzees. Eight of them were fed a 2.5% cholesterol-high fat diet. After a few days on the diet, one of the animals died of hemorrhagic rectocolitis, and we had to procure a substitute for the program. Chimpanzees for sale were not common at that time, and we were very happy to buy from a circus a ten year old female which has recently developed an hemiparesis of the left side after an accident, but was otherwise in excellent health.

Upon introduction into the study and before being fed the atherogenic diet, the cholesterol level of the animal was fairly high (400 mg%) but still in the range of the starting values of the other experimental chimpanzees (220-420 mg%) and of the "normal" levels in the above mentioned colony of captive chimpanzees. After several months on the diet, it died unexpectedly. Autopsy revealed that the cause of death was a large fresh infarction of the anterior wall of the left ventricle, due to an occluding thrombus on stenosing lesions of the anterior descending branch of the left coronary artery (Vastesaeger et al, 1972).

Unfortunately, instead of the expected traumatic cerebral lesion, we found a striato-capsular necrosis as the sequal of an old recanalized thrombotic occlusion of the middle cerebral artery of an atheromatous process with cholesterol crystals. As hemiparesis was pre-existing before the animal was put on the diet, it is easily conceivable that the cerebral lesion developed spontaneously, i.e., before any experimental influence. So, even in the most favorable hypothesis, the diet just accelerated the evolution of spontaneous atherosclerosis, and it may well be that the natural course of the disease was little, or not at all, affected by the diet.

In any case, if by chance, the initial spontaneous cerebral

lesion had had no clinical expression during life, one would not have been able to detect the pre-existence of spontaneous athero-sclerosis in a young adult animal, and the whole post-mortem picture would have been erroneously attributed to the experimental intervention. Of course, in our case, a previous angiography of the brain would have shown the pre-existing occlusion of the middle cerebral artery, but even arteriography of the cerebral or coronary bed does not enable nonstenosing plaques to be detected.

Evidence of hereditary hyperbetalipoproteinemia has been pro-vided in other species of nonhuman primates (Morris and Geer, 1970; Lehner et al., 1971). The precociousness of the sponta-neous cerebral lesions in our hypercholesterolemic female chim-panzee makes plausible the hypothesis of essential hypercholestero-lemia in this animal. If genetic studies on a large scale would confirm the reality of familial hypercholesterolemia in chimpan-zees, then perhaps some breedings could be more or less arbitrari-ly selected as suitable and others excluded as unfit for experimental atherosclerosis.

At the present time, we are not so far, and it is obvious that there may be pitfalls in the interpretation of arterial lesions in chimpanzees kept for many months under an atherogenic diet. Fortunately, there are many other stimulating aspects in feeding chimpanzees such a diet: as shown by Mann (1972), their sterol metabolism, especially as far as catabolism is concerned, is quite similar to that of man.

There are nevertheless some slight differences in the plasma lipoproteinic profile of the two species. In the chimpanzee, the mean absolute and relative alpha-cholesterol value is higher than in man. We have observed a mean alpha-cholesterol of 84 mg% ± 25, i.e., 36% ± 12 of total cholesterol in the above mentioned colony of 63 chimpanzees (Delcourt et al., 1964) as compared with 60 mg% ± 12, or 28% ± 6 in 568 healthy male post-men aged 29-39 years (Vastesaeger et al., to be published).

In both the human and the subhuman species there are sponta-neous variations of total plasma cholesterol in the course of time (Paloheimo, 1961; Thomas et al., 1961; Vastesaeger et al., 1966; Petrovas et al, to be published), reflecting mainly absolute and relative changes of the beta-cholesterol fraction. These spontaneous changes are more pronounced in some specimens of captive chimpanzees than those commonly observed in humans. Absolute and relative participation of the alpha component of total cholesterolemia is also more marked in the apes than in man.

Feeding chimpanzees 2% cholesterol in maize or cotton seed oil does not influence significantly neither the cholesterol nor its fractions (Vastesaeger and Delcourt, 1966). Analogy with human behaviour under the same conditions (Keys et al., 1956) is also evident here.

The results are quite different however when cholesterol is fed with 14% butter (Table 1). After a few weeks under such a diet, there is a progressive elevation of total plasma lipids (up to a mean of + 92% above the control levels) and principally of total cholesterol (mean: + 134%). Phospholipidemia is less influenced (mean + 56%) and triglyceridemia practically unaffected (Table II). These changes are almost exclusively due to a large increase (35%) above the control, according to the method of Walton) in the beta lipoproteins, as shown by agarose gel electrophoresis and by electrochromatography. This experimental hyperlipidemia in chimpanzees may thus practically be considered as a hyper-betalipoproteinemia, the VLDL being unchanged.

Table III summarizes the changes in the average lipid concentrations of alpha and beta lipoproteins. The most striking differences between experimental animals and controls are observed in beta-lipoproteins for total cholesterol, cholesterol esters and phospholipids, disproportionately so that the C/PL ratio increases from 1.3 to 1.7. A more detailed study of the plasma lipoproteins separated by ultracentrifugation demonstrated a higher lipid/protein ratio in the LDL from animals under atherogenic diet than in those of their control counterparts.

If, as did Blaton et al (1974), we compare the plasma lipid pattern and the lipoproteinic profile of "spontaneous" hyperbeta-lipoproteinemia of the human on one hand, and experimental hyperbetalipoproteinemia in the chimpanzee on the other, we see (Figure 1 and Table III) that in both conditions there is a tremendous increase of beta-lipoprotein free and esterified cholesterol. The phospholipid increase is limited and confined to beta-lipoproteins.

Under the atherogenic diet, the oleic/linoleic acid ratio in alpha and beta-lipoproteins increases, mainly in cholesterol

Table I

Lipid and Fatty Acid Distribution of the Basic Control and Atherogenic Diets

Diet[a]	Lipids[b]					Fatty acids													
	CE	FC	FFA	TG	PL	10:0	12:0	14:0	15:0	16:0	16:1	18:0	18:1	18:2	20:0	18:3	20:3	20:4	Total fatty acids
C (gm%)	0.13	0.15	0.38	2.16	0.51	–	0.01	0.05	0.01	0.64	0.07	0.22	0.89	0.87	0.01	0.08	0.01	0.01	2.87
A (gm%)	0.22	3.15	0.76	19.83	0.62	0.34	0.41	1.99	0.34	6.30	0.63	2.13	6.10	1.58	0.04	0.32	0.04	0.04	20.25
C (%)	3.9	4.5	11.4	64.9	15.3	–	0.3	1.8	0.3	22.3	2.5	7.6	31.1	30.3	0.3	2.8	0.3	0.3	–
A (%)	0.9	12.8	3.1	80.7	2.5	1.7	2.0	9.8	1.7	31.1	3.1	10.5	30.1	7.8	0.2	1.6	0.2	0.2	–

[a]C = control diet; A = atherogenic diet.

[b]CE = cholesterol esters; FC = free cholesterol; FFA = free fatty acids; TG = triglycerides; PL = phospholipids.

From Blaton et al; 1974

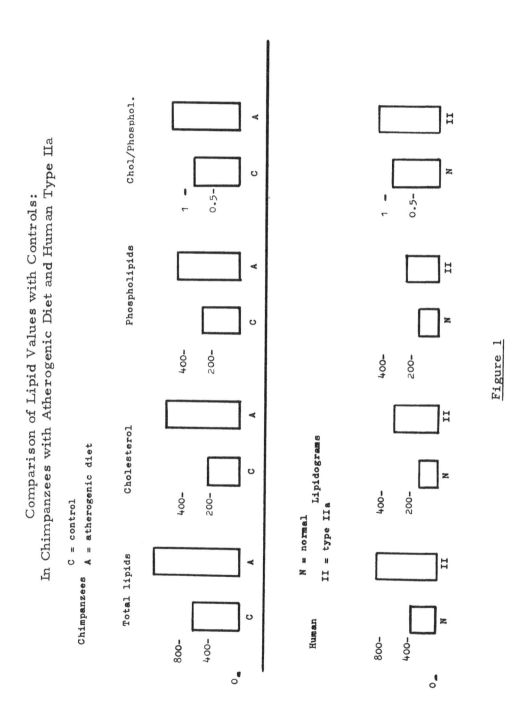

Comparison of Lipid Values with Controls:
In Chimpanzees with Atherogenic Diet and Human Type IIa

Chimpanzees   C = control
              A = atherogenic diet

Human   N = normal   Lipidograms
        II = type IIa

Figure 1

Table II

Percentage Increase Over the Control Lipid Values in Chimpanzees Given An Atherogenic Diet and in Human Type II Hyperlipoproteinemia[a]

(From Blaton et al; 1974)

Parameter	Control values				% increase over control			
	Chimpanzee		Human		Chimpanzee (atherogenic)		Human type II	
	Plasma	Beta LP	Plasma	Beta LP	Plasma	Beta LP	Plasma	Beta LP
Total lipids (mg/100ml)	746	430	430	261	92	157	157	142
Cholesterol (mg/100ml)	259	171	151	108	154	199	125	149
Phospholipids (mg/100ml)	295	129	163	87	55	129	74	106
% Est. cholesterol	75	77	67	66	-3	-5	4	3
C/PL	0.88	1.33	0.92	1.25	49	30	28	19
Sphm/PC	0.25	0.65	0.30	0.28	12	23	27	57

[a]LP = lipoprotein; C = cholesterol; PL = phospholipid; Sphm = sphingomelin; PC = phosphatidylcholine.

Table III

Mean Value ± SE of Plasma and Lipoprotein Lipids in Chimpanzees
Given Control and Atherogenic Diets

Sample	Group	Total lipid	Total Cholesterol	CE	FC	TG	PL	C/PL
Plasma (mg/100 ml)	Cb	746 ± 58	259 ± 21	326 ± 38	65 ± 9	60 ± 10	295 ± 18	0.88 ± 0.02
	Ac	1429 ± 167d	606 ± 76d	741 ± 93d	165 ± 23d	65 ± 16	459 ± 45d	1.31 ± 0.09d
Alpha lipoproteins (mg/100ml)	C	315 ± 21	88 ± 6	104 ± 14	26 ± 3	19 ± 2	166 ± 10	0.53 ± 0.01
	A	322 ± 31	95 ± 10	110 ± 13	29 ± 2	20 ± 2	163 ± 15	0.58 ± 0.03
Beta lipoproteins (mg/100ml)	C	430 ± 40	171 ± 16	222 ± 24	39 ± 7	41 ± 9	129 ± 10	1.33 ± 0.06
	A	1107 ± 157d	512 ± 72d	631 ± 86d	136 ± 23e	45 ± 15	296 ± 42d	1.73 ± 0.11d
Plasma (%)	C			43.5 ± 2.9	8.8 ± 1.3	8.0 ± 1.3	39.7 ± 0.8	
	A			51.6 ± 1.1d	11.4 ± 0.9	4.4 ± 0.7e	32.6 ± 1.4e	
Alpha lipoproteins (%)	C			32.4 ± 2.5	8.7 ± 1.5	6.1 ± 0.8	52.8 ± 0.4	
	A			33.9 ± 1.4	9.2 ± 0.5	6.3 ± 0.5	50.6 ± 1.3	
Beta lipoproteins (%)	C			51.9 ± 3.6	8.9 ± 1.4	9.2 ± 1.8	30.0 ± 0.9	
	A			57.3 ± 1.0	11.9 ± 1.1	3.9 ± 0.9e	26.9 ± 1.1	

a C = control ; A = atherogenic ; CE = cholesterol esters ; FC = free cholesterol ; TG = triglycerides ; PL = phospholipids.

b Number of animals = 4

c Number of animals = 6

d $P \leq 0.01$

e $0.01 < P \leq 0.05$

From Blaton et al; 1974.

esters. In our experimental chimpanzees as well as in human type IIa, we observe an elevation of the sphingomyelin/phosphatidyl-choline ratio, especially in the beta-lipoproteins (Blaton et al., 1974).

Summing up, we must now be aware that no more than any other animal model, the chimpanzee is an open sesame for every aspect of atherogenesis. Indeed the striking resemblance of the lipoproteinic profile of the cholesterol-fed chimpanzee to that of the human type IIa makes of this ape a most valuable tool for the pharmacological investigation of new drugs affecting lipid metabolism. The first steps have already been made in this direction (Vastesaeger et al., 1974).

Nevertheless, the type IIa pattern is only one of the numerous risk factors for coronary heart disease, and at the time being we have not yet succeeded in inducing type IIb or type IV abnormality in the chimpanzee. But, in spite of these limitations and of the fact that we still need further biochemical data on the protein moiety of the lipoproteins in the chimpanzee, it is evident that the balance of advantage lies with this animal as a model for the study of some definite aspects of dietary induced hyperbetalipoproteinemia. This is particularly valid for experimental procedures which, for ethical reasons, are unfeasible in man.

Last but not least, big colonies of chimpanzees are probably the only suitable system for intervention studies of the respective influence of genetic and environmental factors (such as diet and stress) on plasma cholesterol levels and betalipoproteinemia. From this point of view also, these nonhuman primates are certainly unique, since gorillas and orangutans are much more difficult to procure and to breed in large numbers.

REFERENCES

1. Blaton, V., Vastesaeger, M., Van Damme, D. and Peeters, H. Exp. Mol. Path. 20: 132, 1974.
2. Clarkson, T. B., Prichard, R. W., Netsky, M. G. and Lofland, H. B. A. M. A. Arch. Path. 68: 143, 1959.
3. Delcourt, R., Ninane, G., Osterrieth, P. and Vastesaeger, M. Acta Cardiol. 19: 531, 1964.
4. Goodall, J. Nat. Geographic 124, 1963.

5. Keys, A., Anderson, J. J., Fidanza, F., Keys, M. H., and Swahn, B. Clin. Chem. 1: 34, 1955.

6. Lehner, N. D. M., Clarkson, T. B., Bullock, B. C., Lofland, H. B., St. Clair, R. W. and Prichard, R. W. Medical Primatology, 1970. Proc. 2nd Conference Exp. Med. Surg. Primates, New York, 1969. Karger, Basel, 1971, p. 873.

7. Lofland, H. B. In: Comparative Atherosclerosis, edited by J. C. Roberts and R. Straus. Hoeber, Harper and Row, New York, 1965.

8. Mann, G. V. Circulat. Res. 18: 205, 1966.

9. Mann, G. V. Medical Primatology, 1972. Proc. 3rd Conf. Exp. Med. Surg. Primates, Lyon, 1972.

10. Morris, M. D. and Geer, W. E. In: Atherosclerosis. Edited by R. J. Jones, Springer Verlag, Heidelberg, 1970, p. 192.

11. Paloheimo, J. Ann. Med. Exp. Biol. Fenn. 39 (Supplement 8): 1-88, 1961.

12. Petrovas, C., Vanderveiken, F., Blaton, V., Peeters, H. and Vastesaeger, M., to be published.

13. Prichard, R. W. In: Comparative Atherosclerosis, edited by J. C. Roberts and R. Straus. Hoeber, Harper and Row, New York, 1965.

14. Stehbens, W. E. Proc. Royal Soc. London 185: 357, 1974.

15. Thomas, C. B., Holljes, H. W. D. and Eisenberg, F. F. Ann. Int. Med. 54: 413, 1961.

16. Vastesaeger, M. and Delcourt, R. Acta Cardiol. Supplement XI: 283, 1966.

17. Vastesaeger, M., Vercruysse, J. and Martin, J. J. Medical Primatology, 1972, Proc. 3rd Conf. Exp. Med. Surg. Primates, Lyon, 1972. Karger, Basel, 1972.

18. Vastesaeger, M., Blaton, V., Declercq, B., Vercruysse, J., Van Damme, D., Peeters, H. and Mortelmans, J. Acta Zool. Path. Antverpiensia 58: 74, 1974.

19. Vastesaeger, M., Vanderveiken, F., Gillot, P. and Petrovas, C., to be published.

STUDIES ON EXPERIMENTAL ATHEROSCLEROSIS BY

IMMUNOFLUORESCENCE

Kenneth W. Walton

Department of Experimental Pathology, University of
Birmingham, England

It has been established by several investigators (e. g. , Watts,
1959, 1963; Woolf and Pilkington, 1965; Kao and Wissler, 1965;
Walton, 1966; Walton and Williamson, 1968; Walton et al. , 1970),
using the technique of immunofluorescence, that the principal
vehicle transporting lipid into human atherosclerotic lesions, is
serum low-density lipoprotein (LDL).   The purpose of the present
study was to see whether a similar technique could be applied to
the arterial lesions of lipid-fed rabbits.

MATERIALS AND METHODS

Animals

The tissues examined were derived from the same group of
30 rabbits maintained on diets either (a) supplemented with
cholesterol, or (b) semi-synthetic in nature and containing beef-
lard but no added cholesterol (Gresham and Howard, 1962); or
from 6 control animals maintained on a standard pellet-diet, as
previously described (Walton et al. , 1973).

Histological Procedures

Formalin-fixed material was embedded in polyethylene glycols.
In some instances, material fixed in cold ethanol (Saint-Marie,

371

1962) was embedded in paraffin-wax. Fresh, unfixed material
was snap-frozen and cryostat sections prepared as detailed in
earlier communications (Walton and Williamson, 1968; Walton
et al., 1970). Sections of fixed material were examined after
treatment by the same range of conventional staining methods for
lipids and other components which had been previously employed.
Unfixed frozen sections and sections fixed in cold ethanol were
examined by the fluorescent antibody technique using the antisera,
technique and equipment previously described.

In some instances, the immuno-histological and the conventional staining procedures were applied sequentially to the same
section (see Results) to allow detailed comparison of photographs
of the same microscopic fields. The procedure used was that
described by Walton et al (1970; 1973) except that elution of the
labelled antibody from the section prior to its conventional staining was found, from later experience, to be unnecessary and was
therefore not carried out in all cases.

Serum lipids and lipoproteins were estimated by the techniques
previously detailed (Walton et al., 1973).

RESULTS

Relation Between Serum Lipoprotein Changes and Development
of Arterial Lesions

The nature of the dietary lipid supplement influences the pattern of alteration of serum lipids and lipoproteins in the rabbit and
also the rate of which hyperlipidemia develops and its intensity.
Whether rabbits are maintained on a diet supplemented with 2%
cholesterol, or on the semi-synthetic diet supplemented with beef-
fat without added cholesterol, the animals develop a marked hypercholesterolemia and a parallel elevation of total $(S_f 0-400)$ β-lipo-
proteins. The rapidity with which such changes occur and the
intensity of the hyperlipoproteinemia developed is much more
marked in animals on the cholesterol diet (Walton et al., 1973).
Correspondingly, the rate and intensity of development of arterial
lesions reflect the serum lipid and lipoprotein changes, being
more marked in cholesterol-fed animals.

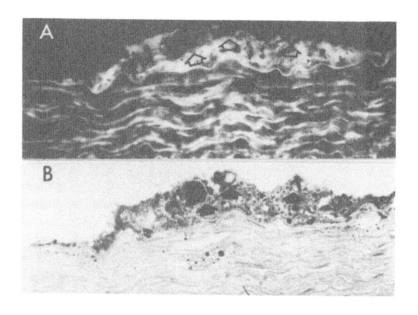

Figure 1: (A) Frozen section of very early aortic lesion from cholesterol-fed rabbit after treatment with fluorescein-labelled anti-rabbit β-lipoprotein antiserum. Note bright specific fluorescence (green in original, white in photograph) in slightly thickened intima, corresponding to extracellular lipid as seen in Fig. 1(B). But weak or absent fluorescence at sites corresponding to fat-filled cells (arrow).

(B) Same field of same section treated with Oil red O and Light Green. Note lipid present both extracellularly and in lipid-filled cells (arrows) in intima (bright-red in original, grey or black in photograph). x 320

Histogenesis of Arterial Lesions

Frozen sections from early arterial lesions were examined after treatment with fluorescein-labelled sheep anti-rabbit lipoprotein. The appearances seen were compared with those found in either the same section, or a consecutive section of the identical lesion, after treatment with Oil red O. Precise correspondence was found between the distribution of specific fluorescence for β-lipoprotein and that of lipid reacting with Oil red O and distributed

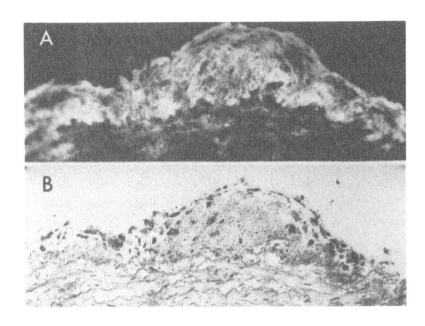

Figure 2: (A) Frozen section of later aortic lesion from rabbit on beef-fat diet after treatment with fluorescein-labelled anti-rabbit β-lipoprotein. Note specific fluorescence in intimal cells, ground-substance of intima and in media. But weak or absent fluorescence in areas corresponding to lipid-filled cells as seen in Figure 2(B).

(B) Same field of same section after treatment with Oil red O and Light Green.   x 320

extracellularly in the intima in early lesions (Figure 1). On the other hand, in later lesions fat-filled cells reacted variably with the labelled anti-β-lipoprotein, some cells fluorescing brightly, some weakly and some failing to react (Figure 2). Similar observations have been made in relation to human arterial lesions (Walton and Williamson, 1968) and spontaneous or induced xanthomata in lipid-fed rabbits (Walton et al. , 1973). They have been interpreted as suggesting that extracellular lipid results from insudation of β-lipoprotein into the ground-substance. The initial immunoreactivity of lipid-filled cells is compatible with uptake of the lipoprotein by phagocytic cells while the progressive loss of

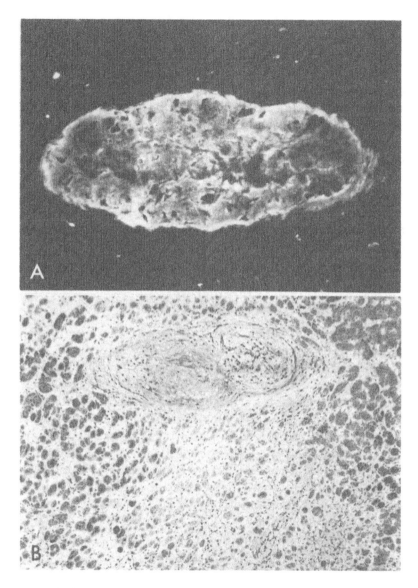

Figure 3: (A) Frozen section of intramural branch of coronary artery in cholesterol-fed rabbit after treatment with fluorescein-labelled anti-rabbit β-lipoprotein. Note complete occlusion of vessel by material giving specific fluorescence (white in picture, green in original). x 320

(B) Fixed section from adjacent block of tissue from same animal stained with hematoxylin and eosin to show area of ischaemic myocaridal fibrosis adjacent to occluded branch of coronary artery. x 160

reactivity in cells, as lesions develop, is suggestive of degradation of the lipoprotein molecule by intracellular proteases which first digest its protein portion (the site of antigenicity) leaving a lipid residue detectable by conventional fat stains.

Essentially similar results were obtained with the lesions resulting from both kinds of lipid-supplemented diet at all sites examined in the arterial tree. But the lesions in cholesterol-fed rabbits contained larger numbers of lipid-filled cells. Further degradation of the lipoprotein with the release of crystalline chole-sterol in areas of immunoreactivity to β-lipoprotein could be de-monstrated by examination of lesions in polarized light. At some sites (e. g. , in coronay vessles) occlusive lipid-filled lesions could be shown to be associated with ischaemic effects similar to those seen in human material (Figure 3).

DISCUSSION

It is submitted that these results in animals maintained on lipid supplemented diets are closely similar, in general, with the findings in human atherosclerosis and are compatible with an in-sudative mechanism for their production. In this sense, the lipid-fed rabbit is indeed a satisfactory model for demonstrating the relation between hyper-β-lipoproteinemia and the arterial lesions of atherosclerosis. It has similarly been shown that this serves as an acceptable model for conditions associated with atherosclerosis and characterized by lipid deposition in tissues, such as the corneal arcus (Walton, 1973a, b, c; Walton and Dunkerley, 1973) and xanthomata (Walton, 1973d; Walton et al. , 1973).

ACKNOWLEDGEMENTS

This work was supported by the British Heart Foundation. A more detailed account of this investigation has been submitted for publication in Atherosclerosis.

REFERENCES

1. Gresham, G. A. and Howard, A. N. : Arch. Pathol. 74: 1, 1962.
2. Kao, V. C. Y. and Wissler, R. W.: Exp. Molec. Path. 4: 457, 1965.
3. Saint-Marie, G. : J. Histochem. Cytochem. 10: 250, 1962.
4. Walton, K. W.: Arch. Mal Coeur, 59, Revue Atheroscler. , 8: suppl. 2, p. 41, 1966.
5. Walton, K. W. : Nutr. Metab. 15: 37, 1973a.
6. Walton, K. W. : J. Path. 111: 263, 1973.
7. Walton, K. W. : In J. C. Brocklehurst (ed.) Textbook of Geriatric Medicine and Gerontology, pp. 77-112, London, Churchill-Livingstone, 1973c.
8. Walton, K. W. : Nutr. Metab. 15: 59, 1973d.
9. Walton, K. W. and Dunkerley, D. J. : J. Path. , in press.
10. Walton, K. W. , Thomas, C. and Dunkerley, D. J.: J. Path. 109: 271, 1973.
11. Walton, K. W. and Williamson, N. : J. Atheroscler. Res. 8: 599, 1968.
12. Walton, K. W. , Williamson, N. and Johnson, A. G. : J. Path. 101: 205, 1970.
13. Watts, H. F. : Amer. J. Path. 35: 719, 1959.
14. Watts, H. F. : In R. J. Jones (ed.) Evolution of the athero-sclerotic plaque, p. 116, Chicago, Chicago University Press, 1963.
15. Woolf, N. and Pilkington, T. R. E. : J. Path. Bact. 90: 459, 1965.

THE EFFECTS OF TOLBUTAMIDE ON THE DEVELOPMENT OF ATHEROSCLEROSIS IN RHESUS MONKEYS FED AN AVERAGE AMERICAN TABLE-PREPARED DIET

R. W. Wissler, J. Borensztajn, A. Rubenstein,
G. Getz and D. Vesselinovitch

Department of Pathology, The University of Chicago,
Chicago, Illinois

Fourteen adult male Rhesus monkeys were followed for 18 months during which they all consumed daily measured portions of a simulated average American diet whose ingredients were based on average food consumption figures for the USA. Seven of these animals, each paired with a comparable control, were also fed 20 mg/kg of Tolbutamide per day. No significant differences in weight gain, glucose tolerance, electrocardiograms or serum lipids were noted on numerous determinations during this period of study.

At the termination of the study the animals were carefully examined with special attention to the quantitation of atherosclerosis in the aorta as well as the carotid, iliac and coronary arteries of each pair. Although the aortic weights were slightly, but not significantly, greater in the Tolbutamide treated animals (2.53 ± 0.1 vs 2.39 ± 0.1 gm) the lesions were slightly less severe in this treated group (0.7 ± 0.3 vs 0.9± .09). The surface area involvement with atheromatous disease (36% ± 10 vs 25% ± 10) as well as the frequency of lesions (68 ± 5.4 vs 63 ± 3.4), which was based on a study of a standard groups of sections of each aorta stained with oil red O, revealed slightly more extensive disease in the Tolbutamide treated animals, but again the results showed no significant differences.

Other facets of this study including the frequency and severity of coronary, iliac and carotid artery involvement have thus far not revealed any notable differences, but are not yet complete.

This study was supported by the Food and Drug Administration Contract number 72-114.

THE COCKEREL AS AN ANIMAL MODEL FOR ATHEROSCLEROSIS RESEARCH

Harry Y. C. Wong

Department of Physiology, Howard University,
College of Medicine, Washington, D. C.

SUMMARY

The chicken is a good animal model for the study of athero-sclerosis research because it is:

1.   Omnivorous.
2.   Small and suitable for prolonged laboratory investigation.
3.   Able to develop spontaneous atherosclerosis.
4.   Capable of producing atherosclerosis after cholesterol feeding with elevated hypercholesterolemia. A diet of 1/4% cholesterol plus 5% cottonseed oil added to starter-grower-mash resulted in aortic atherosclerosis with a slight but significant increase in plasma cholesterol.
5.   Plasma levels of cholesterol and triglyceride are similar to those in humans.
6.   Lipid composition of high and low density lipoproteins as well as chylomicrons resembles those of humans.
7.   Has been noted that there is no essential difference between vascular lesions seen in chickens as a result of cholesterol diet and that of atherosclerosis observed in man.

COCKEREL AS AN ANIMAL MODEL FOR
ATHEROSCLEROSIS RESEARCH

In an attempt to find a model research animal for the study of
atherosclerosis, Dauber and Katz (1) selected the chicken. It was
stated by Fox (2) that "of all animals, birds have arteriosclerosis
more closely resembling human arteriosclerosis." For this reason
the experimental production of arteriosclerosis in chicken was
undertaken by Dauber (3). The reason was that it would be beneficial to reproduce the disease in an animal naturally subject to the
same type of vascular disorder as man. The fact that the chicken,
like man, is omnivorous only added significance to its use as a
research model.

The first descriptive detail of the morphology of spontaneous
atherosclerosis in chickens was reported by Dauber (3). Her
investigations included gross analysis of fresh and Sudan IV stained
aortas and microscopic studies of histological sections. In roosters
she observed that the abdominal aorta was by far the most common
site of change. The spontaneous lesions were characterized as
elevated, smooth, longitudinal, white or yellow ridgelike thickenings
of the abdominal aorta which extended from the interrenal area to
the bifurcation of the iliacs. Occasional small elevated pin-head
size yellow plaques were observed in adjacent orifices of arteries
branching from the aorta. It was further noted by Dauber (3) that
hens produce nodular and ridgelike lesions of the descending
thoracic and abdominal aorta similar to the spontaneous lesions
observed in roosters. In both roosters and hens it was observed
that the spontaneous lesions of the abdominal aorta had similar
microscopic morphology.

The morphology of cholesterol induced atherosclerosis of the
aorta and great vessels has been reported in detail by Dauber and
Katz (1, 4) and Horlick and Katz (5). Studies from our laboratory
(6-12) are in agreement with these observations. In contrast to
spontaneous atherosclerosis in the chicken, Katz and Stamler (13)
reported that the greatest incidence of atherogenesis in cockerel
fed a cholesterol diet was found in the ascending aorta and aortic
arch. Cholesterol in the diet also led to an increased incidence
and severity of gross atherosclerosis of the abdominal aorta.
Chickens fed a cholesterol regimen were characterized by large,
yellowish and elevated longitudinal abdominal aortic lesions resembling the spontaneous plaques of chickens which were not fed

an atherogenic diet. Sometimes small, elevated, pinhead like nodules were found along the abdominal aorta, particularly adjacent to the orifices of aortic branches. Furthermore, irregular plaques resembling those seen in the thoracic aorta as well as raised, rough, granular, yellow transverse lesions were occasionally observed in the muscular aorta of birds with advanced atherogenesis. The smooth, longitudinal, ridgelike lesions observed in the lower abdominal aortas of birds fed atherogenic diet demonstrated a pathologic pattern resembling that of spontaneous lesions. Studies untertaken by Horlick and Katz (5) to quantitate the effects of different amounts of dietary cholesterol on the rapidity, incidence, and degree of atherosclerosis in chickens were performed on four-week old White Leghorn cockerels. Three series of experiments were undertaken lasting 5, 10 and 15 weeks respectively. Each series had 5 groups of 12 birds. In each study controls were maintained on chicken mash. The remaining groups of cockerels were placed on mash consisting of 0.5, 1, 2 and 4% cholesterol suspended in cottonseed oil with the oil making up 20% of the diet by weight. At the end of five weeks on various diets, the following results were obtained (Table 1). It was noted that control birds had no lesions in the thoracic and abdominal aortas while cockerels on 0.5% cholesterol, 3 birds showed gross lesions of the thoracic aorta. The average gross grading of the thoracic aorta for this group was 0.1 and none in the abdominal aorta based on a 0-4 scale. However, 8 of the birds on 1% cholesterol had gross arterial lesions whose grading ranged from 0.5 to 2. Only one bird had a lesion in the abdominal aorta. The average gross grading for this group was 0.7 for the thoracic aorta and 0.1 for the abdominal. Nine birds on 2% cholesterol showed gross intimal lesions in the thoracic aorta of which 4 had gross lesions in the abdominal aorta. The lesions were more extensive and advanced than in the preceding groups. The average gross grading for this group was 1.3 for the thoracic and 0.4 for the abdominal aorta. Birds on 4% cholesterol regimen all had gross lesions of the thoracic aorta which ranged from 0.5 to 4. The average gross grading for this group was 2.0 for the thoracic aorta, and 0.5 for the abdominal aorta. The report showed a progressive increase in the frequency and severity of atherosclerosis as the amount of cholesterol in the diet was increased; that is, for thoracic aorta plaques, cockerels with 0.5% cholesterol, 3 of 12 had lesions; with 1%, 8 of 12 had lesions; in the 2% group, 9 of 12 had lesions; and with 4% cholesterol, 12 of 12 had plaques. There was a similar increase in the incidence of lesions in the abdominal aorta when cholesterol was added to the diet.

Table 1

EFFECT OF FIVE WEEKS OF FEEDING OF CHOLESTEROL

Cholesterol in diet (per cent)	Thoracic Aorta			Abdominal Aorta		
	Birds with lesions (per cent)	Degree of athero-sclerosis	Average grade*	Birds with lesions (per cent)	Degree of athero-sclerosis	Average grade*
Control	0	0	0	0	0	0
0.5	25	0-0.5	0.1	0	0	0
1	66	0.5-2	0.7	8	0-1	0.1
2	75	0.5-2	1.3	33	0-2	0.4
4	100	0.5-4	2.0	33	0.5-2	0.5

* 4 = severe.   From Horlick,L., and Katz, L.N., Amer. Heart J., 38:
                                 336-349, 1949. Reproduced with permission.

Therefore, the severity and incidence of atherogenesis was directly related to the amount of cholesterol in the diet. Lesions of the abdominal aorta were not observed as frequently as thoracic lesions as a response to increased dietary cholesterol. At the end of 10 weeks on a no cholesterol diet, no lesions were observed in the controls (Table 2) but, in comparison, 10 of 12 birds fed 0.5% cholesterol had lesions in the thoracic aorta while the other groups of cockerel fed an atherogenic diet of 1,2 or 4%, 12 of 12 had athero-sclerosis in the thoracic aorta. The severity of atherogenesis was progressively increased according to the amount of cholesterol added to the diet. It was further observed that there was a parallel increase in severity and incidence of atherogenesis as the amount of cholesterol was increased.

However, as in the 5 week study, the severity and number of lesions of the abdominal aorta were not as great as those of the thoracic aorta. In addition, examination of the pulmonary arteries showed that the incidence of these lesions increased as the amount of cholesterol in the diet was increased. Table 3 depicts the influence of 15 weeks on an atherogenic diet as once again was observed

Table 2

EFFECT OF TEN WEEKS OF FEEDING OF CHOLESTEROL

Cholesterol in diet (per cent)	Thoracic Aorta			Abdominal Aorta			Pulmonary Artery
	Birds with lesions (per cent)	Degree of athero- sclerosis	Average grade*	Birds with lesions (per cent)	Degree of athero- sclerosis	Average grade*	Birds with lesions (per cent)
Control	0	0	0	0	0	0	0
0.5	80	1-0.5	1.2	40	0.5-1	0.3	0
1	100	1-4	2.5	80	1-3	1.5	50
2	100	2-4	3.0	100	0.5-3	1.7	70
4	100	1-4	3.4	70	1-3	1.6	100

* 4 = severe

After Horlick, L., and Katz, L.N., Amer. Heart J. 38: 336-349, 1949. Reproduced with permission.

Table 3

EFFECT OF FIFTEEN WEEKS OF FEEDING OF CHOLESTEROL

Cholesterol in diet (per cent)	Thoracic Aorta			Abdominal Aorta			Pulmonary Artery
	Birds with lesions (per cent)	Degree of atherosclerosis	Average grade*	Birds with lesions (per cent)	Degree of atherosclerosis	Average grade*	Birds with lesions (per cent)
Control	0	0	0	10	0.5	0.10	0
0.5	67	0.5-4	1.3	67	0.5-3	1.2	0
1	92	0.5-4	2.4	75	0.5-2	0.9	60
2	92	0.5-4	2.2	83	0.5-3	1.5	50
4	100	0.5-3	2.6	90	0.5-3	1.5	

* 4 = severe

From Horlick, L., and Katz, L.N., Amer. Heart J. 38: 336-349, 1949. Reproduced with permission.

an increased severity and incidence of atherosclerosis with the
high levels of cholesterol. However, please note that the severity
and incidence of the lesions were less after 15 weeks than after
10 weeks of cholesterol feeding. Atherosclerosis was again observed to be more marked in the thoracic aorta than in the abdominal
aorta. Increased amounts of cholesterol in the diet resulted in
significant elevation of plasma cholesterol in most studies. It is
to be noted that atherosclerosis in humans frequently is observed
in the presence of normal or nearly normal plasma cholesterol.
For this reason investigators have questioned the relevance of
experimental atherosclerosis caused by an atherogenic regimen
in chickens or other animals, because they feel that the pathophysiology of cholesterol-fed animals has its counterpart only in
grossly hyperlipidemic man. Since high plasma cholesterol is not
present in most people with clinical atherogenesis, these critics
maintain that atherosclerosis in man is different in the pathogenesis
and etiology from induced lesion from cholesterol regimen in
laboratory animals. To determine whether atheroma by cholesterol
feeding could be produced in cockerels with minimal hypercholesterolemia, Stamler and Katz (1, 4) conducted a long term experiment upon five week old birds which were placed on a cholesterol
regimen consisting of 1/4 cholesterol plus 5% cottonseed oil added
to mash. These cockerels were fed the diet for 35 weeks and the
regimen resulted in minimal hypercholesterolemia. The mean
plasma cholesterol increased from a control value of 99 to 166 mg%
over the 35 weeks of the study (Table 4). Plasma lipids of the
control birds ranged from 68-142 mg% while plasma lipid of experi-
mentals ranged from 116-247 mg%. Although this change in plasma
cholesterol was slight, it was significantly increased. There were
no marked changes in plasma lipid phosphorous levels noted in the
cockerels fed 1/4% cholesterol. It was observed that the plasma
total cholesterol to lipid phosphorous was significantly increased
from the control value of 13.1 to 21.4. In spite of the minimal
changes in plasma cholesterol the addition of 1/4% cholesterol to
the diet had a significant effect on atherogenesis (Table 5). It was
observed that there was a high incidence of severe gross atherosclerosis of the thoracic aorta of the cholesterol fed cockerels.
In contrast, no lesions were observed in the thoracic aortas in the
controls. These lesions were grossly and microscopically typical
of cholesterol-induced atherosclerosis. Both the control and
experimental birds had similar incidences of gross atherosclerosis
of the abdominal aorta, and these plaques were markedly greater
in extent and severity in the cockerels fed 1/4% cholesterol added

Table 4

EFFECT OF FEEDING 1/4% CHOLESTEROL ON
PLASMA LIPIDS IN THE CHICK*

Groups	Total cholesterol mg%	Lipid P mg%	Total cholesterol / Lipid P
Control	99	7.5	13.1
Cholesterol-Fed	166	7.8	21.4

* Chicks fed 1/4% cholesterol - 5% cottonseed oil mash from 5th through 40th week of life.

From Stamler, J., and Katz, L. N.: Circulation
2: 705-713, 1950. By permission of the American
Heart Association, Inc.

Table 5

EFFECT OF FEEDING 1/4% CHOLESTEROL MASH
ON ATHEROGENESIS IN THE CHICK*

	% with lesions	% with grading 1 or >	Average grading of lesions
Thoracic aorta--Controls	0	0	0
Thoracic aorta--Cholesterol fed	42	33	1.1
Abdominal aorta--Controls	50	30	1.0
Abdominal aorta--Cholesterol fed	67	58	1.4
Whole aorta--Controls	50	30	1.0
Whole aorta--Cholesterol fed	83	67	1.8

* Chicks fed experimental diet from 5th to 40th week of life.

After Stamler, J., and Katz, L.N.: Circulation 2:
705-713, 1950. With permission of the American
Heart Association, Inc.

Table 6

MEAN LEVELS OF FREE FATTY ACID, TRIGLYCERIDE AND CHOLESTEROL

Group	FFA (mM/liter)	Triglyceride (mg/100 ml)	Cholesterol (mg/100 ml)
Sesame oil	0.198	27	145
0.1 mg DES	0.975*	1,839*	405*
1.0 mg DES	4.369[+]	10.241[+]	1,145[+]
5.0 mg DES	5.137	12,371[‡]	1,381[‡]

* Exceeds level in the sesame oil group (p < 0.05).

[+] Exceeds level in the 0.1 mg DES group.

[‡] Exceeds level in the 1.0 mg DES group.

After Kudzma, D.J., Et al. : Metabolism 22: 423-434, 1973. Reproduced with permission.

to mash. The chick as a laboratory model for the study of estrogen-induced hyperlipidemia has been recently reported by Kudzma et al (15). Their study characterized the hyperlipidemia of the estrogenized chick in terms of changes observed in the major plasma lipids and the hyperlipoproteinemia that results. They demonstrated qualitative similarities to the condition in estrogenized women and show that the chicken is a suitable laboratory model for more detailed study of the mechanism responsible for this cause of hyperlipidemia. Table 6 summarizes the effect of administration of either 0.1, 1.0, or 5.0 mg of diethylstilbesterol (DES) on mean levels of free fatty acid, triglyceride and cholesterol in five day old Rhode Island chicks of undetermined sex. It was observed that diethylstilbesterol treatment of these birds at all three dose levels produced significant elevation in plasma level of free fatty acid, triglyceride and cholesterol. The concentration of free fatty acids is lower than that normally observed in humans. According to Fredrickson et al (16) the levels of triglyceride and cholesterol in the untreated chicks are similar to those found in young humans.

Table 7

COMPARISON OF LIPID COMPOSITION OF HUMAN
AND CHICK LIPOPROTEINS

Lipoproteins class	Triglyceride*	Cholesterol	Phospholipids	Triglyceride/ Cholesterol
Very low density				
Human	50	18	32	2.8/1
Chick	50	25		2.0/1
			25	
Chylomicron				
Human[+]	-	-	-	11/1
Chick	-	-	-	11/1

* Expressed as percentage by weight.

[+] Reference No. 18.

From Kudzma, D. J., et al.; Metabolism 22; 423-234, 1973. Reproduced with permission.

The triglyceride level was 27 mg% as compared to 61 ± 34 for young human males and 73 ± 34 for young human females according to Fredrickson et al (16). The cholesterol value of 145 mg%/100 ml is close to the levels for young human males and females of 172 and 179 mg% respectively. Table 7 shows the comparison of the lipid composition of human and chick lipoproteins. Kudzma et al (15) also noted that the very low density lipoproteins of human were similar to those of chickens when expressed as percentage of weight. Chicken cholesterol was slightly higher than that of the human while human had higher phospholipid levels. The triglyceride cholesterol ratio was higher in human. It was also observed that the chylomicron level of the human is not significantly different from that of the chicken.

REFERENCES

1. Dauber, D. V. and Katz, L. N. Arch. Path. 34: 937, 1942.
2. Fox, H. In: Arteriosclerosis. E. V. Cowdry, editor, Macmillan, New York, pp. 153-193, 1933.
3. Dauber, D. V. Arch. Path. 38: 46, 1944.
4. Dauber, D. V. and Katz, L. N. Arch. Path. 36: 473, 1943.
5. Horlick, L. and Katz, L. N. Am. Heart J. 38: 336, 1949.
6. Wong, H. Y. C., Johnson, F. B. and Wong, A. K. Circulation 16: 501, 1957.
7. Wong, H. Y. C., Wong, A. K. and Johnson, I. B. Circulation 18: No. 3, 482, 1958.
8. Wong, H. Y. C., Johnson, T. F. and Johnson, F. B. Proc. of 1st International Pharmacological Meeting, Vol. 2, Pergamon Press, Oxford, p.115, 1963.
9. West, W. and Wong, H. Y. C. Proc. of 1st International Pharmacological Meeting, Vol. 2, Pergamon Press, Oxford, p. 99, 1963.
10. Wong, H. Y. C. and Johnson, F. B. Circulation Res. Vol. XI: 843, 1962.
11. Wong, H. Y. C. and Johnson, F. B. Fed. Proc. 26, No. 2: 489, 1967.
12. Wong, H. Y. C., David, S. and Orimilikwe, S. O. Fed. Proc. 32, No. 147: 1973.
13. Katz, L. N. and Stamler, J. Experimental Atherosclerosis. C. C. Thomas, Springfield, Illinois, p. 127, 1953.
14. Stamler, J. and Katz, L. N. Circulation 2: 705, 1950.
15. Kudzma, D. J., Hegstad, P. M. and Stoll, R. E. Metabolism 22: 423, 1973.
16. Fredrickson, D. S., Levy, R. I. and Lees, R. S. New Engl. J. Med. 176: 148, 1967.

INFLUENCE OF PLATELETS ON THE INTEGRITY OF THE VESSEL WALL

H. Hess and M. Marshall

Munchen University, 8 Munchen 15, Germany

Blood vessels and circulating blood form a unit both functionally and existentially. Functionally because the blood supply to the tissue is regulated by the synchrony of vessels and streaming blood - the vessel modifies its lumen, the blood its viscosity. Existentially, the vessel and streaming blood are indispensible to one another. The blood remains a stable suspension so long as it flows in an intact vessel system. The vessel wall, on the other hand, remains intact only so long as the blood it encloses possesses an intact coagulation system, especially with regard to the number of platelets.

The pathophysiology of the vessel is closely connected to the pathophysiology of the platelets. In the streaming blood a platelet is an ellipsoid corpuscle of $2\,\mu$m diameter. In this state of rest it is stable in suspension and has no tendency to aggregate with other platelets or to adhere to the intact vessel wall.

Various physiological substances, among others epinephrine, norepinephrine, prostaglandins - that is to say substances which also cause the contraction of smooth muscular cells - and collagen fibers bring the platelet to an excited form. At the same time it develops pseudopodia by help of which it will be able to aggregate with other platelets or to become adherent to a surface.

We know very little about the physiological significance of platelet aggregation in streaming blood.

On the other hand, it is well known for a long time and

undisputed that it is the business of the platelets to preserve and
to restore the integrity of the vessel wall. In case the vessel
wall is hurt, it is the subendothelial collagen which causes only
the passing platelets to adhere to the lesion and to cover it
instantly.

In a few minutes the metamorphosis of the adherent platelets
and the blood stream for a tight film which in itself is the
material to repair the vessel wall ad integrum.

The immense importance of the platelets being an integral
component of the vessel wall becomes even more evident when a
dacron prosthesis (as vessel) is offered to the streaming blood.
The platelets immediately begin to cover it up and this process
of covering is then supported by secondary coagulating processes
within a few minutes. The platelets, together with the streaming
blood form a coherent primary inside film. This inside film is
indifferent to the streaming blood and becomes endothelialized.
Thus by efficacy of the streaming blood alone an almost constitu-
tional vessel with adventitia, neointima and endothelium is formed.

Physiologically the platelet represents the mobile phase of the
vessel wall and in case of need it must always be available in
adequate number and ready to operate. Adequate number for man,
means about $300,000/\text{mm}^3$, but at least $30,000 \text{ mm}^3$. Ready to
operate means that the platelet must be available in the streaming
blood in a stable form of rest, which by adequate irritations can
be transformed into an exictable form able to aggregate and to
adhere.

The pathology of the platelets exhibits positive and negative
variants with regard to number and/or function.

The clinical pictures of the negative variants are characterized by a prolonged bleeding time and by spontaneous bleedings.

The postive variants of the platelet pathology hold a key
position in the pathogenesis of obliterating arteriopathies in all
of their different courses.

This statement must be proved:

We know a series of factors which are related to the onset of

obliterating arteriopathies in man.   Considering the question
which are the earliest changes of the vessel wall under the influence of those factors, we had to go back to animal models.

We used minipigs and rabbits in these experiments. The
scanning electron microscope has proved very useful for vessel
examinations. It is able to show a surface plastically in a mag-
nification up to 20,000:1 and to explore it systematically.

Model Experiments

The vessels we were referring to in all experiments with the
minipig were the carotid, the femoral and the coronary artery
and with the rabbit the abdominal aorta.

These vessels were prepared under general anesthesia and
taken out intravital for examination according to the method we
have described.

1. In careful examination with the scanning electron microscope we could find no adhesions of elements of the streaming
blood, especially no platelets on the inside surfaces of the vessels
of control animals.

2.   The conditions for the beginning of a cold angiitis in man
were imitated by locally touching an artery segment with ice.
On every concerned vessel of both species of animals after few
minutes of local contact with ice we could regularly find platelet
adhesions on the segment under study.

3.   Inhaling smoking represents, beyond doubt, the most
important risk factor for the thrombangiitis obliterans Buerger.
The experimental animals stayed for several hours in a reasonably ventilated cage into which cigarette smoke was continually
exhausted. We regularly and exclusively found platelet adhesions
on the intact endothelium of the various arteries.

4.   By feeding cholesterol we imitated the conditions for the
beginning of an obliterating atherosclerosis caused by a disturbance of lipid metabolism. In this mode, as well, in both species
of experimental animals, and in all concerned vessels platelet
adhesions were found which resembled those seen in the above
mentioned models.

After just one cholesterol enriched meal we could see sporadic platelets on the otherwise absolutely intact endothelium of various arteries of a rabbit. Such platelet adhesions may, if the stimulus to further depositions does not occur, in the same way be completely integrated into the vessel wall as a single defect of the vessel wall and repaired by a cover of platelets. If, however, the stimulus insists on making the platelets adherent to the vessel wall, for instance when the rabbits were given further cholesterol enriched meals, there happened more and more platelet deposition. Simultaneous blood examinations within these experiments showed a measurably more intensive tendency of the platelets to aggregate as blood cholesterol levels increased.

After two weeks with this feeding we found, apart from wall adherent platelets, fibrin, erythrocytes enclosed in it and leucocytes, that is to say a mixed microparietal thrombosis. Such a microparietal thrombosis can no longer be completely integrated into the vessel wall. If the stimulus to further depositions is stopped, it may be endothelialized and thus be incorporated into the vessel wall or it goes on developing finally to the obliterating thrombus.

Morphologically homogeneous platelet adhesions and microparietal thromboses were always seen in the arteries of men suffering from obliterating arteriosclerosis.

This is good reason to assume that with man, too, there is an irritation of the platelets with a tendency to adhere to the endothelium of intact vessels, when risk factors begin to become effective towards an obliterating arteriosclerosis.

Physiological and pathological adhesions of platelets on the vessel wall can be induced:

    1. by the vessel wall itself,
    2. by primary global modifications of the platelets in the streaming blood, and
    3. mechanically, as platelets aggregate more intensively when they are exposed to higher shear rate.

The following factors are easily combinable with the postulate of a pathogenetic fundamental mechanism which is common to all obliterating arteriopathies in the form of pathologically increased adhesiveness of platelets to the vessel wall.

1.   The rather frequent finding of global pathological aggregation of platelets in patients with obliterating arteriosclerosis.

2.   The appearance of obliterating arteriopathies in persons
with thrombocytosis without further risk factors for an obliterating
arteriosclerosis.   The clinical picture is characterized by repeatedly occurring subacute ischemia and by the evidence of stenosis and obliteration of the vessels.   When the thrombocytosis is
corrected, the ischemic attacks cease immediately.

3.   The favored appearance of a stenosis at the point where
vessels are bifurcating: within the sphere of impetuous streaming
the forces that the platelets collide with one another or with the
vessel wall are particularly strong.   Those conditions push forward
the aggregation and adhesion of platelets, as we have shown.

4.   The localization of obliterating angiopathies mostly in
arteries, seldom in veins (phlebitis migrans): in the fast arterial
stream the shear rate and accordingly the forces effective in
platelet collisions are by far more intensive than in the slow
venous stream.

5.   The formation of arteriosclerotic changes in dacron grafts:
platelets and mixed parietal thrombi are the starting material of
the neointimal as well as of sclerotic plaques.

The various forms of obliterating arteriopathies, as there are
acute, subacute and chronic progress can be explained by initial
platelet adhesions and aggregations.

In addition to the component parts of the streaming blood which
become adherent to the vessel wall, there can be lipid droplets in
case of a disturbance of lipid metabolism.

It is quite clear that the material of the adhesion on the vessel
wall finally coming to incorporation also determines the pathological modifications of the vessel wall.

Finally, depending from the reaction of the individual concerned, the mesenchymal reactions can take different forms.
Hence it does not matter whether these mesenchymal reactions

are caused primarily by the risk factors or secondarily by
irritation from the deposits.

The increased adhesiveness of the platelets is also the
decisive mechanism for the progression of obliterating arteriosclerosis. If it comes to nothing, the disease doesn't proceed.
Examples for this are as follows:

    1. A cold angiitis is limited to the place of the single injury.
    2. An angiopathy caused by thrombocytosis stops as soon as
the primary disease has been successfully treated.
    3. In cases of thrombangiitis obliterans, due only to inhala-
tion; cessation of inhalation of smoke resulted in no further
aggregation.

Our data suggest that the progression of vascular disease is
due primarily to continuous exposure of the vessel to the irritating
causative agent (e. g. smoking).

We understand the pathogenesis of all obliterating angiopathies
no longer exclusively as a primary damage of the vessel wall, but
as the result of a distrubed relation between vessel wall and
streaming blood and thereby first of all the platelet. From this
extended pathogenetic conception we propose new hypotheses for
a causal prophylaxis and therapy of these diseases.

Scope and Organization of a Lipid Clinic and Clinical Trials

SCOPE AND ORGANIZATION OF A LIPID CLINIC AND CLINICAL TRIALS

A. N. Klimov, M. D.

Institute for Experimental Medicine, Academy of
Medical Science, Laboratory of Lipid Metabolism,
Leningrad, USSR

It is well known that in the United States, the single greatest
cause of death before age 65 is myocardial infarction due to coronary artery atherosclerosis. This also appears to be true for
the Soviet Union, at least in its large urban communities. Data
gathered in many countries have indicated that the probability of
development of premature coronary artery disease is increased
when certain "risk factors" are present. The most obvious of
these include hyperlipidemia, cigarette smoking, hypertension,
and diabetes mellitus. Quantitavely, hypercholesterolemia is
perhaps the most important. Not only is extreme hypercholesterolemia associated with high risk, but even the "average" values
believed to be present in Soviet and American populations are
associated with higher risks than are the average levels in certain
less industrialized societies.

The concentrations of cholesterol and triglycerides, another
risk factor, are determined by diet, by caloric balance, and other
environmental factors, and are also under important genetic influences. It has been shown that blood lipid levels can be controlled by changes in diet, way-of-life, and sometimes by drugs.
It is also possible to affect the expression of certain genetic causes
of hyperlipidemia. One of the more important advances is the
recognition of many different causes of hyperlipidemia and, thus,
the diversity of therapeutic and preventive approaches that must
be applied.

There are many questions still to be answered about hyperlipidemia and coronary artery disease. The most important is
whether control of hyperlipidemia actually affects control of
atherosclerosis. It is also the most difficult question to answer
and is being studied in several ways. More data are urgently
needed to assist in such studies. These include better statistics
about the prevalence of coronary artery disease and of hyperlipidemia in different populations, where environmental factors are
not identical. The Soviet and American ways of life offer important comparisons. The perhaps greater diversity among different
population groups within the Soviet Union offer exceptional opportunities for comparison studies. Does diet seem to have the same
influence in both countries? Are there significant genetic differences? Are there risk factors unique to one country? Can common approaches to prevention be utilized?

Fortunately the science of classifying hyperlipidemia (or
hyperlipoproteinemia) has advanced to a stage where standardized
common methodology may be used for such comparisons. The
basic methods have been recommended by WHO as a standard for
all countries. As it is known, such techniques have been set up
in a number of laboratories or clinics in the United States - called
Lipid Research Clinics, supported by the National Heart and Lung
Institute. Common protocols have been developed, data are cen-
trally collected and exchanged, and standardization is supervised
by the WHP center in Atlanta, Georgia.

The lipid clinics (centers) in Moscow and Leningrad were
organized at the beginning of 1974 in accordance with the agreement between the governments of the USSR and the USA on Cooper-
ation in the Field of Medical Science and Public Health. The
Moscow center is located at the Myasnikov Institute of Cardiology
and the Leningrad center - at the Institute for Experimental
Medicine.

The goal of joint USSR-USA trials consists in study of prevalence of different types of the hyperlipoproteinemias and especially their types among defined population and a connection of hyperlipoproteinemias with prevalence of ischemic heart disease.

The tasks of the joint trials are as follows:

a) to determine the frequency of dislipidemias, especially

their types;

   b) to obtain the prevalence of ischemic heart disease in defined population;

   c) to evaluate relationship between prevalence of hyperlipoproteinemias and ischemic heart disease;

   d) to provide the opportunity of testing the influence of the
most active hypolipidemic drugs on normalization of some types
of hyperlipoproteinemia, concerning prevention of ischemic heart
disease.

   The Soviet-American cooperative program is based on the
national research program already in existence in the USSR and
the USA (on phenotyping of lipoproteinemias in the USSR see 1-4).

   Agreement has been reached that the combined USSR-USA
study will be of men, age 40-59 years. On the USSR side,
10,000 subjects will be sampled in Phase 1 and approximately
2,500 in Phase 2. The populations have been randomly selected
from 1974 voting lists of one of the districts in Moscow and in
Leningrad. It is proposed to start the pilot study (the preliminary
investigation of 200 subjects in Moscow and the same number in
Leningrad) at the beginning of 1975. The basic study will begin
in March or April 1975 and will be completed within 2 years.

   We are prepared to use in the USSR the same protocols as
in the American clinics. Standardization is supervised by the
WHO center in Atlanta, Georgia. Phase 1 will consist of the
US Phase 1 plus:

   1. Resting ECG
   2. Rose Questionaire
   3. Blood pressure
   4. HDL cholesterol
   5. Anthropometry.

   The following subjects will be recalled for the Phase 2
examination:

   1. 15% random sample from Phase 1;
   2. 10% upper cholesterol distribution;

3. 5%: upper triglyceride distribution.

The concentration of cholesterol and triglyceride will be determined by Autoanalyzer AA II. The USSR side uses polyacryl-amide gel for lipoprotein electrophoresis. To rule out secondary causes of hyperlipoproteinemia (in Phase 2) some standardized laboratory tests will be used (determination of plasma sugar, serum protein, bilirubin, urea, uric acids, alkaline phosphatase, transaminase). The exchange of data will be carried out period-ically. Data will be transmitted on magnetic tapes. It was stated that each side has the right of publication and other use of its in-formation. Any publication of data or results connected with analysis of joint investigations will be done by mutual agreement.

There can be no doubt that from the USSR-US cooperative program on prevalence of hyperlipoproteinemia and ischemic heart disease in the Soviet and American populations a great bene-fit to both sides and to the world in general is foreseen in this common search for knowledge about a disease which knows no national boundaries.

REFERENCES

1. A.N. Klimov, N.G. Nikulcheva. Types of hyperlipoproteine-mias, their relation to atherosclerosis and treatment. Cardi-ologia 6: 133, 1972 (in Russian)
2. M.V. Bavina, N.V. Perova, N.M. Lobova, and G.I. Koro-pova. The significance of typing of hyperlipidemias for lipo-tropic therapy of atherosclerosis. Cardiologia 3: 27, 1973 (in Russian)
3. I.V. Krivorutchenko, E. Ya. Magracheva, N.G. Nikulcheva, and T.S. Yanushkene. Lipoprotein blood spectrum in patients with ischemic heart disease based on the data derived from electrophoresis in polyacrylamide gel. Cardiologia 9: 21, 1974 (in Russian)
4. A.N. Klimov, N.G. Nikulcheva and I.V. Krivorutchenko. Phenotyping of hyperlipoproteinemias (methodical approaches). Cardiologia 12: 103, 1974 (in Russian)

PORTACAVAL SHUNT IN TWO PATIENTS WITH HOMOZYGOUS HYPERCHOLESTEROLEMIA

E. A. Stein[1,2], C. Mieny[3], J. Pettifor[2], and M. Dinner[2]

[1]Cardiovascular Research Unit, South African Institute for Medical Research, Johannesburg; [2]Lipid Disorders Clinic, Departments of Pediatrics and Pediatric Surgery, University of Witwatersrand and Transvaal Memorial Hospital for Children, Johannesburg; [3]Department of Surgery, University of Witwatersrand and J. G. Strydom Hospital, Johannesburg, South Africa.

INTRODUCTION

Despite the fact that the homozygous form of familial hyperbetalipoproteinemia (HβLP) is exceedingly rare, 17 such patients (from fourteen families) have been seen at a treatment centre for lipid disorders in Johannesburg during the past three years.

The disease in South Africa is confined almost entirely to those of Caucasian origin, and familial HβLP even in the heterozygous form has still to be documented in the Black population. Furthermore it has been our experience that the patients most severely afflicted with the disease, including 16 of the 17 homozygotes, are descendants of the Afrikaans speaking community.

The prognosis for the homozygote is extremely poor, with few surviving the third decade of life.

During the course of the disease the patients often suffer gross disfiguration from xanthomas and crippling arterial disease.

The development of new therapeutic regimes seems to have

altered the course of the disease little, although a few workers
(1, 2) have claimed some amelioration in the clinical and biochemical progression of the disease.   Results of medical treatment in
the Johannesburg centre has, in most cases, been disappointing.

Two deaths have occurred from myocardial infarction in our
group of homozygotes during the past eight months.   The first was
a twelve year old male who had undergone ileal bypass at age three,
and had been on large doses of cholestyramine - up to 48 grams
daily - nicotinic acid and clofibrate, for two years prior to his
sudden death.   The second also died suddenly and had been on intermittent treatment for many years.   Neither of the two patients
had experienced myocardial infarction prior to death, but they had
shown gross ischaemic changes on electrocardiograph.

The publication by Starzl et al (3) of the dramatic and sustained clinical and biochemical improvement in a twelve year old
girl after portacaval shunt, and the recommendations emitting
therefrom, offered hope for some of our patients considered at
high risk.   After careful consideration it was decided to proceed
with portacaval shunt in a limited number of selected high-risk
patients.   We describe here the results of two patients after portacaval shunt.

CASE REPORTS

Patient No. 1

A seven year old male, A. P. , was noted to have xanthoma be-
hind both knees at birth.   At the age of one year he was diagnosed
as having hypercholesterolemia.   At that time his cholesterol level
was 1000 mg/dl.   Xanthoma appeared over the dorsum of his hands,
knees and elbows.   By age four they had increased considerably,
and were noted on his buttocks, the soles of his feet and the palms
of both hands.   From the time of diagnosis until the age of three
he was treated with clofibrate, nicotinic acid and a carbohydrate
restricted diet.   Cholestyramine, 4 grams daily, was added to
this regime for the following two years.   There was no clinical
or biochemical response to the treatment.

He was first seen at the Lipid Disorders Centre in July, 1972, by which time all therapy had been stopped. His cholesterol level at the time was 900 mg/dl, triglycerides were normal, and there was a marked elevation of the β lipoprotein fraction on electrophoresis (87% of the lipogram). Treatment with low cholesterol, low fat, and increased polyunsaturated fat diet was commenced, with a mild response. Cholestyramine was again administered at a dose of 12 gm daily, and increased slowly to 42 grams per day. To this regime, nicotinic acid, 2 gm daily, was added. A moderate response was observed (Figure 1). During this period there was no amelioration in the growth or formation of new xanthoma.

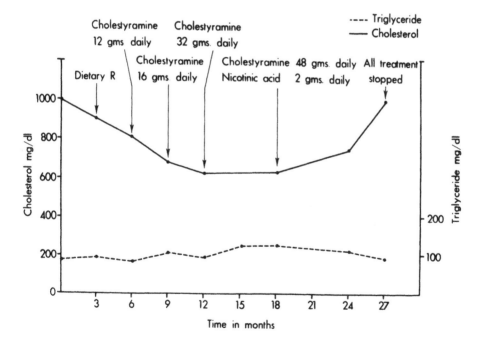

Figure 1: Cholesterol levels during 30 months medical treatment in patient A. P.

Toward the latter half of 1973 the patient began to experience episodes of left-sided chest pain. Although an ejection systolic murmur, compatible with aortic stenosis was present together with generalized carotid, abdominal aortic, renal and femoral bruits, both resting and effort electrocardiographs failed to reveal ischaemic changes.

Investigations for carbohydrate intolerance and thyroid malfunction proved negative. The patient had an elevated sedimentation rate, at all times greater than 50 mm per hour and raised SGOT levels (50-60 units).

Kindred studies (Figure IIA) revealed both parents to be heterozygotes for hypercholesterolemia. His father experienced a myocardial infarct at the age of thirty-seven, he had no xanthoma, but arcus juvenilis was present. When first seen at the Lipid Disorders Centre, his cholesterol was 476 mg/dl. Hypercholesterolemia was confirmed in all the father's siblings. Two paternal uncles died from premature coronary artery disease. A. P. 's mother presented with marked achilles tendon xanthoma and an ejection systolic murmur radiating into the neck, compatible with aortic stenosis. Her cholesterol was 489 mg/dl. Both her mother (A. P. 's maternal grandmother) and one brother were confirmed hypercholesteremics with serum cholesterol levels of 500 and 540 mg/dl respectively.

The patient's eldest sister aged fifteen had achilles tendon thickening and a serum cholesterol of 328 mg/dl.

The kindred studies together with the patient's total and low density lipoprotein (LDL) cholesterol levels, the presence of xanthoma prior to age ten, and the suggestion of ischaemic heart disease so early in life, were sufficient to verify the presence of true homozygous familial hyperbetalipoproteinemia.

The patient was removed from all drug therapy, and after one month, baseline parameters were measured. The patient was then hospitalized for hyperalimentation prior to performance of a portacaval shunt.

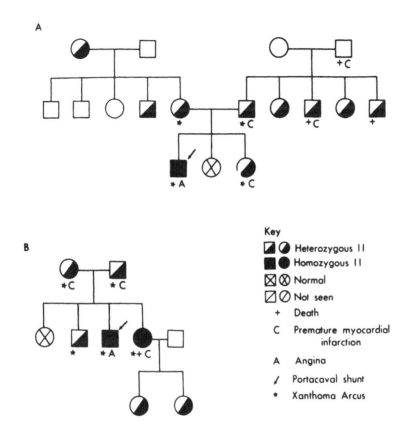

Figure II (a-b): Investigation for lipid abnormalities in the families of the two patients subjected to portacaval shunt.

Patient No. 2

A twenty-seven year old married man, C. J., had no lesions at birth, but within the first year of life xanthoma appeared on his hands and buttocks, slowly increasing in size and becoming more generalized during the next few years. No medical advice was sought until the age of seven when the xanthoma were biopsied and hypercholesterolemia diagnosed. No treatment was instituted, and the patient, who then lived on a farm, pursued a diet rich in dairy and meat products. In 1965, at the age of eighteen, xanthoma were removed surgically from both elbows. The only treatment used was clofibrate in intermittent doses. At the age of twenty-two, with further increase of the xanthoma, C. J. underwent an ileal

bypass. There was no sign of improvement, and the bypass was
corrected in 1971 as the patient experienced intractable diarrhea.

The patient first attended our Lipid Disorders Centre at the
beginning of 1972. His height was 172 cms and he weighed 90 kg.
Prominent arcus juvenilis, surrounding almost the entire cornea,
was present. Pendulous xanthoma had regrown over his elbows,
and his hands, palms, knees, feet, buttocks and achilles tendons
were involved to a greater or lesser degree. A grade 3/6 ejection
systolic murmur was present over the aortic area and radiated
into his neck. Generalized bruits were also present. Hepatosplenomegaly was found, however this had been present for a number of
years. Previous investigations for the hepatosplenomegaly, including sternal bone marrow biopsy, had proven negative. He
came from a bilharzia area, and subsequent investigations for bilharzia proved positive. Portal hypertension was not present.

He had experienced angina on effort the previous 4-5 years.
At the time of his first visit his effort tolerance was 200 metres
or two flights of steps, limitation being due to angina. Although
there was no history of myocardial infarction, his electrocardiograph showed ischaemic changes after mild exercise.

A low cholesterol, low modified fat diet was instituted and the
patient was advised to stop smoking, which he did. Cholestyramine, 24 grams daily, gradually increasing up to 36 grams per
day, Clofibrate, 2 grams daily, and nicotinic acid, 3 grams daily,
were added to the regime. Angina still persisted, and the patient
was hospitalized in December, 1973 in an attempt to ensure weight
reduction. A weight loss of 15 kg was achieved during the following
4 months. The patient's effort tolerance increased to 500 metres
or three flights of steps. Anginal attacks became less frequent.
During the period of treatment the patient's cholesterol remained
between 600-700 mg/dl, having dropped from a pre-treatment
level in the region of 1000 mg/dl.

An interesting feature was a persistent elevation of plasma
triglycerides, varying between 370 and 505 mg/dl while on treatment. On the withdrawal of medication and after the 15 kg weight
loss, the patient's triglyceride values fell below 200 mg/dl.

Early in 1974 the patient underwent a second operation to remove the regrown pendulous xanthoma on his elbows. This

operation was undertaken privately despite advice from the Lipid
Centre to the contrary. Following this operation the angina increased in frequency and duration. The patient had discontinued
all lipid lowering treatment except the diet. Three months after
stopping treatment he was admitted for hyperalimentation and
portacaval shunt.

Both the patient's mother and father have been shown to be
hypercholesterolemic (Figure IIB). His father, who has refused
medical advice for the past six years, had a serum cholesterol
of 525 mg/dl. Although now in his late sixties, he has suffered
from ischaemic heart disease since age fifty, including myocardial
infarction. C. J.'s mother, now age forty-nine, has experienced
angina since age thirty-five. She has a cholesterol level of 455
mg/dl, normal triglycerides, elevated LDL cholesterol (368 mg/
dl), and elevated β fraction on electrophoresis.

An elder sister of the patient died at the age of twenty-six
from myocardial infarction. She too presented with xanthoma and
elevated plasma cholesterol levels early in life. During her life
she gave birth to two children, both heterozygous for hypercholesterolemia. A younger brother aged twenty-three, has achilles
tendon thickening and a serum cholesterol of 395 mg/dl. A
younger sister is normal. Although no further relatives have
been seen at our centre, some are receiving treatment for hypercholesterolemia at other centres.

METHODS

A. Hyperalimentation

Both patients prior to portacaval shunt (PCS) had a one month
period free of medical treatment to establish baseline data. The
patients were then submitted to three weeks of total parenteral
alimentation. During the first two weeks they received a casein
hydrolysate, dextrose, electrolyte and vitamin infusion. The
protein and calorie intake was varied according to body weight and
age. A fat emulsion (Intralipid 10%) was administered together
with the above infusion for the third week. The daily amount of
the fat emulsion was gradually increased to 2 gms/kilogram body
weight.

B. Operative Procedure

On the completion of three weeks alimentation, an end-to-side portacaval shunt was performed. In patient A. P. interrupted sutures were used for the vascular anastomosis in order to allow for future growth of the vessels. During the operative procedure, skin and a wedge liver biopsy were taken for histology and biochemical studies, the results of which will be reported in a later communication.

C. Investigations

Both patients were subjected to regular hematological, electrolyte and liver function investigations. Serum lipid and insulin levels were measured twice weekly during the pre-operative and immediate post-operative periods and later at monthly intervals. Serum cholesterol and triglycerides were measured on Technicon AAII.

RESULTS

Total cholesterol levels decreased during hyperalimentation (Figures III, IV), however, in patient A. P. this reduction was not sustained and during Intralipid administration, serum cholesterol rose slightly (Figure III).

After portacaval shunt, cholesterol levels rose during the following 25-45 days compared to alimentation levels. Cholesterol levels have since this period, undergone a gradual decrease. Triglyceride levels have remained normal in patient A. P. , and in patient C. J. in whom mild hypertriglyceridemia was present pre-operatively, triglyceride values have fallen to normal levels.

Clinically a diminution in eruptive xanthoma has been noted post-operatively, however there has been a significant difference between the two cases. Patient C. J. showed a dramatic reduction in superficial skin xanthoma over his knees within two weeks of the operation. Furthermore, since portacaval shunt, he has experienced a marked improvement in effort tolerance with a concomitant reduction in the frequency and severity of anginal attacks. C. J. 's ejection systolic murmur has decreased in intensity and there has been a reduction in the bruits over the large arteries.

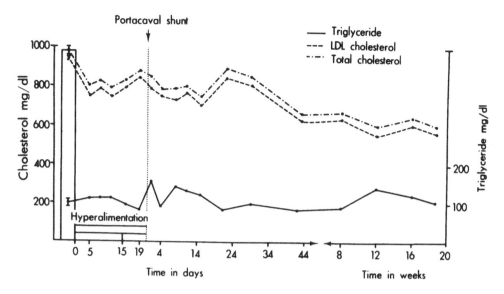

Figure III: Lipid Changes during alimentation and after portacaval shunt in patient A. P.

Patient A. P., who experienced less cholesterol reduction during alimentation has responded slower post-operatively. Reduction in xanthoma only became clinically apparent 6 weeks post-operatively. Although there has been no reduction in the intensity of his aortic murmur or large vessel bruits, A. P. has experienced no further episodes of chest pain and his activity has increased markedly.

DISCUSSION

The recent communication by Ahrens (5) and Starzl et al (3) have suggested a conservative approach at present, to the use of portacaval shunt for the treatment of homozygous hypercholesterolemia. For this reason only well documented homozygotes, considered as "high risk" candidates for myocardial infarction were considered for the procedure. A motivating factor for the use of portacaval shunt in the patients described in this report, was the sudden death of 2 homozygous patients, aged 12 and 13, after protracted medical treatment and with no history of previous

myocardial infarction.   Both of the patients in this series have
had extensive genetic validation of their disease (Figure II), and
in most cases three generations have been studied.   In addition,
the patients have conformed to the major and minor criteria, as
laid down by Fredrickson (6), for the establishment of the homozygous condition.   At present no facilities exist in our unit for the
study of fibroblast skin cultures.   Intensive medical treatment had
in both cases been unsuccessful in retarding the clinical progression
of the disease, and only marginal improvements had been recorded
in the serum cholesterol levels.   Patient C. J. had also failed to
respond to ileal bypass.

Both patients had clinical evidence of ischaemic heart disease
which was deteriorating despite treatment.   Myocardial infarction
had not been recorded in either of the patients prior to hyperalimentation.   The patients were therefore considered to be true
homozygotes who did not respond to medical therapy and were at
high risk for myocardial infarction in view of their age, history
or clinical findings.   The decision to commit the patients to portacaval shunt under these circumstances is in keeping with the belief
of Starzl et al (7) that the procedure should be carried out "hope-
fully prior to myocardial infarction."

The response to hyperalimentation was similar to that reported
by Starzl (3), however, differences between the 2 cases were
found.   A. P. responded less rapidly and to a lesser extent (Figure
III) than did the other patient (Figures IV).   During the Intralipid
phase the serum cholesterol rose in the case of A. P. , while a continued decrease was noted in the other patient during the same
phase.   No clinical or biochemical differences could be detected
to explain this variation in response to Intralipid.

Post-operatively, both patients experienced a slight rise in
serum cholesterol especially between days 25 and 45.   A similar
rise in cholesterol was noted in Starzl's patient between the
twentieth day and the third month.

Patient C. J. has experienced a 50% reduction in serum
cholesterol over pre-alimentation levels, however his cholesterol
level has remained above 600 mg/dl.   Serum cholesterol in A. P.
has fallent to two-thirds of pre-treatment levels.

The most dramatic clinical improvement has been observed
in C. J. in whom there was a decrease in the size and number of

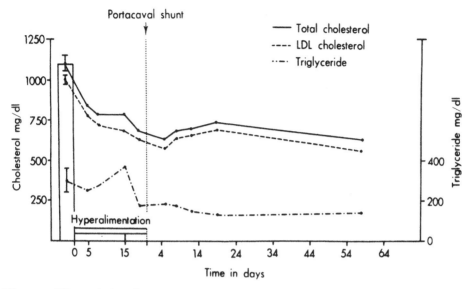

Figure IV: Lipid changes during alimentation and after portacaval shunt in patient C. J.

eruptive xanthoma on his knees and buttocks within 2 weeks of portacaval shunt. His ejection systolic murmur and generalized bruits are now less audible. Angina occurs only on extreme effort and his electrograph shows minimal ischemic changes on effort.

The other patient has shown a far less rapid clinical response post-operatively, however there has been some reduction in xanthoma.

Neither of the patients have suffered any ill effects post-operatively. Growth has been maintained. Liver function, hema-tological and electrolyte studies have remained normal. The patients remain only on dietary therapy.

In view of the continued clinical improvement in both patients, the fact that serum cholesterol has risen slightly or remained static after the initial post-operative reductions, has not caused undue concern.

Further information as to the mechanisms involved and even the short term effects of portacaval shunt on the vascular complications of the disease are needed. The role of hyperalimentation with and without Intralipid, as a prognostic test prior to operation, still needs clarification.

At this stage, therefore, portacaval shunt for the treatment of homozygous hypercholesterolemia should only be considered in patients with myocardial ischemia who have not responded to medical therapy.

REFERENCES

1. Levy, R. I., Fredrickson, D. S. and Shulman, R. Ann. Intern. Med. 72: 267, 1972.
2. Moutafis, C. D., Myant, N. B. and Mancini, M. Atherosclerosis 14: 247, 1971.
3. Starzl, T. E., Chase, H. P., Putnam, C. W. and Porter, K. A. Lancet 2: 940, 1973.
4. Laboratory Methods Committee. Manual of Laboratory Methods, Lipid Research Clinics Project. Lipid Metabolism Branch of the National Institutes of Health, Bethesda, 1973.
5. Ahrens, E. H., Jr. Lancet 2: 449, 1974.
6. Stanbury, J. B., Wyngaarden, J. B. and Fredrickson, D. S. The Metabolic Basis of Inherited Disease, McGraw Hill, New York, 1972, p. 565.
7. Starzl, T. E., Chase, H. P., Putnam, C. W., and Nora, J. J. Lancet 2: 714, 1974.
8. Dietschy, J. M. and Wilson, J. D. Lancet 1: 1128; 1179; 1241; 1970.

PLANNING THE TYPE II CORONARY PRIMARY PREVENTION TRIAL OF THE LIPID RESEARCH CLINICS (U. S. A.)

Daniel Steinberg, M. D. , Ph. D.

Division of Metabolic Disease, Department of Medicine, University of California, San Diego School of Medicine, La Jolla, California

One of the important potential functions for an organized system of cooperating lipid research clinics is to serve as a framework for large-scale intervention studies, studies beyond the scope of any individual clinic. The Lipid Research Clinics in the United States, sponsored by the National Heart and Lung Institute, are already embarked on such a large-scale study and the experience gained in the planning stages may be helpful to other groups contemplating related studies. My purpose today is to share with you some examples of the problems that were encountered rather than attempt a complete review of that study. This is the report not of an epidemiologist but a physician and it will be more anecdotal than analytical.

In July 1971, shortly after the Lipid Research Clinics were first established in the U. S. , I was asked to co-chair, with Dr. John W. Farquhar of Stanford University, a committee whose charge it was to design a feasible study to test the "lipid hypothesis," i. e. , the hypothesis that intervention to reduce serum cholesterol levels does reduce risk of clinically manifest coronary artery disease. Indications were that the National Heart and Lung Institute was now prepared to finance such a test. However, it was also clear that the level of support was not unlimited and that pragmatic consideration would have to be given to costs and therefore sample size. Data were already available from several intervention studies (1-6) that tended to support the lipid hypothesis but it was felt that the case had not yet been made in unassailable fashion. Some of the reported studies were weak because the control group was not selected and studied in truly parallel fashion; some were not done double-blind; there were ambiguities in some with respect to end-point definition; some had raised questions regarding excess mortality from malignancies and/or failure to reduce overall mortality. In short, it was felt that before there could be the basis for an all-out, community supported attack on hyperlipidemia as a risk factor, there would have to be a definitive confirmation of this lipid hypothesis.

Our Committee encountered many knotty problems in designing what has developed to be an enormously complex mass experiment - some theoretical problems, some ethical problems and some highly pragmatic problems. The discussions of our Intervention Committee spanned almost a two-year period. In the course of that time I learned a great deal from my colleagues and I want to thank them publicly for that and for their conscientious and earnest devotion to a difficult task. The make-up of the original committee is shown in Table 1. Additional members were added later, at the

Table 1

Intervention Committee, Lipid Research Clinics, 1971

LRC Representatives

Daniel Steinberg, U. of Calif. San Diego, Chairman

John W. Farquhar, Stanford U., co Chairman

William R. Hazzard, U. of Washington

Edmond A. Murphy, Johns Hopkins U.

Al Oberman, U. of Alabama

Richard D. Remington, U. of Texas

Data Coordinating Center Representatives

Dale Williams, U. of North Carolina

James E. Grizzle, U. of North Carolina

NHLI Staff

Robert I. Levy, NHLI

Basil Rifkind, NHLI

Table II

LRC Intervention Committee
Current Membership

John W. Farquhar, Stanford University, Chairman

William E. Connor, University of Iowa, Co-Chairman

G. William Benedict, John Hopkins University

C. E. Davis, University of North Carolina

Ronald W. Fallat, University of Cincinnati

Antonio M. Gotto, Jr., Baylor University

Richard C. Gross, University of California, San Diego

William R. Hazzard, University of Washington

Donald B. Hunninghake, University of Minnesota

John C. LaRosa, George Washington University

Maurice Mishkel, McMaster University

Gustav Schonfeld, Washington University

L. Thomas Sheffield, University of Alabama

Thomas F. Whayne, Jr., University of Oklahoma

Richard J. Havlik, Program Office Representative

end of the first year, when 6 more Lipid Research Clinics were
established.   Table II lists the current membership of the Committee.   I should add that we also had invaluable help from many other
NHLI staff members and from a number of expert ad hoc consul-
tants in biostatistics, epidemiology and clinical medicine.   Special
recognition should be accorded the Chairman of today's panel, Dr.
Basil Rifkind, for his tireless staff work, and Dr. Robert I. Levy,
Chief of the Metabolism Branch, under whose patient and capable
direction this program was initiated and nurtured.

Let me start by pointing out some of the constraints the
Committee imposed on itself.   First, we decided that we wanted to
do a primary rather than a secondary prevention study.   One of the

purposes was to show that prevention was possible in clinically well persons. Hence, the many exclusions (e. g. , clinical coronary heart disease, congestive heart failure, hypertension, diabetes, hepatic or renal disease). Second, the study was to be done in a free-living population so that the result would not have to be extrapolated from a closed to open population. Third, we agreed that the study must be of a double-blind design. A double-blind design is, of course, always preferable when possible but here it was felt to be absolutely essential if the enormous effort involved was to have any chance of yielding an unimpeachable result. Finally, we elected to study patients with elevation of low density lipoprotein (Type II) and to use cholestyramine as the hypolipidemic agent (with diet prescription for both control and treatment groups).

Although we were not wholly unprepared for it, our first shock came when we grappled with the size of sample needed. When dealing with any chronic disease entity with a relatively low incidence rate the numbers of subjects required will be large, even assuming a reasonably large treatment effect on incidence. One thing that was immediately apparent was that we simply could not seriously consider a study in a random, open population given the constraints imposed on manpower and money power.

There are many factors that enter into sample size estimations some of which I only learned to fully appreciate during my service on this Committee. Many of you are much more familiar with these matters than I and I don't propose to go deeply into biostatistics. But one of my major points is to underscore the necessity for cooperative research protocols in order to study preventive therapy in chronic disease like coronary heart disease. For that reason it may be useful to review briefly the factors that determine the large sample sizes we are talking about. Some of the key factors are listed in Table III.

One needs to decide the confidence limits one insists on - α, the chance that a no-effect regimen will <u>falsely</u> be considered to be beneficial, and β, the chance that an effective regimen will falsely be concluded to have had <u>no</u> effect. The higher the level of certainty you insist on, the larger the sample size required.

Drop-out rate is very important in determining sample size. It is difficult to predict and may be importantly influenced by the

Table III

Factors Entering Into Determination of
Sample Size (n) Required

1. **Confidence limits desired**
    α- the probability of a false positive result
    β- the probability of a false negative result

2. **Anticipated drop-out rate**

3. **Duration of study**

4. **Incidence rate with chosen end-point**

5. **Predicted reduction of incidence with intervention**

6. **f-factor — the number of years before full treatment
    effect is realized**

rigor of the regimen the patients are asked to accept.

Obviously, the sample size varies inversely with the duration of the study. The level of risk - the anticipated yearly incidence in the untreated group - is an important factor and this is determined by the chosen endpoint. As you will see, we were ultimately driven to select a group with a much higher than average risk. Only in this way could the sample size be kept down. The predicted effectiveness of the treatment is one of the flabby figures; obviously, if we knew it we wouldn't be doing the study. What we did was to use the data of the NHLI-sponsored Framingham Project (7) to estimate incidence in the control group. Then we assumed - rightly or wrongly - that a given reduction in plasma cholesterol would reduce incidence to that of people normally characterized by the new, lower cholesterol level.

Finally, we came to another flabby figure, the f-factor, which is the time before the full impact of the treatment regimen on incidence of endpoints is reached. It is most unlikely that the instant a man reduces his cholesterol level, say from 300 to 200 mg%, his risk of a myocardial infarction drops to that characteristic of a population of men that have always had cholesterol levels of 200 mg%. But how long does it take? We have to admit ignorance and guess. From the positive results reported by Leren (2), by Dayton et al (4), by Turpeinen et al (5) and by others (1, 3, 6), one

can guess that it is less than 5 years at any rate! Arbitrarily, we
have assumed an f-factor of 3 years.

The National Heart Institutes Diet-Heart Panel had been
through this kind of exercise previously (8) and Table IV gives an
example of their sample size estimate for a particular protocol.
The values for α and β are those commonly employed in epidemiologic studies of this kind - 0.01 and 0.10, respectively. The predicted drop-out rate - 8% year - may have been on the pessimistic
side. No one happily faces a study extending beyond 5 years so
they elected this magic figure. The study population had to be
males above 40 and with cholesterol levels above 240 mg% if the
numbers required were to be kept down. A 25% reduction in incidence was hoped for from adherence to a low-cholesterol, low-
saturated fat diet. Now, even if the treatment effect were maximum from the onset of the study (i. e. , f = 0), 22,500 men would
have had to be enrolled! If the treatment effect took 3 years to

Table IV

Estimation of Sample Size (n) Required for a Hypothetical Diet-Heart Study

α - the probability of a false positive result:	0.01
β - the probability of a false negative result:	0.10
Drop-out rate:	~8%/year
Duration of study:	5 years
Study population:	Men, 40-59; cholesterol >240 mg%
Endpoint:	MI or CHD death
Reduction in incidence due to treatment:	25%
f - number of years before full treatment effect is realized:	0 years

Then, n = __22,500!__

If f = 3 years, then, n = __47,000!!__

(Diet-Heart Review Panel, 1969)

become maximal (f = 3), not an unreasonable possibility at all, 47,000 men would have been needed!!

These are the sobering realities regarding the definitive testing of therapeutic regimens in coronary heart disease - or any similar chronic disease. The numbers can be reduced by using closed populations, prisons for example, where the drop-out rate should be low! Or one can limit the study population to subjects at very high risk. But each such compromise also compromises the legitimacy of extrapolating the result in order to justify an expensive, large-scale program of preventive medicine for the general public. Unless we are willing to resign ourselves to "flying blind," we have no choice but to be prepared to meet the challenge of large-scale trials. And that probably means government-funded, multi-center studies. The Lipid Research Clinics represent a start in that direction taken in the United States.

Let me return to our own study as it evolved. To hold the sample size down we elected to study males only, ages 35-59 and with significant hypercholesterolemia. In other words, we selected a group with a considerably higher-than-average expected incidence of the chosen endpoints - myocardial infarction and coronary heart disease death. In view of some of the published evidence indicating that coronary heart disease becomes clinically manifest earlier in men with essential hypercholesterolemia than in men with hypertriglyceridemia or mixed hyperlipidemia and to define a population that could be all treated the same way, the prime requirement was an LDL cholesterol above the 95th percentile and a triglyceride value below 300 mg%, corresponding to phenotypes IIa or "IIb minus." After much discussion of the various treatment regimens open to us - and I don't have time to review this or to justify our choices - we elected to use cholestyramine plus diet. A placebo very difficult to distinguish from the resin was an essential and that is being provided. We are assuming a 25% reduction in cholesterol level which, if the premise stated above is correct, should reduce the incidence of events (myocardial infarction or coronary death) by about 50%. Finally, we agreed to commit ourselves to a 7-year study, if necessary, hoping that a significant result may be achieved sooner in which case the study will be terminated. Table V recapitulates the skeleton outline of the protocol with a sample size of 3,600 men required. We are excluding patients with clinically manifest coronary disease and patients with several other categories of disease but I won't take

Table V

Parameters for the LRC Type II Intervention Study

α: 0.01

β: 0.10

Predicted drop-out rate: 5%/year

Duration of study: 7 years (maximum)

Study population: Males, 35-59, without clinical coronary heart disease;
LDL cholesterol > 175 mg%

End points: Myocardial infarction or coronary heart disease death

Anticipated reduction in cholesterol level:

   In the placebo group (diet only) <5%
   In the treatment group (cholestyramine plus diet) >25%

f: 3 years

$$n = 3,600$$

---

time to review the strategies for randomization and stratification
or the complex mechanics of this 12-center trial. The final protocol book is about an inch thick!

Before leaving the theoretical issues, let me say that we are
fully aware that there are real limitations on the extent to which
any result coming out of this study can be generalized. First, our
study population is selected - males 35-59, at high risk because
of hypercholesterolemia. Second, our intervention is of a particular kind - cholestyramine treatment. This may - or may not -
be equivalent to cholesterol-lowering regimens of other kinds.
Finally, we have limited ourselves to men with a particular lipoprotein pattern. For these reasons, this study will not yield any
totally generalizable result. Only the totally random open population study would do this (and still only with regard to the specific intervention elected) and we have seen the numbers that make
it most unlikely that such a study will ever be done in a controlled
fashion.

Now I want to say a few words about an ethical issue we faced and which other groups will have to face. Should the control group be followed with no treatment whatever? The easy answer is the following: If we do not know the answer - that is, do not know if lowering serum cholesterol levels constitutes meaningful therapy - then there is no ethical problem. But like so much else in medicine the situation is not black and white but some uncertain shade of gray. From what we know about experimental atherosclerosis from available prospective epidemiologic data and from the positive although not unchallenged intervention trials already completed, we really have - at least some of us - a certain degree of conviction that the treatment will work. The higher the level of that conviction, the more difficult the ethical question becomes for us. It could be argued that if they weren't enrolled in the study, the men on placebo would be unlikely to receive meaningful treatment anyway. I don't think we can lean too heavily on that argument. After much discussion - we ultimately opted for dietary treatment of the control group rather rather than no treatment. This decision resulted in a requirement for a significantly higher "n" so it was not an easy one.

Finally, a few words about pragmatic problems. In a multicenter trial there must be the strictest possible comparability in all methodology from center to center in order to justify pooling of results. Dr. Rifkind and Dr. Noble have discussed some aspects of this problem and I only have one thing to add. I believe one of the main reasons we have managed as well as we have on this score is that all the personnel in all the clinics - not just the Directors - were very much involved in the elaboration of the common protocol. If it were not for this participation - if a protocol had been drawn up arbitrarily by any select group without constant consultations with those at the clinic and at the bench - the machinery might be creaky and the results sloppy. I would urge any group embarking on this sort of venture to keep in mind the importance of involvement and shared responsibility.

Another difficult problem is that of recruitment. Here we were somewhat overly optimistic and underestimated the amount of effort necessary to identify and bring into the study the number of subjects we need. The recruitment process is going along reasonably well now but we have had to learn new approaches to make it go. Some of the devices explored and reduced to practice may be useful in guiding others in future studies.

The list of practical problems is very long - from one as serious as how to define endpoints objectively to one as trivial as whether or not to provide free coffee and doughnuts to subjects coming in to give a fasting blood sample. I hope that we will eventually publish the list and report on our experience with both the serious and the trivial ones. Meanwhile, I'm sure Dr. Rifkind or Dr. Levy at the National Heart and Lung Institute stand ready to answer questions or give interim reports where they would be useful to others in any country.

The study is under way. It is costing many man-years of professional and non-professional effort and many, many dollars. We only hope that a definitive result will emerge.

REFERENCES

1. Christakis, G. , Rinzler, S. H. , Archer, M. et al: Amer. J. Public Health 56: 299, 1966.
2. Leren, P. : Acta Med. Scand. Suppl. 466, 1966.
3. Bierenbaum, M. L. , Green, P. P. , Florin, A. et al: J. Amer. Med. Assn. 202: 1119, 1967.
4. Dayton, S. , Pearce, M. L. , Hashimoto, S. et al: Circulation 40: Suppl. II, 1969.
5. Turpeinen, O. , Miettinen, M. , Karvonen, M. J. et al: Amer. J. Clin. Nutr. 21: 255, 1968; Miettinen, M. , Turpeinen, O. , Karvonen, M. J. et al: Lancet 2: 835, 1972.
6. Dewar, H. A. and Oliver, M. F. : Brit. Med. J. 4: 784, 1971.
7. Truett, J. , Cornfield, J. and Kannel, W.: J. Chron. Dis. 20: 511, 1967.
8. Report of the Diet-Heart Review Panel of the National Heart Institute American Heart Association Monograph No. 28, The American Heart Association, Inc. , New York, 1969.

CONCLUDING REMARKS

Hugh Sinclair

Magdalen College, Oxford, England

THE HUNTING OF THE PLAQUE

During two weeks in September there were three International Conferences on Lipids in Milan, each lasting about a week (and therefore two being concurrent), and all presided over by Rodolfo Paoletti. Hurrying between papers in different buildings kept the Congressists on their toes and reminded them when they had caught their breath that exercise is good for you. All Conferences and Congressists) discussed atherosclerotic plaques. Exactly a century earlier, in the summer of 1874, a mathematics don in the second best College of Oxford - Christ Church - took a young girl for a walk. It (or rather, she) was not Alice Liddell who had earlier gone through the looking-glass; for the Rev. Charles Lutwidge Dodgson was a polygynaepaedophiliac; her name was Gertrude Chattaway. For her he wrote a splended poem - The Hunting of the Snark - worthy to lie beside Land of Hope and Glory or Eskimo Nell. For those who were not properly brought up, I might mention that the Snark was hunted with diverse methods by a motley team with a frequent refrain: "Just the place for a Snark." Had "Lewis Carroll" been in Milan a century later he would have noted the atherosclerotic plaque being hunted with diverse methods by a motley team including even a surgeon who quoted from Leviticus (7, 22) Jehovah's instructions to the Israelites: "You shall not eat the fat of any ox, sheep or goat;" but he was not aware that He considered the saturated fat of these ruminants to be the best food which should be reserved for sacrifice, the Celestial Lipid Metabolism

427

differing from ours.   We mortals at the Congress were advised
to decrease mortality by eating Japanese mushrooms.

"Just the place for a Congress, " Rodolfo exclaimed,
    "Now our 5th Drug Symposium's due;
Since Milan, which for beauty is widely acclaimed
    Has a fine University too. "

"We will gather a team that is harmonius,
    Representing each subject there is;
We will settle how drugs lower lipids, and thus
    Both treat and prevent heart disease. "

The team he selected included Bill Holmes,
    Dan Steinberg, Lars Carlson, and Dave
To edit proceedings in two costly tomes
    For which we must all start to save.

They hunted the plaque by the light of the moon;
    They sought it in Japanese quail;
They searched for a plaque in an aged baboon,
    In opossums, in snakes and a snail.

"Just the place for a plaque" the Pathologists cried
    As they scraped the aorta with care;
"Just the place for a plaque where the vessels divide
    If the intimal wall is laid bare. "

"You may seek it with forceps, and seek it with care
    As the intimal wall you explore
With scanning EM; when the plaque is laid bare
    You may stain it with Sudan IV. "

"Just the place for a plaque" Dick Havel declared
    As he stained his chromatogram;
"In this coloured strip of the gel I've prepared
    The lipids I'll easily scan. "

"Just the place for a plaque" Joe Goldstein believes;
  "Where the fibroblast's no binding site;
7-keto-cholesterol enters, and leaves
  Inhibited enzymes aright. "

"Just the place for a plaque, " Dr. Buchwald's team hope,
  "For an ileal bypass we'll make;
"After surgical plumbing - much better than dope -
  You can feast, and no fats need forsake. "

"Just the land for a plaque, " Steins and Eisenberg claimed,
  "Where honey and milk freely flow,
And dietary fats - by <u>Leviticus</u> blamed -
  Cause intimal lesions to grow. "

"Not a plaque you'll find here" said a man from Japan,
  "For with Japanese mushrooms for tea
Triglycerides fall, and the chromatogram
  Shows that all the cholesterol's free. "

They sought it with test-tubes, they sought it with care,
  With immuno methods and hope,
The centrifuged fractions with gels to ensnare
  And inspect it in a big microscope.

A plaque won't be present if all that you ate
  Is some fat with the right double bonds
And chlor-benzyl-oxy-fluor-nicotinate
  Which to "AZ 19" corresponds.

So join in the hunting of plaques if you're still
  Young and strong; when you're old, then reverse
The plaque with a pharmacological pill
  To conquer this prevalent curse.

THE EFFECT OF SOME DRUGS ON LIPID METABOLISM IN EXPERIMENTAL LIVER
AND INTESTINAL PATHOLOGY

N. K. Abdullaev

Tashkent, USSR

The intestine and liver play a prominent role in lipid metabolism. It seemed reasonable then to study the effects of pathology of these organs on lipid metabolism.

White rats (130-200 g) were used. One group (270) was given subcutaneous injections
of the alkaloid heliotrin (2, 5 or 10 mg/100 g) in order to produce toxic hepatitis and liver
cirrhosis. Another group (35) was given 3 mg/100 g of aminophenol to induce coecal
ulceration The remaining 30 rats were kept as controls.

The effects of a number of compounds (among them ATP, methionine, chlorpropamide,
insulin, vitamin C and biotin) on lipid metabolism in blood, liver and adipose tissue were
studied

A STUDY BY ELECTRON MICROSCOPY OF SOME ENZYMATIC AND STRUCTURAL
CORRELATIONS ON PLASMA LIPOPROTEINS

B Agostini

Max-Planck-Institut fur medizinische Forschung, Abteilung Physiologie, 6900 Heidelberg,
Germany

Structure of plasma lipoproteins and lipolytic activity in serum are closely related.
Triglyceride lipase in post-heparin plasma has been considered to be identical with
lipoprotein lipase, an enzyme present in adipose tissue and several organs, which hydrolyzes triglycerides of chylomicrons and very low density lipoproteins (VLDL). Electron
microscopy of negatively stained plasma shows that intravenous administration of heparin
to fasting healthy humans results in a rapid degradation of VLDL   These are also rapidly
digested by post-heparin lipolytic activity, when serum from non-heparinized subjects or
suspensions of isolated VLDL are incubated at 27° in vitro with postheparin serum of
fasting controls. When pre-heparin serum of fasting humans is incubated with post-
heparin plasma in the presence of protamine sulfate, which is known to inhibit extrahepatic triglyceride lipase activity of post-heparin plasma a smaller proportion of VLDL
particles is digested In addition degradation of chylomicrons by post-heparin lipolytic
activity is diminished when post-prandial serum is incubated with post-heparin plasma
added with protamine sulfate.

These results provide evidence that chylomicrons are first metabolized by the action
of extrahepatic triglyceride lipase, while liver triglyceride lipase appears to act pre-
ferentially on further steps of lipoprotein catabolism. Moreover observation in the electron
microscope of the changes in the structure of lipoprotein particles after incubation with
lipolytic enzymes offers another possibility of investigating the mechanism of lipoprotein
catabolism.

EFFECT OF DIETARY FATTY ACIDS ON DRUG METABOLISM

E. Agradi and C. Galli

Institute of Pharmacology and Pharmacognosy, University of Milano, 20129 Milano, Italy

Isocaloric semisynthetic diets containing 10% fat (w/w) of different fatty acid composition have been fed to growing male rats from the last week of pregnancy up to three to four months of age. Liver microsomes were prepared by ultracentrifugation and the basal activity of hydroxylating enzymes (benzpyrene and aniline hydroxylation) and the levels of cytochrome P-450 were determined.

Considerable modifications of these parameters were observed under the different dietary conditions. More specifically remarkable reduction of cytochrome P-450 and of benzpyrene hydroxylation without a decrease of aniline hydroxylation is observed in animals fed an essential fatty acid deficient diet. The dissociation in the effects of the dietary treatment on aniline and benzpyrene hydroxylation is observed also in animals fed diets with varying fatty acid composition.

SOME EFFECTS OF A NEW DRUG (3-METHYL-4-PHENYL-3-BUTENOIC ACID DIETHYLAMIDE) ON LIPOLYSIS IN MAN

P. Avogaro, G. Cazzolato and C. Capri

Ospedale Regionale Venezia, 30122 Venezia, Italy

Eight patients received 2 g of the drug per os at 8 a. m. after a light meal (g 30 bread and g 20 butter). The FFA level lowered 45% with a nadir between 60 and 120 min. The decrease was minor compared to the one obtained with Nicotinic Acid 750 mg (57%) and with propranolol 60 mg (52%). The difference versus placebo was significant.

Seven normal subjects received an intravenous infusion of nor-epinephrine (1 g/Kg/min x 30').

Before N. E. infusion each patient received 2 g of the drug at -30' and -15'. Some days later 5 patients out of 7 received the N. E. infusion without drug. During N. E. infusion FFA increased 200% with a zenith at 30 min. In subjects receiving N. E. plus drug FFA increased 95%.

FFA and TG behaviour in the first 24 h after the onset of an acute myocardial infarction has been followed in 11 infarcted people. Seven patients out of 11 received 0. 5 g of the drug per os every 6 hours. In treated people the FFA level decrease was significantly greater than in non-treated people. TG behaviour was meaningless.

CHLOROQUINE NEUROPATHY: A MODEL OF A DRUG INDUCED LIPIDOSIS

A. Bischoff

University of Bern, Switzerland

A 65 yr. old female developed muscle weakness in the thighs following chloroquine therapy for chronic polyarthralgia. The symptoms started three months after treatment with 250 mg daily of Resochin (Chloroquine phosphate). The neurological examination revealed a marked paresis of the lower extremities. The upper limbs were affected to a lesser degree. Sensory disturbances were only moderated. Electromyography demonstrated findings of a neuropathy. Bioptic specimens of the rectus femoris muscle showed a neurogenic atrophy.

The evaluation of the disease was achieved by electron microscopical investigation of a sural nerve biopsy. There was a moderate axonal degeneration and in addition a storage of lipidic inclusions in the Schwann cell cytoplasm. These inclusions evidently were of lysosomal origin and revealed a paracristalline structure indicating a high content of a lipidic material which would represent a ganglioside. The finding is corresponding with analogous findings in animal experiments.

HYPERLIPEMIA INDUCED BY STEROID CONTRACEPTIVES AND EFFECT OF SOME HYPOLIPEMIC DRUGS

A. Bizzi, A. M. Tacconi, C. Valenti, E. Veneroni and S. Garattini

Istituto Mario Negri, Milan, Italy

It is well established that contraceptive therapy induces hypertriglyceridemia. Data are presented which show that rats are a very sensitive model to use in the study of the effect of contraceptives on lipid metabolism. In fact, an antifertility dosage of 1/20 is capable of enhancing plasma triglycerides and a dosage of 1/60 still decreases plasma cholesterol. Concomitantly a sharp decrease in liver triglycerides suggests that this effect may be very complex and may involve also some step in lipid transport. Conversely, in mice only liver triglycerides are decreased and in guinea pigs hypotriglyceridemia was observed after treatment with contraceptive compounds. The hypertriglyceridemia observed in rats involves mainly VLDL, however triglycerides in chylomicrons, in LDL and even in HDL were also affected. It is interesting to note that cholesterol was decreased only in HDL fraction.

A number of hypolipemic agents with different mechanisms of action have challenged the hyperlipemia induced by contraceptives in rats. The results will be discussed in view of possible practical application and of a better understanding of the mechanism of action.

COMPARATIVE PROPERTIES OF PLASMA LIPOPROTEIN POLYPEPTIDES IN PRIMATES

V. Blaton and H. Peeters

Simon Stevin Instituut voor Wetenschappelijk Onderzoek, B-8000 Brugge, Belgium

In previous work a comparison of the lipid moiety of the lipoproteins from human plasma and from plasma of the non-human primates was described. In this paper the apopolypeptides of high density lipoproteins (HDL) in the chimpanzee, the baboon and the Maccacus Rhesus are compared to the human data.

Our studies have shown that the two major polypeptides of serum HDL from the primates, apo-A(I) and apo-A(II) can be isolated by the same techniques developed for the human products. In the non-human primates apo-A(I) is the main apopolypeptide, similar to their human counterpart in molecular weight ($\pm$ 30,000) in microheterogeneity which is clearly documented by isolectric focusing, as well as in the NH_2 (asparagine) and COOH-terminals (glutamine). However there are differences in apo-A(I) between the animal species. These differences concern mainly the glutamic acid content.

It is of particular interest that apo-A(II) exists in a monomeric form in the baboons and in the maccacus rhesus, unlike human apo-A(II) which contains dimers of two identical monomers linked by a single disulfide bridge. This structural difference was found to be related to a substitution, in position 6, of cysteine (human apo-A(II) by serine (rhesus and baboon). The chimpanzee, an ape close to the human family, contains apo-A(II), which consists also of a dimeric form with cystein in position 6. Differences in the methionine content in apo-A(II) are observed between the animal species.

The observed significant structural differences in the polypeptide composition are of main importance from the phylogenic standpoint and provide useful structural information on the lipoproteins in as far as non-human primates are used as model of experimental dyslipidaemia.

THE EFFECT OF 4-METHYLPYRAZOLE ON ETHANOL-INDUCED CHANGES IN LIVER LIPID METABOLISM IN THE RAT STUDIED IN VIVO AND IN VITRO

R. Blomstrand

Department of Clinical Chemistry, Huddinge University Hospital, S-141 86 Huddinge, Sweden

A single large peroral dose of ethanol caused a three-fold increase in liver triglycerides, while no effect was demonstrated on the amounts of total phospholipids or distribution of individual phospholipids. The relative amounts of palmitic and myristic acids in the liver triglycerides were increased by ethanol.

In rat liver slices incubated with oleic acid-1-^{14}C, ethanol decreased production of labeled CO_2 and aceto acetic acid, increased incorporation of radioactivity into liver triglycerides and increased the β-hydroxybutyrate/acetoacetate ratio. Ethanol had no effect on the amounts of radioactivity incorporated into β-hydroxybutyrate and liver phospholipids from oleic acid-1-^{14}C.

All the ethanol-induced changes demonstrated, both in vivo and in vitro, were prevented by 4-methylpyrazole which indicates that the different effects were due to oxidation of ethanol and not due to ethanol per se.

Some results on the metabolism of 4-methylpyrazole in man will be given. Furthermore different derivatives of pyrazole have been investigated with regard to their inhibitory effect on LADH in vivo.

DIFFERENTIATION OF LIPASES

J. Boberg, J. Augustine, M. Baginsky, P. Tejada and W. V. Brown

Department of Medicine, School of Medicine, University of California - San Diego, La Jolla, California, USA

A quantitative method has been developed for applying earlier-described techniques to purify and separate the hepatic lipase (H-TGL) and lipoprotein lipase (LPL) activities of post-heparin plasma. Two ml of post-heparin plasma was applied to small heparin-Sepharose columns and their respective activities were eluted by step-wise addition of 0.005 M veronal buffer containing 0.75 M NaCl (H-TGL) and 1.5 M NaCl (LPL). The recovered enzyme activities were compared to the lipase activity in the original post-heparin plasma when assayed under conditions optimal for H-TGL (pH 8.8, 0.75 M NaCl) or LPL (pH 8.2, 0.13 M NaCl). The recovery of H-TGL was 88 ± 14% and for LPL 81 ± 8. Thus, the method provides a rapid and precise assay for the independent measurement of the two lipase activities. Values for the two activities in ten healthy subjects ranged from 10 to 35 moles/ml/hour for H-TGL and from 4 to 12 μmoles/ml/hour for LPL activity. The importance of the concentrations of the two enzymes in patients with hypertriglyceridemia is presently under investigation.

EFFECTS OF LONG TREATMENT (16 MONTHS) WITH COLESTIPOL (U, 26, 597A) ON SERUM LIPIDS IN FAMILIAL TYPE II HYPERLIPOPROTEINEMIA

G. Briani, R. Fellin, P. Balestrieri, G. Baggio, M. R. Baiocchi and G. Crepaldi

Clinica Medica, Policlinico, Universita, 35100 Padova, Italy

Twenty-three patients with familial hyperlipoproteinemia Type II (3 homozygotes, 12 Type IIA, 8 Type IIB) were given 15 g Colestipol (U, 26, 597A) for 12 months (5 g t. i. d.) and a double dose for a further 4 months (10 g t. i. d.). Placebo was given during 6 weeks before treatment with bimonthly checks. All patients were maintained on a low cholesterol

(< 300 mg/day) polyunsaturated:saturated (1. 8:1) fat diet throughout the study. Mean serum cholesterol (SC) decreased from 456 ± 27 to 422 ± 35 mg/dl after a twelve month treatment. At the end of the 4 months with double dose the mean value was 388 ± 26 mg/dl. Mean SC decrease was 42 ± 18 mg/dl at the 12th month and 69 ± 17 mg/dl at the 16th month. The decreases with respect to the mean basal value are significant (P < 0. 025 and P < 0. 0005 respectively). During the first 6 month therapy the mean serum triglycerides (TG) showed a constant moderate increase from 187 ± 16 to 221 ± 26 mg/dl at the 6th month with a mean increase of 33 ± 15 mg/dl (P < 0. 05). The mean TG values were almost the same as the basal ones at the 12th and 16th month (189 ± 18 and 185 ± 24 mg/dl respectively).

In the three homozygous patients SC showed a constant progressive decrease from 679 ± 16 to 566 ± 10 mg/dl at the 14th month (P < 0. 01), with a mean decrease of 113 ± 26 mg/dl (P < 0. 025). SC decrease in 12 Type IIA heterozygotes and in 8 Type IIB patients was almost the same in both groups (from 423 ± 29 to 350 ± 27 mg/dl at the 16th month in Type IIA and from 423 ± 40 to 361 ± 22 mg/dl at the 16th month in Type IIB). In Type IIA TG showed a slight increase; in Type IIB there was a marked increase from 247 ± 16 mg/dl to a maximum value of 369 ± 25 mg/dl at the 6th month (mean increase of 94 ± 25 mg/dl; P < 0. 005).

These results show that Colestipol significantly reduces SC in Type II, both homozygotes and heterozygotes. However in Type II a significant TG increase was observed at the 6th month of treatment. Constipation was the most prevalent side effect (17 our of 23 patients). Nausea and bloating were observed in about one-third of the subjects. No other important chemical or laboratory signs were noted.

THE EFFECTS OF DERIVATIVES OF CLOFIBRATE, HALOFENATE AND FENFLURAMINE ON THE SYNTHESIS OF GLYCEROLIPIDS BY RAT LIVER

D. N. Brindley and M. Bowley

Biochemistry Department, The Medical School, University of Nottingham, University Park, Nottingham NG7 2RD, U. K.

Using homogenates of rat liver, p-chlorophenoxyisobutyrate (CPIB) and halofenate had little effect on the synthesis of glycerolipids from glycerol phosphate and palmitate. Clofenapate at 1. 6 mM and (P-chlorophenyl) (m-trifluoromethyl phenoxy) acetate (HFA) at 1. 5 mM gave 50% inhibitions of total lipid (mainly phosphatidate) synthesis. The equivalent concentrations required for a 50% inhibition of glyceride synthesis were 0. 7 mM and 0. 5 mM respectively. Fenfluramine and hydroxyethylnorfenfluramine did not inhibit phosphatidate synthesis until about 5 mM but both produced 50% inhibitions of glyceride synthesis at 1. 3 mM.

The simultaneous synthesis of glycerolipids from glycerol phosphate and dihydroxy-acetone phosphate was studied with rat liver mitochondria. Clofenapate inhibited the esterifaction of dihydroxyacetone phosphate at concentrations where the esterification of glycerol phosphate was not affected.

Phosphatidate phosphohydrolase was assayed directly by measuring the conversion of membrane-bound ^{3}H-phosphatidate to diglyceride. The concentrations required in order to obtain a 50% inhibition were as follows: CPIB (> 20 mM), clofenapate (6.8 mM), HFA (7.8 mM), fenfluramine (0.8 mM) and hydroxyethylnorfenfluramine (0.4 mM). Work with tissue slices indicated that the inhibitions of glyceride synthesis produced by fenfluramine were caused by an inhibition of phosphatidate phosphohydrolase.

It is concluded that CPIB and halofenate have little direct effects on glycerolipid synthesis in the systems in vitro which were studied. Clofenapate and HFA appear to inhibit an early reaction in phosphatidate synthesis, probably at the level of glycerol phosphate and dihydroxyacetone phosphate acyltransferase. Fenfluramine and its derivatives appear to inhibit glycerolipid synthesis through phosphatidate phosphohydrolase, an enzyme which may be important in the physiological regulation of glyceride synthesis.

ALTERATIONS OF LIPID METABOLISM IN THYROIDECTOMIZED RATS

E. Burdino, P. A. Milillo, O. Danni, G. Ugazio and L. Sena

Istituto di Patologia Generale, 10125 Torino, Italy

Surgical thyroidectomy lowers down the secretion rate of both triglycerids and phospholipids from liver into plasma compartment. However, the pool size of hepatic precursors of the lipids which are to be secreted is normal. Esterified sterol output is higher than in the controls, as indicated by the sterol to neutral lipid ratio observed in serum.

Qualitative composition of very low density and low density lipoprotein lipid moiety is altered in thyroid devoid animals, while a T_3 treatment almost completely reverses the changes observed in the hypothyroidism state.

Radioactive experiments demonstrate that a remarkable increase in the incorporation of free fatty acids into esterified sterols occurs after thyroidectomy without any significant change in cholesterogenesis.

These findings give support to the hypothesis that qualitatively altered lipoproteins can represent the most suitable precursors for the lipids which have been found to accumulate in the atheromatous arterial wall.

HEPATIC CHOLESTEROL BIOSYNTHESIS IN RAT FOETUS: EFFECT OF DIETARY CHOLESTEROL

S. Calandra, M. Montaguti and G. S. Quartaroli

Istituto di Patologia Generale, Universita degli Studi di Modena, Modena, Italy

In the normal adult liver of all mammalian species cholesterol biosynthesis is under the control of dietary cholesterol. This feed-back mechanism is regarded as a specialized function of the normal hepatocytes which is lost in primary liver tumors. In view of the possible similarities between the functions of the neoplastic liver and the foetal liver, we have studied cholesterol biosynthesis in rat foetus at term to assess whether the control of hepatic synthesis of sterols was present in rat foetus. Under normal dietary conditions foetal liver was found to be capable of synthetizing cholesterol from acetate in vitro; the rate of incorporation of acetate into cholesterol, fatty acids and CO_2 in foetal liver greatly exceeded that found in the maternal liver.

Cholesterol feeding reduced the sterol synthesis in maternal liver to 50% but it did not have any appreciable effect on the foetal liver. In order to investigate whether this lack of feed-back control in foetal liver could be attributed to an impairment of the placental transfer of dietary cholesterol from the mother to the foetus, radioactive cholesterol was administered to the pregnant rats and its distribution in maternal and foetal tissues was studied.

The ratio of foetal to maternal plasma cholesterol specific activity was persistently below 0.200 indicating that the transfer of cholesterol from mother to foetus occurs at a very slow rate. On the other hand the ratio of liver to plasma cholesterol specific activity in rat foetus approached unity and even exceeded it after cholesterol feeding.

These findings indicate that: 1) foetal liver is capable of taking up dietary cholesterol transferred from the mother; 2) the amount of cholesterol transferred from the mother to the foetus at term is not sufficient to inactivate the control mechanism of cholesterol biosynthetic pathway in the foetal liver.

ABNORMAL LOW DENSITY LIPOPROTEIN IN PLASMA OF RAT WITH BILIARY OBSTRUCTION: A CHEMICAL AND MORPHOLOGICAL STUDY

S. Calandra, I. Pasquali-Ronchetti, M. Montaguti, M. Cambi, and P. Caccone

Istituto di Patologia Generale, Universita degli Studi di Modena, 41100 Modena, Italy

Although the association of hypercholesterolemia with experimental biliary obstruction is well documented in rat, less attention has been paid to the plasma lipoprotein changes which occur in this experimental condition. In the present study we have separated the plasma lipoproteins of biliary obstructed rats and we have characterized both their lipid composition as well as their ultrastructure. The great elevation in plasma free cholesterol and phospholipids in obstructed rats is related to the increase of the lipoproteins which were separated in the density range of 1.006-1.063 g/ml. This fraction has been purified by agarose gel filtration and it was found to contain 63% phospholipid, 21% unesterified cholesterol, 3.3% triglycerides, 1.2% cholesteryl ester and 11% protein. Lecithin was the major phospholipid present in this fraction. In view of its high free cholesterol and lecithin content this abnormal LDL has been tested in its ability to act as a substrate for the enzyme plasma lecithin-cholesterol acyltransferase (LCAT). The assay of LCAT showed that this abnormal LDL is capable of acting as a substrate for the enzyme.

All lipoprotein fractions were examined under the electron microscope both in negative staining and after sectioning and some of those obtained from obstructed rats showed a peculiar particulate component. The analysis of sectioned material revealed the vesicle-like shape of these lipoprotein particles. The fine structure and size of the vesicles have been defined by the use of a double-negative staining combination technique. The great majority of LDL from obstructed rats consisted of vesicles, about 500 A diameter, as compared to the 200 A diameter of normal LDL. The class distribution of diameters revealed a tremendous decrease of the lowest diameter classes in the obstructed rats and a coming out of classes of 600 to 1500 A diameter.

EFFECT OF DIPHOSPHONATE ON PLASMA CHOLESTEROL AND TOTAL LIPIDS IN MAN

A. Caniggia and C. Gennari

Institute of Medical Pathology, University of Siena, Italy

In 18 bone disease patients a 3 or 6 months treatment with diphosphonate (sodium etidronate) resulted in a statistically significant decrease of total plasma cholesterol. An acute trial on 4 additional inpatients demonstrated that the decrease of plasma cholesterol, total lipids and prebeta-lipoproteins began within few days. This effect was not evident in a case of hypercholesteremia due to obstructive jaundice. The results may support the concept that patients with increased plasma cholesterol level should be treated with diphosphonate.

REDUCTION OF HYPERLIPIDEMIA IN HUMANS WITH DH-581 (PROBUCOL)

F. L. Canosa, A. M. Aparicio, and E. Boyle, Jr.

Miami Heart Institute, Research Division, Miami Beach, Florida 33140, USA

To determine the effectiveness of PROBUCOL in reducing serum cholesterol and triglycerides, 116 hyperlipidemic patients were given 500 mg of the drug orally b. i. d. Twenty-seven of these patients have completed two years, and 81 have completed one year of treatment. Examinations were done at monthly intervals for two months and every two months thereafter. No dietary changes were requested of the patients. No toxicity or changes in body weight were observed. Marked xanthelasma and xanthoma reductions were noted in some subjects. Evaluation was made by comparison of pre-treatment control values of cholesterol and of triglycerides with treatment values up to twenty-four months. For the total group of 116 patients, a reduction in serum cholesterol from 301 to 262 mg% ($P < .0001$) was observed after one month, and the cholesterol did not vary significantly from the reduced levels in subsequent months, being relatively more effective in Phenotype II than in IV. Triglyceride response was erratic and inconsistent.

It is concluded that PROBUCOL is effective in reducing cholesterol in hyperlipidemic humans with no significant side effects.

ULTRASTRUCTURAL MODIFICATIONS OF THE RAT LIVER AFTER ADMINISTRATION OF HYPOLIPIDEMIC AGENTS

F. G. Caramia, A. Conforti, and G. Ceccarelli

Istituto di Patologia Generale dell'Universita di Roma, II Cattedra, Italy

The effect caused by the protracted administration by peritoneal route of some hypolipidemic agents (Tibric Acid, Clofibrate) has been studied in the rat.

In all of the animals a modest, but constant, hepatomegaly more substantial and frequent in the young male rat was observed after 15-21 days.

Optical microscope examination showed an increased volume of hepatocytes containing scarce quantities of glycogen. A considerable increase of mitochondria and microbodies, so thickly crowded in cytoplasm as to have the hepatocyte assume the aspect of oxyphilic cells was observed at the ultramicroscope together with the reduced quantities of glycogenic particles.

Calculations effected on about 50 hepatocytes gave an increase, in comparison to the control group, of about 90% for mitochondria and of about 136% for microbodies; planimetric measurements brought this variation to global values of + 87% for mitochondria and of + 327% for microbodies respectively.

These data are discussed and interpreted in relation to their possible significance

HYPOLIPIDEMIC TREATMENT IN SECONDARY PREVENTION OF CORONARY HEART DISEASE - STUDY OF SURVIVAL

C. Caruzzo

Clinica Medica Generale, Universita di Torino, Italy

Five hundred thirty-five patients with CHD, i. e. myocardial infarction and/or angina pectoris, have been treated for a period from 1 to 20 years with a symptomatic therapy and the correction of main coronary risk factors.

Hypolipidemic treatment, subject to typing, has been applied only to a part of subjects both continuously and irregularly.

The multiple linear regression analysis has been applied to 72 patients, dead from cardiovascular diseases, to investigate the influence on survival of the following variables: duration of hypolipidemic therapy, initial diagnosis, expected survival, blood pressure at the beginning of the study, degree of angina at the beginning and at the end of observation.

The results show that: 1) Hypolipidemic therapy modifies in positive but not statistically significant way the observed survival, which is, on the contrary significantly (P = 0. 05) related with the expected survival obtained from ISTAT Mortality Tables. 2) The angina at the end of observation has some negative, but not statistically significant influence on observed survival. 3) Initial diagnosis (infarction or angina), degree of angina and blood pressure at the beginning have not a significant influence on survival. 4) Therapy significantly reduces angina at the end of the observation and the angina is negatively related with survival, but because of the lack of a positive mutual relation between therapy and survival, this result may be considered as a placebo effect.

The possible interpretation of this behaviour is under discussion.

STUDIES ON THE METABOLISM OF ^{125}I LABELLED LIPOPROTEINS IN NORMAL AND HYPERCHOLESTEREMIC RABBITS

A. Catapano*, J. Rodriguez**, and C. R. Sirtori*

* Center "E. Grossi Paoletti" for the Study of Metabolic Diseases and Hyperlipidemias, University of Milan, 20129 Italy; ** Esl. de Bioquimica Facultad de Ciencias, Universidad de La Habana, Cuba

Lipoproteins from normal and hypercholesteremic rabbits were separated and labelled with ^{125}I according to the MacFarlane's technique as modified by Bilheimer et al. (Biochem. Biophys. Acta 260: 212, 1972). After reinjection into normal animals and rabbits which had been on cholesterol containing diets for 8-10 weeks, plasma radioactivity was monitored and the animals were sacrificed at intervals to detect tissue radioactivity levels. Main findings were:

1. Disappearance of labelled VLDL was significantly slower in hypercholesteremic rabbits as compared with normals; while the rate of disappearance of LDL did not differ between the two groups.

2. Atherosclerotic aortas showed an increased uptake of labelled VLDL in the first 48 hrs after injection of lipoproteins; while the uptake of LDL was significantly more marked only early after injection.

3. Liver uptake of VLDL in hypercholesteremic animals was reduced, while that of LDL did not differ.

Preliminary data will be provided on the identification of the labeled apo-protein moieties entering the different tissues.

STUDIES ON THE HYPOTRIGLYCERIDEMIC ACTION OF HALOFENATE (MK-185)

R. J. Cenedella* and W. G. Crouthamel**

Department of Pharmacology* and the School of Pharmacy**, West Virginia University, Morgantown, West Virginia 26506, USA

Halofenate (MK-185), 2-acetamidoethyl (p-chlorophenyl) (M-trifluoromethylphenoxy) acetate, given to male rats (Wistar) at 0.10% of the diet (fat free) for 14 days decreased both plasma triglycerides and total cholesterol levels by 50-60%. These lipids were also lowered by about 25% with 0.02% halofenate. At the higher dose, the drug appeared to slightly decrease hepatic cholesterol and triglyceride levels while producing a significant 15-20% increase in liver size.

Kinetic measurements were made of the serum appearance and disappearance of ^{3}H-labeled triglycerides after i.v. injection of 2-^{3}H-glycerol (75 µCi/kg) into control and treated rats. Halofenate at 0.02 and 0.10% of the diet produced about 40 and 70% reductions, respectively, in the total amount of serum ^{3}H-triglyceride formed. Also, serum clearance of the ^{3}H-triglyceride was significantly slower in treated rats ($T_{1/2}$ for clearance = 22 min at 0.02% and = 29 min at 0.10%) as compared with control animals ($T_{1/2}$ = 13 min). Thus, the reduction of plasma triglyceride levels produced by halofenate is not due to a net increase in the rate of clearance of triglyceride from the circulation. Rather, its hypotriglyceridemic action appears due to a reduced serum entry of triglyceride from the liver and (or) intestines, the only tissues recognized to contribute triglycerides to the circulation. Further, since halofenate did not increase the concentration of hepatic triglycerides, it appears likely that this drug lowers serum triglycerides by inhibiting hepatic triglyceride synthesis at an early stage versus inhibiting the release of triglycerides from the liver. (Supported by a grant from the Merck Institute for Therapeutic Research.)

OCCURENCE OF PRE-FORMED PROSTAGLANDINS IN THE AORTIC TISSUE AND THEIR BIOSYNTHESIS FROM ARACHIDONIC ACID BY NORMAL RABBIT AORTA

G. Ciaceri and G. DiMaggio

University of Catania, Italy

In order to extend the actual knowledge about the occurence of prostaglandins in tissues and particularly to penetrate their suspected influence on haemodynamic regulation, experiments have been carried out for identification and estimation of these lipid fractions in normal rabbit aorta. The procedure for the detection included the thin layer chromatographic separation and the conclusive stage was the quantitative determination using biological assay (rat fundus). The findings show that prostaglandins of the E and F series are present in the aortic tissue at levels of about 15 ng/ml lysate (ratio 1:4).

Parallel trials were performed in an attempt to demonstrate the capacity of the aortic tissue for achievement of prostaglandin biosynthesis from arachidonic acid. There has been clear evidence that neogenesis of prostaglandins occurs in the arterial tissue and at a significant rate, the found amounts for PGE and PGF being between 30 and 40 ng /ml lysate.

The obtained results suggest some considerations and among other things it seems justified to emphasize, that a deviation concerning the prostaglandin content of vessel tissue or the prevailing formation of a fraction as compared to another may be involved in the development of vascular injuries and especially in the etiology of atherosclerotic disease. On this regard researches are in progress and a following paper could give information for elucidating the problem.

EFFECTS OF THE PROSTAGLANDIN ANTAGONIST POLYPHLORETIN PHOSPHATE (PPP) ON THE METABOLISM OF RAT ADIPOSE TISSUE

P. B. Curtis-Prior

Pharmacology Department, The Wellcome Research Laboratories, Langley Court, Beckenham, Kent, England

Basal and noradrenaline-stimulated lipolysis in isolated fat cells obtained from fed and fasted rats were enhanced by a low but not by a high molecular weight fraction of polyphloretin phosphate (PPP). Since PPP (low MW) is known to antagonize the effect of PGE_2 on the isolated bird colon and of PGF_{2a} on rabbit blood pressure (Eakins, 1971), it is suggested that the enhancement of lipolysis that is produced, is mediated by antagonism of endogenous adipose cell PGs. Such a conclusion would be compatible with the hypothesis that PGs have a physiological role as natural regulators of fat cell lipolysis. They may act through a negative feed-back inhibition.

PPP (low mw) (1 mg/ml) also reduced basal and insulin-enhanced incorporation of $[U-^{14}C]$-glucose into the lipid of fat cells obtained from fed or fasted rats.

OXANDROLONE TREATMENT IN A FAMILY WITH TYPE I HYPERLIPOPROTEINEMIA

F. Damgaard-Pedersen, J. Dyerberg and P. Nilson-Ehle

University Hospital, DK-2100 Copenhagen, Denmark

Type I hyperlipoproteinemia or familial hyperchylomicronemia is believed to be a recessive disease in which low lipoprotein lipase activity as well in adipose tissue as in post-heparin plasma is a typical finding. The low lipoprotein lipase activity is accepted as responsible for the hyperchylomicronemic conditions.

We have investigated a family, which include father, mother and 4 children. Three children are typical type I patients as described by Fredrickson. The whole family was treated with oxandrolone for 14 days, and results of quantitative lipoprotein measurements, serum lipids, post-heparin-lipolytic-activity, (PHLA) lipoprotein lipase activity in adipose tissue before and after treatment are presented.

In all family members PHLA increased to normal or more than normal level after treatment, but the hyperchylomicronemia was not corrected. Further investigations of post-heparin plasma indicated that the PHLA increase was caused as well by increase in lipoprotein lipase as increase in hepatic triglyceride lipase activity. The origin of this lipoprotein lipase activity will be discussed.

THE CHRONIC EFFECT OF DH-581 (PROBUCOL) ON PLASMA LIPIDS IN 20 PATIENTS WITH PRIMARY HYPERLIPOPROTEINEMIA

J. Davignon, A. Gattereau, M. Chretien and R. Collin

The Clinical Research Institute of Montreal, Montreal H2W 1R7, P. Quebec, Canada

The effect of DH-581 (1 gm/d) on plasma lipids and uric acid was studied in 20 ambulatory patients (10 males, 10 females; mean age 41.7 years) with primary hyper-lipoproteinemia (HLP) using a single blind design. The study totaled 598 patient weeks of observation on the drug.

There was a significant fall in plasma cholesterol in 17 patients. The mean fall was not different in the 9 subjects with type IIa HLP (-14.8%) from that of the 6 type IIb patients (-15.6%). Of the 4 subjects with type III HLP, 2 showed a significant fall in plasma cholesterol as did the patient with type IV.

The effect on plasma triglycerides was less predictable and in most cases non-significant; in 3 subjects there was a highly significant increase in plasma triglycerides. In one patient this increase was tentatively ascribed to the concomitant administration of a contraceptive drug.

In 11 patients DH-581 was compared with Clofibrate, each patient serving as his own control. In 7 of 10 type II patients the fall of plasma cholesterol was greater with DH-581 than with Clofibrate (2 gm/d). DH-581 did not share the triglyceride-lowering effect of Clofibrate.

Several parameters were monitored (blood pressure, plasma uric acid, LDH, SGOT, alkaline phosphatase, urea, WBC, hemoglobin...) and found to be unaffected by DH-581. Urinary 24 hour 17 Ketosteroids were significantly decreased after 16 weeks or more on DH-581, but in only one instance were abnormally low levels reached. Side effects were rare and mostly gastrointestinal.

STUDY BY GAS CHROMATOGRAPHY OF BLOOD BEHAVIOUR OF CLOFIBRATE IN
MIXED HYPERLIPIDEMIA (M. H.) RESISTANT TO THIS TREATMENT

J. L. de Gennes and J. Truffert with technical collaboration of J. P. Lagarde

Clinique Endocrinologique, Hopital de la Pitie, 75634 Paris Cedex-13, France

Twenty-two patients with mixed hyperlipidemia (type IIb) under Clofibrate treatment
at the daily dosage of 2 grams, were studied by gas chromatography analysis of fatty
acids, comparing profile of 12 cases well controlled by treatment and 10 cases with
primary resistance to the same treatment, and staying with high blood triglyceride
levels. Fasting blood samples were collected after an overnight fasting, the last
Clofibrate ingestion at the dinner time (12 hours before). Lipids were extracted by
chloroform methanol (2/1) extraction, after centrifugation and evaporation of the liquid
phase. Gas chromatography was done on a B. D. S. column at a temperature of 180°C.
Temperature of injection, and of the detector, was 190°C. The nitrogen pressure was
1. 4 B.

On chromatographic profiles, a special peak located between the C_{14-0} and C_{16-0}
fatty acids was individualized. Its identity as p-Chlorophenoxy isobutyric acid was confirmed by checking that the in vitro addition to a normal serum (free of this peak) of a
soluble Clofibrate salt, gives the same peak after the same technical procedure.
Coupling thin layer chromatography of lipids from these treated patients, the Clofibrate
special gas chromatography peak was located in phospholipids migrating specifically
with lecithins. Coupled study of these serums by preparative ultracentrifugation showed
the Clofibrate peak is found in the VLDL layer floating at the density of 1. 006. There
was a striking and significant difference between the importance of Clofibrate peak in
M. H. resistant, and its s i z e i n M. H. sensitive to the drug. This finding opens new
perspective in the way of pharmacological action of Clofibrate.

ACTION OF CINNARIZINE ON THE HYPERLIPAEMIA OF EXPERIMENTAL IMMUNE
COMPLEX DISEASE

T. Di Perri, S. Forconi, A. Auteri and A. Vittoria

Istituto di Semeiotica Medica dell'Universita, Siena, Italy

Immune complex disease was produced in rabbits by injecting horse serum at the
dose of 0. 175 mg/kg of protein every 72 hours i. v. The observation period was 28 days.
During this period the serum complement activity progressively decreased to very low
titer while serum total lipids, total cholesterol, triglycerides and gamma globulins
significantly increased. A group of 10 NZ rabbits was treated with Cinnarizine before
and after the onset of immunization. Cinnarizine has shown a strong inhibitory power on
the activation of the complement system. While this substance is known to be an anti-
histaminic drug, it shows marked inhibitory effect on the development of hypocomplemen-
temia and hyperlipaemia in rabbits treated with heterologous serum. In these animals
only the gamma globulin titer increased in the serum at the same level as in the control,

thus suggesting a normal antibody formation.   Therefore the action of Cinnarizine must
be localized on the formation of active antigen-antibody complex, perhaps at the phase
of the complement fixation.   The development of hyperlipaemia in immune complex disease
can be therefore considered as secondary to the inflammatory reaction.   The lipid lowering action of the tested drug in this experimental model seems to be   secondary to its
anticomplementary-anti-inflammatory activity.

EFFECT OF PROPRANOLOL ON TRIGLYCERIDEMIA IN MAN

W. Donadon, G. Ambrosio, A. Corgniati, A. Pessina, E. Tonolli, and C. Dal Palu

Clinica Medica, Policlinico di Borgo Roma, 37100 Verona, Italy

Two groups of hypertensive patients with normal or elevated plasma triglycerides
were studied before and after 10 days treatment with propranolol.   In the former a
consistent increase in triglycerides fasting levels was observed while in the latter there
was a slight fall compared to pretreatment values.   In both cholesterol levels fell to a
similar extent.   These results were not statistically significant.

In ten patients with normal triglyceridemia propranolol induced a significant
increase in lipemia measured at 180 and 240 minutes after a fatty meal.

Glucose-induced insulin secretion was not uniformly affected by the treatment.

The mechanism whereby beta-blocking agents produce these effects will be discussed.

RELATIONSHIP BETWEEN HORMONE-INDUCED LIPOLYSIS AND ATP LEVELS IN RAT
EPIDIDYMAL FAT

P. Dorigo, M. Prosdocimi, R. M. Gaion and F. Bonazzi

Department of Pharmacology, University of Padua, 35100 Padua, Italy

Tissue levels of ATP and cyclic AMP, together with glycerol release, were followed
during the incubation of rat epididymal fat under aerobic and anaerobic conditions in the
presence and absence of 10^{-5}M noradrenaline.

In air, after 180 min of incubation the ATP level in untreated tissue did not change
from the initial value of 160 ± 10 nmoles/g fresh tissue.   In the presence of noradrenaline,
the ATP level decreased rapidly in the first 30 min (to 50%), more slowly between 60-120
min of incubation, and then again rapidly, reaching 35% of the control after 180 min.

The time-course of glycerol release and of ATP consumption under hormonal stimulation was perfectly corresponding, and the two curves reached the plateau at the same time.

In anoxia, the initial ATP level in the control (89 ± 16 nmoles/g fresh tissue) rapidly declined to 50% after 30 min of incubation. In the presence of noradrenaline a still more rapid fall of ATP than in the control was found. Cyclic AMP was increased, but lipolysis was not stimulated.

Thus, under anaerobic conditions the two phases of the lipolytic process, (a) the cyclic AMP synthesis and (b) the final FFA release, were separated through the lack of ATP supplied from aerobic sources. The separation is held only after cyclic AMP synthesis.

Finally, a different behaviour of the time-course in ATP consumption was found in the presence of β or α antiadrenergic drugs (D(-) INPEA and phentolamine.

A THREE YEAR REPORT ON MORTALITY AND MORBIDITY IN A CONTROLLED MULTICLINIC TRIAL OF COLESTIPOL HYDROCHLORIDE (COLESTID, UPJOHN)

A. E. Dorr, W. B. Martin and W. A. Freyburger

The Upjohn Company, Kalamazoo, Michigan 49001, USA

Approximately a fourth of 2,100 patients entering a multiclinic, random assignment, placebo controlled study on the hypo cholesterolemic efficacy and safety of the bile acid sequestrant, colestipol hydrochloride, had an antecedent history of cardiovascular disease. Randomization procedures resulted in this high risk population being apportioned equally between the placebo and colestipol groups. Of the 41 deaths that have occurred during the first three years of this study, there were 27 in the placebo group and 14 in the drug group (p < 0.05). Twenty of the deaths during placebo treatment and eight during colestipol treatment (p < 0.05) can be attributed to coronary heart disease. The placebo/drug ratio for other deaths was: cerebrovascular 2/1, congestive heart failure 0/2, uremia 2/1, pulmonary embolism 1/1, peritonitis 1/0, acute hemorrhagic pancreatitis 1/0, unknown 0/1.

Of the non-fatal major medical events in the study there have been 41 coronary events in the placebo group and 33 in the colestipol group. The mortality and morbidity data will be presented in relation to age, sex, race, diabetic status, type of hyper-lipoproteinemia, and previous history of cardiovascular disease.

THE EFFECT OF COLESTIPOL PLUS CLOFIBRATE ON SERUM LIPIDS IN FAMILIAL TYPE II HYPERLIPOPROTEINEMIA

R. Fellin, G. Baggio, P. Balestrieri, G. Briani, M. R. Baiocchi and G. Crepaldi

Clinica Medica, Policlinico, Universita, Padova, Italy

Colestipol 15 g/day and Clofibrate 2 g/day were given for six months to 20 subjects with familial hyperlipoproteinemia (13 Type IIA and 7 Type IIB). These patients had been previously treated with Colestipol, 12 months with 15 g/day and 4 months 30 g/day. All patients were maintained on a low cholesterol (< 300 mg/day) polyunsaturated: saturated (1. 8:1) fat diet throughout the study, as in the previous 16 months in which they were treated with Colestipol alone. Mean serum cholesterol (SC) showed a further slight decrease from 372 ± 22 mg/dl to 363 ± 18 mg/dl at the 6th month of the combined treatment. The figure obtained after a 16 month Colestipol treatment was taken as mean basal value. However serum triglyceride (TG) levels showed a rapid and significant decrease from 194 ± 25 to 132 ± 15 mg/dl (P <0.05) after one month treatment; and this decrease was maintained during the following 5 months. The mean TG decrease after 6 months of combined treatment was 63 ± 21 mg/dl (P < 0. 005). Serum cholesterol levels (mg/dl) at months 0, 3 and 6 were: 373 ± 22, 354 ± 18 and 363 ± 18, respectively. Triglyceride levels at those times were: 194 ± 25, 115 ± 13 and 130 ± 15. Mean SC decrease was significant in Type IIA patients only at the 1st, 3rd and 4th month. Instead TG decrease was always significant during the study. The hypotriglyceridemic effect of this therapy was particularly evident in Type IIB patients. Mean TG fell from 307 ± 30 to 210 ± 17 mg/dl at the 1st month and to 164 ± 19 mg/dl at the 6th month (Δ TG were -97 ± 32 mg/dl and -158 ± 39 mg/dl respectively; P < 0. 0125 and P < 0. 005).

These results show that Colestipol + Clofibrate treatment is very effective in familial Type II hyperlipoproteinemias and because of its marked hypotriglyceridemic effect seems to be particularly indicated in the treatment of Type IIB patients.

ISOLATION AND ANALYSIS OF HUMAN PLASMA LIPOPROTEINS ACCUMULATING POSTPRANDIALLY IN AN INTERMEDIATE DENSITY FRACTION (d 1. 006-1. 019 g/ml)

R. Fellin, D. Siedel, B. Agostini and W. Rost

Clinica Medica, Policlinico, Universita, Padova, Italy

Plasma lipoprotein patterns have generally been determined in the fasting state. However there is evidence from turnover and dietary studies for short living "remnants" or "intermediate particles" accumulating postprandially. In this study we have been able to identify, isolate and partially characterize by immunochemical, chemical and ultrastructural means, at least two different lipoprotein populations accumulating 6 hours postprandially in the intermediate density fraction d 1. 006-1. 019 g/ml of healthy volunteers. The immunochemical and structural results of our study suggest that at 6 hours postprandially the intermediate density fraction (d 1. 006-1. 019 g/ml) of healthy volunteers contains at least two different lipoprotein populations of different sizes and different protein portions. The smaller particles up to to 250 A contain only Apo-B, the larger particles (probably those ranging from 350 up to 600 A) designated Intermediate Lipoprotein (I. L. P.) carry all major apolipoproteins. The I. L. P. in both double immunodiffusion and immunoelectrophoresis showed a precipitin line of complete identity with antibodies to Apo-A, Apo-B and Apo-C. This finding clearly indicates that Apo-A, Apo-B and Apo-C are part of the structure of this plasma lipoprotein. The polyacrylamide pattern of tetramethylurea treated I. L. P. revealed all bands typical for the three apolipoprotein C peptides. I. L. P. isolated from 6 healthy volunteers was protein, 22. 1 ± 2. 2; total cholesterol,

26. 1 ± 1. 4; cholesterol % ester, 62;64; triglyceride, 33. 5 ± 2. 3; and phospholipid, 12. 1 ± 1. 9

It differs significantly from fasting VLDL, fasting LDL and fasting HDL. The intermediate nature of I L. P. between VLDL and lipoproteins of higher density is suggested by the unique lipid composition and precipitation behaviour with polyanionic compounds of this fraction. Since the d 1. 006-1. 019 g/ml density fraction isolated from fasting subjects seems to contain only lipoproteins in form of "association products" consisting of Apo-B and Apo-C, the apparent differences to the postprandial state as demonstrated in this study may reflect different ways of conversion of VLDL to LDL. This possibility is supported by recent turnover studies of VLDL apolipoproteins.

STRUCTURE-ACTIVITY RELATIONSHIP OF THE HYPOLIPIDEMIC PHENYLACETALS OF GLYOXYLIC ACID

J. Fischer, J. Borsy, T. Fodor, J. Rakoczi and A. Maderspach

Pharmacochemical Works and Pharmaceutical Research Institute, Budapest, Egyt, Hungary

Among the phenylacetals of the glyoxylic acid one of the most prominent hypolipidemic compounds is bis/4-chlorophenoxy/acetic acid whose activity has been discovered by Griot in 1966. Its cholesterol- and triglyceride-lowering activity is about ten times higher than that of Clofibrate. We have investigated the derivatives of bis/4-chlorophenoxy/acetic acid in order to get more active and less toxic compounds.

EFFECT OF ANTI-INFLAMMATORY, ANTI-5-HYDROXYTRYPTAMINIC AND ALPHA-ADRENOLYTIC DRUGS ON PLATELET AGGREGATION AND ON EXPERIMENTAL THROMBOSIS

G. B. Fregnan, T. Chieli and S. Brunet

Lusofarmaco, Istituto di Ricerche, 20132 Milano, Italy

Numerous drugs, characterized by different mechanism of action, were tested for their properties to antagonize the rabbit platelet aggregation induced in vivo and in vitro by ADP, epinephrine, 5-hydroxytryptamine (5-HT), collagen and thrombin. The effect of the same drugs was also studied either on acute thrombosis of the blood vessels of rats and rabbits, caused by electrical and chemical means, or on the bleeding time from the mouse tail. All the antagonists tested in vivo were administered by gastric gavage in awake animals and by duodenal route in anesthetized animals.

Non-steroidal anti-inflammatory drugs were quite effective in inhibiting the platelet aggregation induced by collagen and thrombin but were almost ineffective against ADP,

5-HT and epinephrine aggregation. They were also effective in preventing and in re-
solving the arterial thrombosis caused by electrical means but were inactive against
venous thrombosis caused by sodium salicylate. Moreover, they prolonged the bleeding
time in the mouse. Their activity was generally demonstrated at doses well below those
effective in the experimental inflammatory processes. Dose-response curves were obtained for almost all the anti-inflammatory agents and the strongest activity was elicited
by some anthranolic acid derivatives.

Anti-5-hydroxytryptaminic drugs showed significant anti-aggregating properties in
vitro and in vivo against all the aggregating agents used (especially against 5-HT), while
were scarcely active in the other tests.

α-adrenolitic drugs readily antagonized the platelet aggregation induced by epinephrine,
but were completely inactive in all the other tests.

HYPOLIPIDEMIC ACTIVITY OF 18, 19-BISNOR-PROSTANOIC ACID DERIVATIVES

R. Fumagalli*, S. Gorini, C. Omini*, U. Valcavi and G. B. Zabran

* Institute of Pharmacology and Pharmacognosy, University of Milan, and Research
Laboratory of Istituto Biochimico Italiano, Milan, Italy

The synthesis of some derivatives of 18, 19-bisnor-prostanoic acid is described.
These compounds, although structurally different from naturally occurring prostaglandins,
show prostaglandin-like action at some pharmacological and metabolic levels.

Particularly the sodium salt of 9-hydroxy-18,19-bisnor-prostanoic acid, tested on
several preparations of isolated organs, exerts actions qualitatively comparable to those
of PGE_2. This is the case using guinea-pig tracheal smooth muscles and the stomach
fundus preparation.

The substance when tested in vivo shows a slight hypotensive effect and a spasmolytic
activity similar to that exerted by PGs.

This compound differs from type E prostaglandins for several metabolic effects. It
does not show in vivo antilipolytic activity, but it retains the hyperglycemic action.

Furthermore, it appears to have hypolipidemic properties in dietary induced hyperlipemia in rats.

HYPOLIPIDEMIC ACTIVITY OF SOME PHENYL ALKANOIC ACIDS

R. Fumagalli*, S. Gorini, C. Pezzini, C. Sirtori* and U. Valcavi

*Institute of Pharmacology and Pharmacognosy, University of Milan, and Research
Laboratory of Istituto Biochimico Italiano, Milan, Italy

The synthesis and hypolipidemic action of a series of esters and amides of the 3-methyl-4-phenyl-3-butenoic acid is described.

The hypolipidemic action of derivatives of the above mentioned structure substituted in the side chain and in the aromatic ring has also been tested.

Hypertriglyceridemia has been induced either with fructose or with ethanol. Among the various structures analyzed, the diethylamide of the 3-methyl-4-phenyl-3-butenoic acid (C_{11}) has shown a remarkable activity on the experimentally induced hypertriglyceridemias.

These results, along with the lack of side effects in acute and chronic administration, indicate compound C_{11} as a new possible agent for the control of hypertriglyceridemias.

EFFECT OF CLOFIBRATE AND OTHER HYPOLIPIDEMIC PHENOXYACETIC ACID DERIVATIVES ON CYCLIC AMP SYNTHESIS IN ADIPOSE TISSUE

R. M. Gaion, P. Dorigo, G. Fassina, and J. J. Kabara*

Institute of Pharmacology, University of Padua, Padua, Italy; * Michigan State University, College of Osteopathic Medicine, East Lansing, Michigan 48823, USA

Some phenoxyacetic acid derivatives were shown to act as hypolipidemic and hypocholesterolemic drugs. They produce a wide range of metabolic effects, and inhibit cholesterol biosynthesis with the same action mechanism. All of them inhibit ATP production in mitochondria.

The influence of these drugs on cyclic AMP levels was studied taking into consideration the relationship between hormone-stimulated lipolysis, oxidative phosphorylation and cAMP synthesis. Clofibrate, Halophenate, SaH 42348 and Nafenopin were tested in vitro on rat epididymal fat, both in basal conditions and under hormone stimulation. The opposite effect of Sodium Clofibrate and Clofibrate Ethyl Ester on the oxidation of different substrates in mitochondria suggested the comparison between the two different forms of the drug.

While Sodium Clofibrate increased cAMP basal level without influencing the stimulation produced by noradrenaline plus theophylline, Clofibrate Ethyl Ester inhibited this stimulation. SaH 42348 enhanced cAMP level both in basal conditions and in the presence of noradrenaline plus theophylline. Halophenate increased only hormone-induced cyclic nucleotide synthesis. Nafenopin had no effect.

Such a different kind of action shows the lack of correlation between the hypolipidemic activity of these drugs and their influence on cAMP. Therefore this nucleotide which is shown to play an important role in nicotinic acid mechanism of action, is not an evident factor here in regulating the pharmacological effect of phenoxyacetic acid derivatives.

EFFECT OF TETRAHYDROPAPAVEROLINE ON CYCLIC AMP SYNTHESIS AND
LIPOLYSIS IN ADIPOSE TISSUE

R. M. Gaion, M. Prosdocimi and G. Fassina

Institute of Pharmacology, University of Padua, 35100 Padua, Italy

Tetrahydropapaveroline (THP) is an alkaloid present in P. sonniferum as precursor
of papaverine and morphine. It is structurally related to the catecholamines, and can
be biosynthesized from dopamine in the presence of liver mitochondria.

THP exerts, in vivo and in vitro, beta-sympathomimetic effects and a papaverine-
like spasmolytic activity. Experiments on lipolysis indicated an affinity of THP for the
same receptor as isoprenaline. Therefore the effect of THP was studied on cyclic AMP
level in rat adipose tissue in basal conditions, in the presence of theophylline, and of
papaverine. The effect of THP on lipolysis and on cAMP was compared to that of noradrenaline (NA).

The level of cAMP was strongly increased by THP, more than by NA. In contrast,
the potentiating effect of theophylline on cAMP accumulation, was lower in the presence
of THP than for NA. Papaverine did not affect the action of THP on cAMP level, as in
the case of noradrenaline. Thus, the actions of THP and of NA on lipolysis are very
similar, both at the level of the initial steps of the process (affinity to the same beta-
receptor, stimulation of adenylate cyclase and cAMP increase) as well as on the final
triglyceride hydrolysis. These similarities, and quantitative differences, could be
significant because of a possible role of THP as a false adrenergic transmitter in the
brain and peripheric level, and in post-intoxication states of alcoholism, as previously
proposed and investigated by other authors.

THE NORMALIZING EFFECT OF POLYUNSATURATED PHOSPHOLIPIDS (PPL) ON
PLASMA FATTY ACIDS

H. Geoffroy, H. Choisy, and H. Fornet

Clinique Medicale A, Centre Hospitalier Universitaire, F-51100 Reims, France

Since November, 1973, we have been using PPL in a dosage of 2.1 gms p. d. (two
LIPOSTABIL caps. t. i. d.) during a minimum of 60 days in all our patients with dyslipid-
emia types IIa, IIb, or IV of the Fredrickson classification.

Laboratory tests were done before the patients' admittance to the trial and repeated
between three and five weeks following the beginning of treatment as well as at its end.

Testing comprised repeated determinations of total lipids, free and total cholesterol,
and of fatty acids in total lipids by gas-chromatography.

In most of the cases evaluated so far, we have seen, besides a normalization of plasma lipids, a normalization of plasma fatty acids characterized by a marked decrease of oleic acid and a corresponding increase of linoleic -; linolenic- ; and arachidonic acid.

Further confirmation of these results seems warranted and work on this project is being continued at our departments.

THE EFFECTS OF "DIETARY FIBRE" ON FAT ABSORPTION IN MAN

D. V. Goff, L. M. Castell, J. I. Jensen, A. R. Leeds, C. Newton, and D. J. A. Jenkins

University Laboratory of Physiology, Oxford, and the M. R. C. Gastroenterology Unit, Central Middlesex Hospital, London N. W. 10, England

Much publicity has been given to the role of so-called "dietary fibre" in lowering the serum cholesterol. It has been suggested that the non-absorbable carbohydrate constituents of certain foods may have ion exchange properties resulting in the binding of bile salts and thus diminished fat absorption.

We have looked at the effects of wheat bran, apple pectin and guar gum in man on the blood levels for vitamins A and E and triglyceride as chylomicra (measured by nephelometry) over a 5 or 7 hour period after taking a liquid test meal containing these substances.

Comparing test and control experiments in the same individual, bran reduced the vitamin A level at 5-hour by 17% (9pairs $P < 0.05$) while having no other effect.

Pectin increased the chylomicroanemia at 3 hours by 46% (N = 7, $P < 0.05$). Guar, however, though increasing the rate of absorption at 1-1/2 and 3 hours, resulted in vitamin A levels which were over 20% lower at 5 and 7 hours ($P < 0.02$, N = 9, and $P < 0.05$, N = 4, respectively) and lower chylomicra levels at 7 hours (by 67%, $P < 0.01$, N = 4).

Of the substances tested guar had the most pronounced effect on fat absorption and the lower levels of vitamin A and chylomicra seen at 7 hours suggesting that this substance may be the most rewarding in further long-term studies on the lipid lowering effects of "fibre".

INFLUENCE OF TIBRIC ACID ON HUMAN HYPERLIPIDEMIA

R. C. Gross, R. C. Cornell and P. E. Pool

Department of Medicine, University of California -San Diego, La Jolla, California 92037, USA

Tibric acid (CP-18,524) is a dimethyl-piperidino-sulfonyl-benzoic acid derivative which lowers plasma triglycerides. Twenty-four patients with hypertriglyceridemia have been treated for up to 2 years with doses ranging from 225 mg to 1000 mg per day. These included 15 males and 9 females from 26 to 68 years of age. Twenty-three had Type IV lipoprotein patterns and 1 had a Type IIb pattern. All patients were advised on a modified fat, controlled carbohydrate diet prior to study.

Plasma triglycerides and cholesterol levels were analyzed biweekly, and parameters for toxicity were obtained monthly. Electrocardiogram and slit-lamp examinations were performed every 4 months.

Mean triglyceride level for the group was 428 mg/dl at baseline, falling to 331 and 330 mg/dl during the first 6 months and 12 months of treatment, respectively. Mean cholesterol was 264 mg/dl initially, and fell to 228 and 231 mg/dl at 6 months and 1 year. After 1 year overall reductions averaged 23% for triglycerides and 12% for cholesterol. These changes were statistically significant ($p < 0.01$).

Ten of 24 subjects, and 10 of 20 subjects had triglyceride reductions of 20% or more after treatment for 6 and 12 months, respectively. However, only 1 of 24 had reduction of triglycerides by more than 30% after 6 months, while 7 of 20 had a 30% or greater reduction after 12 months. This may be due to a higher mean dose of drug during the second 6 months. Twelve of 24 and 8 of 20 subjects had cholesterol reductions of 10% or more after treatment for 6 and 12 months, respectively.

No significant adverse reactions due to tibric acid were observed. Two subjects had elevations of CPK, and 1 had a small increase in alkaline phosphatase; none of these changes was accompanied by symptoms, and no patient withdrew because of side effects.

Tibric acid appears to be a safe, well-tolerated drug, which has significant lipid lowering effects.

INVESTIGATION OF COMBINED TREATMENT OF COLESTIPOL AND β-SITOSTEROL ON HYPERCHOLESTEROLEMIA

K. Gundersen, W. A. Phillips and J. C. Schneider, Jr.

Pharmaceutical Research and Development, The Upjohn Company, Kalamazoo, Michigan, 94001, USA

Nine subjects with Type II hyperlipidemia (3 type IIa, 6 type IIb) were treated with colestipol HCl (Colestid) and colestipol HCl plus sitosterol to ascertain any possible additional benefits of the combination on serum cholesterol levels. Colestid, an anionic exchange resin, at a daily dose of 15-20 grams, lowered initial serum cholesterol levels from a mean of 396 mg% to a mean level of 326 mg% during a 4 month period. The addition of sitosterol at a dose of 3 grams t. i. d. to this therapy resulted in an additional lowering of cholesterol levels by an average of 24 mg%. Two patients did not respond to the combination therapy. Serum cholesterol response to therapy did not seem to depend on serum triglyceride levels, but rather on adherance to diet and drug therapy. There were no ill effects of the combination therapy.

Gas liquid chromatography of serum sterols before and at 5 months of sitosterol therapy showed no significant amounts of either campesterol or β-sitosterol (< 2 mg%), indicating little or no absorption of these plant sterols.

PLATELETS AND THE INTEGRITY OF THE VESSEL WALL

H. Hess

Munchen Universitat, 8 Munchen 15, Germany

Platelets are an integral component of the arterial wall. They are sensitive to a number of physiological and pathological stimuli which cause them to aggregate and to become adherent. Any disturbance to the platelet system will disturb the integrity of the vessel wall. Pathology of blood lipids causes platelets to aggregate and to adhere to both defective and intact endothelium. The vessel wall can absorb platelet aggregates to a certain extent, but if the tolerance is exceeded deposits will appear. These deposits begin as platelets but may become clots. The clots along with lipid droplets and cholesterol crystals adhere to the endothelium and are eventually incorporated into the vessel wall. Vessel wall deposits along with primary and secondary mesenchymal reactions complete the picture of an arteriosclerotic plaque.

SECHOLEX AND CLOFIBRATE IN DIFFERENT TYPES OF HYPERLIPIDEMIA

A. N. Howard and R. I. C. Evans

Department of Investigative Medicine, University of Cambridge, Addenbrooke's Hospital, Cambridge CB2 2QQ, England

Previous work has shown that an anion exchange resin, Secholex (formerly known as DEAE Sephadex), was able to decrease serum cholesterol and the effect could be greatly potentiated by the addition of Clofibrate. In a continuation of these studies, Secholex (15 g/day) was given to 20 hypercholesterolaemic patients for one year, and a mean decrease of 21% achieved; 17 patients given placebo were unchanged. Nine patients with type IIa hypercholesterolaemia gave a mean decrease of 32% when treated with Secholex (15 g/day) and Clofibrate (1.5 g/day) for one year. The chief side effect of Secholex was constipation, which occurred in about 15% cases. No significant abnormalities were seen in routine haematological and biochemical tests.

In another experimental series, patients after a baseline examination were classified as type IIa, IIb, or type IV, divided into five groups and treated for eight weeks as follows: Group I, type IIa, treated with Secholex (15 g/day); Group II, type IIa, treated with Secholex (15 g/day) and Clofibrate (1.5 g/day); Group III, type IIb, treated with

Secholex; Group IV, type IIb, treated with Secholex and Clofibrate; Group V, type IV, treated with Clofibrate. Secholex alone reduced serum cholesterol and low density lipoproteins but not triglycerides. Clofibrate alone reduced serum cholesterol, triglycerides and very low density lipoproteins. The combination of Secholex with Clofibrate reduced serum cholesterol, gave a greater decrease in low density lipoproteins and lowered serum triglycerides and very low density lipoproteins. It is concluded that Secholex alone is of value in the treatment of moderately affected type IIa and the combination with Clofibrate in severely affected type IIa and type IIb hyperlipoproteinaemia; Clofibrate alone is of value in type IV.

THE INFLUENCE OF A LOW FAT DIET ON DECREASED SUSCEPTIBILITY TO THROMBIN AND COLLAGEN AGGREGATION IN MAN

J. M. Iacono, R. A. Binder, M. W. Marshall, N. W. Schoene, J. Jenks and J. F. Mackin

Lipid Nutrition Laboratory, Nutrition Institute, U. S. Department of Agriculture, BARC-East, Beltsville, Maryland 20705, and Georgetown University Medical School, Washington, D. C. 20007, USA

With a view toward investigating the relationship between dietary fats and the tendency to thrombosis in man, this study reports the effect of feeding a low fat diet (25% fat calories, P/S ratio 1. 0) on the susceptibility of blood platelets to thrombin and collagen induced aggregation. Results showed an average decrease of plasma cholesterol of 15% after 40 days on the low fat diet and this cholesterol level was maintained during the feeding of a diet containing 35% fat calories, P/S ratio 1. 0, for an additional 40 days. Average triglyceride levels increased by 15% after the low fat dietary period and fell to the initial levels at the end of the 35% fat calorie period. Twelve of 17 subjects, both males and females in the 40-60 age group, showed a marked reduction in thrombin and collagen induced aggregation of blood platelets at the end of the low fat dietary period and these values returned to the pre-dietary level at the end of the 35% fat calorie period No significant changes were observed in ADP or epinephrine aggregation of platelets during the experiment. It is concluded that a lower level of fat calories in the diet exerts a beneficial effect on platelet aggregation tests.

EFFECTS OF APPETITE SUPPRESSANT, MAZINDOL, ON OBESITY AND HYPERLIPIDEMIAS

S. Ishikawa, Y. Ehata, N. Nakaya and Y. Goto

Department of Medicine, Keio University Hospital, Shijuku, Tokyo 160, Japan

Thirty-nine obese patients over 20% of relative body weight were treated with an appetite suppressant, Mazindol, at out-patient clinic. 3 mg of Mazindol was prescribed, which, in case the dose turned out ineffective, was increased to 6 mg. All the patients were allowed to eat at libitum at home and examined every two weeks. Out of 39 patients, seventeen took medicine regularly for 5 to 18 months. Nine stopped visiting clinic for the reasons not related to medication, six took drug sporadically, and six dropped out because of the side effects: fatigue 3, palpitation 1, vomiting 1 and sweating 1. One patient lost his motivation for loss of weight by drug. All the patients except two reported loss of appetite within 4 weeks, and lost their body weight by 13% on the average, ranging from 6 to 20% The major decrement in the body weight occurred in the first 3 months with further slight reduction until 9 months. 13 out of 17 patients had hyperlipidemias, and on the average serum cholesterol level fell by 5% and triglyceride by 3% after body weight reduction. Lipoprotein electrophoresis on cellulose acetate membrane showed no significant changes, and serum uric acid remained unchanged. Blood pressure lowered in 3 cases, but the rest showed no significant alteration. The possible mechanisms for the unparalleled reduction in body weight and blood lipid concentrations are discussed.

TREATMENT OF PATIENTS WITH HYPERLIPIDEMIA WITH CLOFIBRATE AND β-PYRIDYLCARBINOL

C. Keller, N. Zollner, and G. Wolfram

Medizinische Poliklinik der Universitat, 8 Munchen 2, Germany

Fourty-six patients with primary hyperlipidemia of the mixed type and 13 patients with idiopathic hypercholesterolemia were treated with two different preparations of Clofibrate (1.5 g per day) and with β-pyridylcarbinol (1.2 g/day) each of these drugs was given for eight weeks, the periods of treatment were interrupted by placebo periods of two weeks. Three different sequences of the drugs were followed and the patients were assigned to these three sequences according to the order of their admission to the hospital. Therefore, the distribution was at random.

Serum-lipid levels were determined in two or four week intervals, routine laboratory examinations were done at the beginning and the end of the study.

The sequence of the drugs did not influence their effect on the serum lipid levels. The serum cholesterol levels of the patients with hypercholesterolemia showed the same decrease (average 50 mg/100 ml) whether treated with the preparations of Clofibrate or with β-pyridylcarbinol. In mixed type hyperlipidemias serum cholesterol was slightly lowered by the preparations of Clofibrate, while β-pyridylcarbinol was not successful in all cases. The triglyceride levels of the mixed type hyperlipidemias were lowered to the same extent (average 40%) by the two preparations of Clofibrate, but β-pyridylcarbinol had less effect.

Biochemical side reactions to the different treatments were not noticed.

THE EFFECT OF A β-BLOCKER ON PLASMA LIPOPROTEIN METABOLISM IN
SPONTANEOUS HYPERTENSIVE RATS

N. Kimura, S. Nambu, H. Toshima, M. Ageta, and H. Gohoda

The Third Department of Internal Medicine, Kurume University, School of Medicine,
Kurume-shi, Kyushu, Japan

A high concentration of plasma lipids has been recognized as one of the principal
risk factors in the development of ischemic heart disease (IHD) in man. But although
we found the presence of patients with IHD in the absence of hyperlipidemia in Japan,
many of them include hypertension frequently. According to these facts, abnormal
lipoprotein metabolism with hypertension is important as a risk factor of IHD in Japan.

In the present study in male spontaneous hypertensive rats (SHR) and normotensive
Wistar rats (NTR) on a commercial diet was determined a relationship between abnormal
lipoprotein metabolism and hypertension. In SHR, VLDL-triglyceride (TG) and LDL-TG/
cholesterol (TC) were high level, but LDL-TG and TC in HDL2/HDL3 were low level.
These findings suggested the presence of a characteristic lipoprotein metabolism,
abnormal behavior from VLDL to LDL, in SHR. However, after 21 days administration
of beta-adrenergic blockade, pindolol 0.1 mg/kg subcutaneously, these differences in
lipoprotein fraction became to be not apparent between SHR and NTR. On the other hand,
incorporation of ^{3}H-glycine into each lipoprotein fraction was different between the two
groups as follows: VLDL-^{3}H-protein increased with a decrease of LDL-^{3}H protein, in
NTR, but these changes in SHR were not found. These results indicated the possibility
that this lipoprotein metabolism was produced by a catecholamine related to the beta-
adrenergic receptor which was different from that in NHR. Therefore, this abnormal
lipoprotein metabolism suggested one of the risk factors in the development of IHD with
hypertension.

PURIFICATION OF HUMAN ADIPOSE TISSUE LIPOPROTEIN LIPASE AND HUMAN
LIVER LIPASE - A COMPARATIVE STUDY WITH TWO POST-HEPARIN PLASMA LIPASES

G. Klose, R. DeGrella, B. Walter and H. Greten

Klinisches Institut fur Herzinfarktforschung der Medizinischen Universitatsklinik,
69 Heidelberg, Germany

Two triglyceride lipases were characterized after purification from human post-
heparin plasma. The two lipases were eluted stepwise with 0.75 M and 1.5 M NaCl
from columns containing Sepharose with covalently linked heparin and were further
purified by Conconavalin A chromatography and antibody affinity chromatography. Animal
experiments with hepatectomized dogs indicated that the first lipase activity originates
from liver. Human adipose tissue was obtained following surgery and human liver was
obtained immediately after death. Lipase activities from both tissues were purified
applying virtually the same purification procedure as for plasma lipases. It could be
demonstrated that lipase activity from human liver had the same characteristics as the

first plasma lipase (0. 75 M NaCl eluate) while purified human adipose tissue lipoprotein lipase was similar to the second plasma lipase (1. 5 M NaCl eluate). Comparative studies were performed (1) by addition of various inhibitors (NaCl, $CaCl_2$, protamin sulfate, heparin, Triton WR-1339); (2) by evaluating temperature decay of isolated enzymes; (3) by determining pH optima and (4) by determining activation and inhibition of these lipases with human plasma proteins. These results indicate that the two human plasma lipase activities originate from liver and adipose tissue. Their role in lipoprotein catabolism will be discussed.

BINDING OF BILE ACIDS AND BILE SALTS BY FIBER

D. Kritchevsky, S. A. Tepper, and J A. Story

The Wistar Institute, Philadelphia, Pennsylvania 19104, USA

The role of non-nutritive fiber in lipid metabolism has been studied in several laboratories. It has been shown that dietary lignin and guar gum may be hypolipidemic.

One possible mechanism by which fiber lowers lipids may involve binding of bile salts, thus inhibiting absorption of cholesterol and other lipids. We have found that alfalfa, wheat straw and bran (substances used as fiber in animal diets) bind appreciable amounts of sodium taurocholate and sodium cholate; on the other hand, cellulose and cellophane (the most common sources of fiber in semi-purified diets) bind very little of these substances. A variety of food substances among them curry powder, oregano and lettuce residue also bind bile salts. Dietary experiments in which alfalfa is substituted for cellulose in an isocaloric diet show the alfalfa-fed animals to have somewhat lower serum lipids and to excrete considerably more of a single dose of orally administered labelled cholesterol. Different agents have been found to bind individual bile acids or salts to varying extents. Thus, anionic exchange resins bind more taurocholic than glycocholic acid whereas natural substances (alfalfa, wheat straw, sugar beet pulp) bind more glyco than taurocholic. Similarly alfalfa binds more taurocholic acid than taurodeoxycholic acid.

THE EFFECT OF MK-185 ON SERUM LIPID LEVELS IN SUBJECTS WITH DIABETES MELLITUS

L. H. Krut, H. C. Seftel and B. I. Joffe

Department of Medicine, Baragwanath Hospital, P. O. Bertsham, Johannesburg, Republic of South Africa

A double blind trial was conducted in subjects with maturity onset diabetes mellitus who had hyperlipaemia of varying degree and type.

After a pre-treatment control period of up to 8 weeks selected subjects were given either MK-185 (M. S. D.) or Clofibrate at recommended dosage and maintained on these drugs for 96 weeks, in addition to any other medication they may have been receiving. The groups were matched in respect of age, sex, duration and severity of diabetes and degree and type of hyperlipaemia.

The subjects were examined clinically every four weeks throughout the period of trial and serum triglyceride, cholesterol and uric acid estimated at these times.

Possible toxic effects of these drugs on hepatic, haematologic and renal function was assessed at regular intervals by laboratory and clinical criteria and possible adverse effects on other systems evaluated clinically.

The effect of MK-185 on serum and uric acid levels was determined in the subjects on this drug and compared with the effect of Clofibrate on these parameters.

The findings will be presented.

REMOVAL OF ENDOTHELIUM ENHANCES TRANSFER OF PLASMA LOW AND VERY LOW DENSITY LIPOPROTEIN CHOLESTEROL INTO ILIAC ARTERIES

H. Lengsfeld, P. Brand and H. R. Baumgartner

F. Hoffmann-LaRoche and Co., Ltd., 4002 Basel, Switzerland

In 14 rabbits one iliac artery was denuded of endothelium by means of a balloon catheter, the other one served as intact control (Microvasc. Res. 5:167, 1973). Twenty-four hours later each animal received 0.35 mg 4-^{14}C-cholesterol (50 µC) in 10 ml of a triolein-sucrose-protein emulsion orally. At various time intervals labelling of plasma free and esterified cholesterol and of plasma lipoproteins was determined in ear vein blood. Fourty-eight hours after ^{14}C-cholesterol ingestion aorta and distal arteries were perfused with ice cold saline and the rabbits simultaneously exsanguinated. Completeness of endothelial removal was controlled morphometrically. Esterification of ^{14}C-cholesterol (extracted with chloroform:methanol from freeze-dried intact as well as denuded arteries) was below 5%. De-endothelialized iliac arteries (DIA) accumulated 2-5 times more ^{14}C-cholesterol than control iliac arteries (CIA). Cholesterol deposition in arteries was calculated from the mean specific radioactivity of plasma cholesterol during the experimental period. Cholesterol deposition in CIA correlated to the cholesterol concentration of high density lipoproteins (R = 0.49; p < 0.05) but not to plasma cholesterol. In contrast, cholesterol deposition in DIA correlated with cholesterol concentration of low and very low density lipoproteins (LDL + VLDL), (R = 0.57; p < 0.05). The ratios of ^{14}C-cholesterol in DIA/CIA correlated to the cholesterol concentration of LDL + VLDL (R = 0.72; p < 0.01).

The results indicate that LDL and VLDL cholesterol more readily enter an arterial wall which is denuded of endothelium. Thus intact arterial endothelium may function as a barrier.

RESPONSE OF PRIMARY HYPERLIPIDAEMIAS TO TREATMENT ACCORDING TO A
SIMPLIFIED THERAPEUTIC CLASSIFICATION

B. Lewis and S. Tabaqchali

Department of Chemical Pathology, Royal Postgraduate Medical School, Hammersmith
Hospital, London W12 OHS, England

To facilitate the large scale treatment of hyperlipidaemic patients, a simplified
classification has been sought; this was intended not as a fundamental means of dis-
tinguishing disease entities, but to allocate patients to a minimum number of groups
each with different optimal therapies.

The series consisted of 57 consecutive adult lipid clinic referrals, representing the
"mix" of hyperlipidaemic seen at a general hospital, slected on the basis of having 2
cholesterol levels exceeding 300 mg/dl, and/or 2 triglyceride concentrations exceeding
180 mg/dl. Laboratory data reported to the clinic were cholesterol and triglyceride
concentrations, visual appearance of stored serum, and investigations for underlying
disease (thyroid, liver, renal function). History, examination and these investigations
were the bases for therapeutic classification. At 1 year, responses were related to
formal classification of plasma lipoprotein patterns, carried out on the initial sample
by electrophoresis and, where appropriate, preparative ultracentrifugation; this data
was not reported to the clinicians.

Patients were classified into three groups: hypercholesterolaemia (28), endogenous
hypertriglyceridaemia (11), and combined hyperlipidaemia (16) Pure chylomicronaemia
was not represented in this series. Two patients had secondary (alcoholic)lipaemia.

Primary hyperlipidaemias were treated by weight reduction, followed by modified-
fat diet (P/S ratio 1.4, cholesterol 300 mg/day). Residual hypercholesterolaemia was
treated mainly with cholestyramine or D-thyroxine, and hypertriglyceridemia with
Clofibrate. Of 55 patients, 49 had attained cholesterol levels < 270 mg/dl, and triglyceride < 160 mg/dl within 12 months, both values being less than 95th percentile for
healthy Londoners.

THE "IN VIVO" ACCUMULATION OF L-^{3}H-NOREPINEPHRINE IN RAT EPIDIDYMAL
ADIPOSE TISSUE AND ITS MODIFICATIONS BY DRUGS

F. Luzzani and L. Manara

Istituto di Ricerche Farmacologiche "Mario Negri", Milano, Italy

One hour after intravenous administration of a tracer dose of L-^{3}H-norepinephrine
(L-^{3}H-NE) (0.53 g/kg) to male Sprague-Dawley rats its concentration was measured in
plasma, heart and epididymal adipose tissue (EAT) by liquid scintillation radioassay after
purification of the samples on Al_2O_3. The tissue/plasma ratios of L-^{3}H-NE were re-
markably high (150-200) for the heart and only slightly superior to unit (about 1.5) for the

EAT. These findings are in reasonable agreement with the figure which can be anticipated for the EAT based on endogenous catecholamine concentration and relative blood flow (Kopin, Gordon and Horst, Biochem. Pharmacol. 14:753, 1965). When drugs were administered (1/2 hour prior to L-^{3}H-NE) desipramine (10 mg/kg I. P.) reduced markedly the tissue plasma ratio of L-^{3}H-NE both for the EAT and heart, while 5-carboxy-3-methyl-pyrazole (15 mg/kg I. P.) lowered significantly such a ratio only for the EAT. Nicotinic acid (50 mg/kg I. P.) and Na-α-parachlorophenylisobutyrate (100 mg/kg I. P.) had no effect on either EAT or heart.

INFLUENCE OF ARYLOXY ACIDS ON SERUM LIPID FATTY ACIDS

R. Maier and K. Muller

Research Department, Pharmaceuticals Division, CIBA-GEIGY Ltd., CH-4002 Basel, Switzerland

Clofibrate and CIBA 13437-Su, two aryloxy acids, were compared with L-thyroxine and nicotinic acid for their effect on total serum and liver lipids. The lipid extracts were resolved into lipid classes and the fatty acid composition determined. The two aryloxy acids elicited a marked increase in oleic acid and a reduction of the linoleic acid content, whereas L-thyroxine and nicotinic acid showed no such changes. The shift was most obvious in the triglycerides, and somewhat less so in the cholesterol esters of both serum and liver lipids.

Alteration of fatty acid composition appears to be a feature of the aryloxy acid type of drugs and is not a common effect of all hypolipidemic drugs.

COLESTID, A TWO YEAR REPORT OF A PLACEBO CONTROLLED TRIAL

W. B. Martin, K. Gundersen, A. E. Dorr and J. C. Schneider

The Upjohn Company, Kalamazoo, Michigan 49001, USA

Colestipol hydrochloride (Colestid, Upjohn), an insoluble polymer of diethylenetriamine with 1-chloro-2,3-epoxypropane, sequesters bile acids preventing their reabsorption, thereby increasing their excretion. In response, catabolism of cholesterol to bile acids is increased and the serum cholesterol (SC) is lowered.

In a multiclinic, random assignment, placebo-controlled study with about 2,100 patients enrolled, approximately equal numbers of patients were treated with colestipol hydrochloride 5 g three times a day or with placebo (microcrystalline cellulose). The prime requirement for entry into the study was a SC consistently in excess of 250 mg/100 ml. Approximately half of each group were men; the age was 53 years; 82% were white Eighty percent of the patients in each group were presumptively Type II hyperlipoproteinemics by estimation of the LDL concentration using the SC and the serum triglyceride (TG) at initial time.

The purpose of the study was to assess long term effects of the polymer on serum lipids, particularly cholesterol and triglycerides. The average initial SC level in the colestipol group was 313 mg/100 ml and in the placebo group it was 308 mg/100 ml. The average SC decline in the colestipol group was 35 mg/100 ml. This decline was seen by the end of one month of treatment; and from month 1 through month 24 there was no significant difference in the effect of colestipol over time. At any evaluation period, approximately forty percent of the colestipol group and twelve percent of the placebo group had a 15% or greater reduction in SC.

TG were not specifically affected; the mean in the placebo group rose from 158 at initial time to 229 mg/100 ml at month 24, and from 160 to 216 mg/100 ml in the colestipol group over the same time period.

Side effects from colestipol were entirely gastrointestinal, primarily constipation. Eleven percent of the colestipol and 5% of the placebo group reported a side effect resulting in discontinuation in 4% and 0. 7%, respectively.

INFLUENCE OF PLANT STEROLS ON CHOLESTEROL ABSORPTION

F. H. Mattson

The Procter and Gamble Company, Miami Valley Laboratories, Cincinnati, Ohio 45239 USA

Thoracic duct cannulated rats were fed by stomach tube an emulsion type diet containing ^{14}C-cholesterol. Lymph was collected for the 48 hours following the feeding and the amount of ^{14}C-cholesterol in the lymph was determined. Stigmasterol, β-sito-sterol, or campesterol, either as the free alcohol or as the oleate or as the acetate ester, was added to the emulsion diet. All three plant sterols, whether administered as the free alcohol or as the ester, were equally effective in decreasing the absorption of dietary cholesterol.

HORMONAL INFLUENCES ON THE RATE OF BILE ACID BIOSYNTHESIS IN RATS

D. Mayer

Institut fur Klinische Biochemie und Physiologische Chemie der Medizinischen Hochschule Hannover, D-3000 Hannover, Germany

Cholesterol-7α-hydroxylase, the rate limiting enzyme of bile acid biosynthesis is subject to circadian variations level and amplitude of which are modified by the bile acid level in the enterohepatic circulation. The influence of hydrocortisone, thyroxine, and insulin is investigated in rats. To see the response of enzyme activity not only under normal conditions rats of parallel series of experiments are treated additionally with Cholestyramine (enzyme induction) or cholic acid (inhibition of enzyme activity). The determinations are done twice a day at times of low and high activity. Hydrocortisone effects an increase of enzyme activity in all cases. The Cholestyramine induced increase of about 75% rises further for 40% after administration of hydrocortisone. Deficiency of thyroxine (^{131}I-) causes a depressed rhythm (level and amplitude), the Cholestyramine induced increase is less pronounced than in normals (-25%). The influence of insulin is investigated first in short-time and long-time experiments in normal and diabetic rats (onset of diabetes induced by streptozotocin 7 days before). An immediate effect of insulin (2 hr stimulation) is not to be seen in either animal. In contrast, a 4 day insulin treatment lowers the enzyme activity in all animals though normal blood-sugar levels at the time of investigation. In the untreated diabetic rats the enzyme induction caused by Cholestyramine remains unchanged whereas it is depressed (about 30%) in normal and diabetic rats after long-time insulin treatment. The results are compared with those of similar investigations concerning HMG-CoA reductase done by this and other laboratories.

LONG TERM USE OF PROBUCOL IN PATIENTS WITH HYPERCHOLESTEROLEMIA

D. McCaughan

Veterans Administration Hospital, West Roxbury, Massachusetts, USA

Fifty-nine patients with pre-treatment cholesterol levels greater than 250 mgm% (range 261-445) were followed for a period of 37 to 41 months. Probucol was given in daily dose of 0.5 gm b.i.d. Cholesterol levels were determined at two monthly intervals. Cholesterol change was calculated from the average of all determinations during the follow-up periods and compared with the average of three pretreatment values. Fifty-eight patients showed an average decline of 20%. One patient showed a slight rise of 2%. Types 2a, 2b and type IV responded effectively.

Toxicity studies done at two monthly intervals showed no change in urinalysis, complete blood counts, SGPT, bilirubin and BUN. Tolerance was excellent; one patient experienced loose stools requiring discontinuing the medication at intervals.

Although the study was not designed to show the effect of cholesterol-lowering in cardiovascular disease, there has been a reduction of angina in several subjects together with a reduction of xanthelasma and xanthomata. No mortality has occurred since the first year. Probucol appears to be an effective cholesterol-lowering agent. Preliminary findings indicate that further studies to determine the long term effectiveness in preventing morbid events appear to be warranted.

EARLY ARTERIAL LIPIDOSIS IN RELATION TO GROWTH AND DIFFERENTIATION OF THE ARTERIAL TUBE

W. W. Meyer and J. Lind

Karolinska Hospital, 104 01 Stockholm 60, Sweden

In the arteries of children and adolescents, the lipid deposits initially arise from special structures, which develop in the arterial intima during the growth and obviously represent an accommodation to the higher haemodynamic load. An additional haemodynamic load is supposedly present at the arterial branchings and in the curved arterial segments. But even in some straight portions of the arteries, the opposite sectors of the arterial tube may be exposed to a different tensile strength, as evidenced by their different structural features. In the common carotid artery, for example, the lipids selectively appear in the differentiated musculo-elastic intimal layer, which develops in the predisposed anteromedial arterial wall long before the lipid accumulation becomes visible grossly or microscopically. In the other arterial provinces, the lipid deposits remain also initially limited to the special preformed arterial structures. Thus, at least the initial localization and the gross pattern of the early lipid deposits are obviously determined by the local structural and haemodynamic factors. The selective development of lesions in the special arterial structures which are probably continuously exposed to a higher mechanical strain, may rather be interpreted as a manifestation of the local metabolic insufficiency of the arterial intima as the consequence of some general metabolic disturbances.

EFFECT OF CLOFIBRATE ON THE REMOVAL OF INJECTED ARTIFICIAL TRIGLYCER-IDE - PARTICLES FROM THE BLOOD

H. Micheli and D. Pometta

Unite de Diabetologie, Departement de Medicine, Hopital Cantonal, 1211 Geneve 4, Switzerland

The fractional removal rate (K2) of an artificial fat emulsion Intralipid has been used to assess the effect of clofibrate on the disappearance of exogenous triglycerides from the blood. The reproducibility of the intravenous fat tolerance test (IVFTT) was first assessed in 20 normo- and hyperlipemic subjects. K2 value was more reproducible ($r = 0.89$) than the evaluation of fasting serum triglycerides (TG) ($r = 0.79$). The IVFTT was performed in 14 patients receiving clofibrate (1.5 g daily) during one to three months. The control IVFTT without medication was performed before treatment in 7 patients and more than 4 weeks after clofibrate withdrawal in the 7 other patients.

Clofibrate increased the mean elimination rate K2 from 3.98 ± 0.36 (SEM) to 5.43 ± 0.62 per cent per minute ($p < 0.001$) while the mean TG decreased from 2.33 ± 0.39 mmol/l to 1.57 ± 0.29 ($p < 0.001$). Thus the mean individual change of K2 was a 36% increase while the mean individual TG decreased by 26% during treatment.

Another drug, nafenopin, increased K2 by 44% after 1 to 3 month treatment and decreased TG by 39% (n = 16). Conclusion: the hypotriglyceridemic effect of clofibrate may partly be explained by an increased activity of the removal of triglyceride-rich particles from the blood.

SECHOLEX AND CHOLESTYRAMINE IN HYPERLIPOPROTEINAEMIA TYPE II

T. Miettinen, E. Nikkila and A. Lanner

Department of Medicine, University of Helsinki, Helsinki, Finland

The bile acid sequestrants Secholex (PDX chloride) and cholestyramine were evaluated for their effects on serum cholesterol (CH) and other variables in type II patients.

STUDY I: In a short-term metabolic ward trial, Secholex (15 g/day) and cholestyramine (16 g/day) significantly reduced CH. Fecal bile acids and fecal total sterols were significantly increased, whilst serum methylsterol levels, although more than doubled, were not significantly changed.

STUDY II: Secholex (15 g/day) was given to 21 patients for 60 weeks and cholestyramine to 9 patients for 24 weeks. CH fell by 9-21% and 14-26%, respectively, during the first 24 weeks. The effect of Secholex sustained the whole period. The reductions obtained were similar in IIA and IIB patients. The effect on triglycerides varied considerably with both drugs.

STUDY III: In a cross-over study, 7 of the cholestyramine treated patients were switched to Secholex for 24 weeks. Both drugs lowered CH by a mean of 21%. In another cross-over study 9 of the Secholex therapy thereafter. When on cholestyramine CH increased insignificantly, whilst on switching back to Secholex CH fell by 9% (P < 0.05). Almost all patients preferred Secholex to cholestyramine.

STUDY IV: Nine patients were treated at random with Secholex 3 g, 4 g, and 5 g t.i.d. for 8 weeks at each dose level. CH was reduced by 12, 12 and 15%, respectively.

Results indicate: Secholex and cholestyramine lower elevated CH by 15-20% and the initial effect is sustained. The effect of Secholex 5 g t.i.d. is as good as or slightly better than that of cholestyramine 4 g q.i.d. Increasing the dose of Secholex had no significant effect. When comparing the effect of two lipid lowering drugs, a cross-over technique should be used instead of comparing two separate groups.

RELATIONSHIP BETWEEN THE HEPATIC "PEROXIDATIVE BALANCE" AND THE
HALOGENOALKANE-INDUCED TOXICITY

P. A. Milillo, O. Danni, E. Burdino and G. Ugazio

Istituto di Patologia Generale, 10125 Torino, Italy

According to the "peroxidative balance" hypothesis, the extent of the oxidative decom-
position of membrane lipids is directly proportional to both the actual efficiency of pro-
oxidant factors and the concentration of polyunsaturated fatty acids. Therefore, lipo-
peroxidation is expected to occur at a lower rate when cellular content in antioxidants
and saturated fatty acids is enhanced.

Surgical partial hepatectomy, as well as chemical partial hepatectomy, has been
found to protect against otherwise lethal doses of halogenoalkanes. Both these preliminary
treatments leave a regenerating liver made predominantly by immature cells which are
provided with a deficient drug metabolizing enzyme system. These alterations render
much milder the peroxidative attack by the poison which has been suggested as a pathogenetic factor of CCl_4 lethality.

Feeding rats on a diet devoid of polyunsaturated fatty acids for two months causes a
severe decline in the concentration of these fatty acids in liver microsomal phospholipids,
while the level of drug metabolizing enzyme system is practically unchanged. Nevertheless, these alterations do not succeed in protecting against the lethal effect of carbon
tetrachloride.

In our opinion, these results offer evidence that toxicity induced by halogenated
hydrocarbons depends mainly on the rate of metabolism of the poison. Alternatively,
we can assume that specific microregions of the microsomal membrane surface, made
by unsaturated fatty acids, but possibly not affected by essential fatty acid deficiency,
are the target for the peroxidative attack.

REDUCTION BY CLOFIBRATE OF THE SEVERITY OF ACUTE MYOCARDIAL ISCHAEMIC
INJURY IN DOGS

N. E. Miller, M. F. Oliver and O. D. Mjos

Lipid Research Laboratory and Department of Cardiology, Royal Infirmary, Edinburgh,
Scotland

The effect of clofibrate on myocardial ischaemic injury following acute coronary
artery occlusion has been studied in dogs. Ischaemic injury was measured as the sum of
ST segment elevations (ΣST) in epicardial ECG recordings from 10-13 sites. ΣST during
coronary occlusion alone averaged 26 ± 5.7 mV (mean ± SEM, n = 9 dogs). Intravenous
administration of clofibrate (20 mg/kg) 30 minutes before repeating the occlusion reduced
ΣST to 13 ± 3.2 mV (P < 0.025). In other experiments an intravenous infusion of isoprenaline (0.2 μg/kg/min) increased occlusion-induced ST to 74 ± 10.7 mV (n = 8;

P < 0.001). This augmentation of ΣST by isoprenaline was substantially reduced by the prior administration of clofibrate (ΣST = 40 ± 7.2 mV; P < 0.005). These effects of clofibrate occurred in the absence of any changes in mean aortic blood pressure or heart rate.

Clofibrate reduced arterial concentration of free fatty acids (FFA_a) from 466 ± 41 to 221 ± 44 µEq/l (P < 0.001). When isoprenaline was given FFA_a increased to 1966 ± 183 µEq/l. After prior treatment with clofibrate, isoprenaline-elevated FFA_a were reduced to 1429 ± 209 µEq/l (P < 0.001). The FFA-lowering effect of clofibrate was shown in other studies to be associated with a proportionate reduction in the myocardial extraction of FFA.

It has been previously shown that the antilipolytic agents, nicotinic acid and β-pyridyl-carbinol can reduce the severity of an experimental myocardial infarction, probably by decreasing myocardial oxygen demand. The present findings suggest that clofibrate may have a similar effect.

EFFECT OF CHONDROITIN POLYSULFATE ON SERUM LIPID OF ATHEROSCLEROTIC PATIENTS

K. Nakazawa and K. Murata

Department of Medicine and Physical Therapy, University of Tokyo, School of Medicine, Tokyo 113, Japan

The clinical effects of chondroitin polysulfate (CPS) on atherosclerotic subjects were investigated by peroral administration. Forty-six atherosclerotic subjects were selected as follows: 1) 18 subjects at aged home, 2) 10 inpatients with apoplexia for rehabilitation exercise, and 3) 18 outpatients with arteriosclerosis, hypertension and myocardial infarction. CPS 3 gm, daily, was given perorally to the half numbers in each group. At the 6 to 36 months after the peroral administration of CPS, the following results were obtained.

Total cholesterol in serum decreased by CPS 10 to 20% of the control values at one to four months after the starting of the treatment in group 1 and 3. Serum triglycerides showed a significant decrease about 30% of the controls at one to three months after the administration of CPS in the treated groups. Serum phospholipid decreased after the treatment in comparison with controls. Thrombus formation time, which was measured by a modified method of Chandler's rotating loop's technique, prolonged 150% over the value of the control after the three months of CPS. It took 12.1 min in CPS treated group, while 7.8 min were given in placebo control group.

One patient who had angina pectoris had marked improvement of ST on electrocardiogram one month after the CPS treatment. No side effects were observed by the administration of CPS. Thus antiatherosclerotic effects were suggested at the points of anti-lipemic and anti-thrombongenic activities of CPS.

CLINICAL EXPERIENCES WITH DH581: A NEW CHOLESTEROL LOWERING COMPOUND

D. T. Nash

Upstate Medical Center, Syracuse, New York, USA

DH581, a new cholesterol lowering drug, was studied in thirty adults for over one year in a double blind study. There were seventeen females and thirteen males. Seven were studied initially with placebo for three months. The mean of three fasting cholesterol and triglyceride determinations prior to therapy was used as the baseline. Monthly determinations of lipids, physical examinations and screening test for hematological, renal, and hepatic toxicity were performed prior to and after three months of therapy. All patients on therapy received 500 mg of DH581 twice a day.

There was an approximately 15% drop in cholesterol for the entire group studied on DH581. Twenty-two of the patients experienced a cholesterol drop of 12% or more and are considered responders. Their average response was 19%. Eight non-responders averaged a 3% drop in cholesterol. There were no significant weight changes. The effect on triglyceride values was unpredictable. The effect on cholesterol was unrelated to lipoprotein electrophoretic type.

No pattern of toxicity to the drug has been seen, either clinical or hematologic. Only one patient had to discontinue the study because of a drug related complaint.

EFFECTS OF ALIMENTARY HYPERLIPAEMIA ON HUMAN PLATELETS

A. Nordoy, E. Strom and K. Gjesdal

Department of Medicine, Institute of Clinical Medicine, University of Tromso, Norway

To study the effect of a fatty meal on platelets, 30 healthy male subjects were given isocaloric meals composed mainly of saturated (cream) or unsaturated fats (soybean oil).

All subjects had turbid plasma 2 hrs after the meal. Plasma TG increased significantly, and the TG fatty acids reflected the dietary fatty acids. Thus, the cream induced increases in palmitic, stearic and oleic acids, whereas soybean oil increased the content of linoleic acid. Platelet TG did not correlate with plasma TG in the fasting state, but during alimentary hyperlipaemia a significant correlation between TG in the two compartments was established.

Total FFA in plasma and platelets remained unchanged, but FFA 18:0 and 18:1 in platelets increased after the cream. Total cholesterol and phospholipids were constant.

PF-3 activity of PPP and PRP were unchanged, but the availability after kaolin exposure or platelet disruption, was decreased after the saturated fats. PF-4, which is a release marquer, increased in PPP after the cream.

The results showed that a fatty meal influences the lipid composition of platelets.

Saturated fat induced significant changes in the clotting function of platelets, and probably to some extent induced a release reaction. Unsaturated fat did not give these effects.

THE PREVENTION OF POST-OPERATIVE THROMBOSIS BY EARLY ADMINISTRATION OF EITHER LOW DOSE HEPARIN OR OF DEXTRAN: AN EXPERIMENTAL STUDY

W. Obolensky, J. Arendt, H. Hubner, F. Maire and F. Willausch

Dept. Obstet. Gynaec., Kantonsspital CH 4410 Liestal, Switzerland

The prevention of post-operative thromboembolic disease is a question of major concern in gynecology. Recent investigations confirm, that the thrombi are formed during the operation itself. It seems therefore appropriate to start antithrombotic therapy intra-operatively, provided no adverse reaction occurs. The purpose of this paper is to investigate whether the frequency of fibrin agglomeration - i.e. thrombosis - in the post-operative phase may be reduced by drugs given pre-operatively.

Material and Methods: Sixty patients comparable in age and weight undergoing major gynecological operations, all with equal technique of narcosis and with equal general care, were divided into three groups: the first had the usual post-operative care with early ambulation only, the second was given additionally 500 ml Macrodex with the initiation of narcosis and during the next 4 days, while the third had instead 5,000 U b.i.d. heparin (Liquemin) by s.c. route starting 2 hours before operation. On the 5th post-operative day, routine anticoagulation was initiated always.

The incidence of thrombosis was studied by the Pittman isotope monitor using labeled fibrinogen.

The results were evaluated with appropriate statistical measures and the following conclusion is drawn: though the incidence of manifest post-operative thrombosis is low with conventional measures, one of the 2 early therapies is recommended to replace later prophylactic cumarin medication with its hazards of late wound bleeding.

EFFECT OF CHOLESTYRAMINE ALONE AND IN COMBINATION WITH CLOFIBRATE ON SERUM LIPOPROTEINS IN PATIENTS WITH TYPE II HYPERLIPOPROTEINEMIA (HLP)

A.G. Olsson, L.A. Carlson, L. Oro and S. Rossner

King Gustaf V Research Institute and Department of Medicine, Karolinska Hospital, S-104 01 Stockholm 60, Sweden

The effect of cholestyramine (Questran) 4 g q.i.d. alone and in combination with clofibrate (Atromidin) 1 g b.i.d. on serum lipoproteins was studied in 15 subjects with type IIA HLP and 6 subjects with type IIb HLP after treatment in 2 month periods. Mean total cholesterol value before treatment was 382 ± 18 (SEM) mg per 100 ml and decreased to 284 ± 16 mg per 100 ml ($p < 0.001$) on cholestyramine and 273 ± 15 mg per 100 ml on cholestyramine + clofibrate the additional decrease on combination being unsignificant. The triglyceride (TG) concentration was 2.10 ± 0.28 mmol/l before therapy, 2.02 ± 0.19 mmol/l (n. s.) on cholestyramine and 1.42 ± 0.13 mmol/l ($p < 0.005$) on combination.

On only cholestyramine serum low density lipoprotein (LDL) concentration fell from 283 ± 19 mg/100 ml to 190 ± 16 mg/100 ml ($p < 0.001$), very low density lipoproteins (VLDL) and high density lipoprotein (HDL) concentrations were unchanged. The magnitude of the decrease in LDL cholesterol level was weakly positively correlated to the initial LDL concentration ($r = 0.52$, $p < 0.025$). No significant changes in mean VLDL-TG levels occurred on cholestyramine alone. However, the change of individual VLDL-TG concentrations by cholestyramine correlated negatively with initial VLDL-TG levels ($r = .75$, $p < 0.001$, $y = 0.48X + 0.54$).

During combination of cholestyramine and clofibrate VLDL-TG concentrations decreased from 1.04 ± 0.13 mmol/l to 0.55 ± 0.08 mmol/l ($p < 0.001$) and VLDL cholesterol fell from 30 ± 5 to 16 ± 2 mg/100 ml ($p < 0.001$). Serum LDL cholesterol remained unchanged when clofibrate was added (185 ± 15 mg/100 ml). On the other hand, serum HDL cholesterol increased from 54 ± 3 mg/100 ml to 59 ± 4 mg/100 ml ($p < 0.02$).

Conclusions: The decrease in serum total cholesterol concentration by cholestyramine alone is completely a reflection of an effect on serum LDL cholesterol level. Addition of clofibrate results in a decrease in VLDL cholesterol and an increase in HDL cholesterol, the latter partly hiding the effect on VLDL levels when looking only at effects on total cholesterol concentration.

IN VITRO PROTEIN BINDING INTERACTION BETWEEN A NEW HYPOLIPEMIC AGENT, TIBRIC ACID, AND VARIOUS DRUGS

G. Pagnini, A. Crispino and G. Ceccarelli

Istituto di Farmacologia dell'Universita di Torino, Torino, Italy

Studies have been made on protein binding interactions between a new hypolipemic agent 2-chloro-5-(3, 5-dimethylpiperidinosulfonyl) benzoic acid (tibric acid) and various drugs.

Serum albumin protein binding of chlorpropamide, sulphaethyltaizole and tibric acid was calculated as a percentage of bound-drug in comparison to the amount of drug placed in contact with albumin or as drug moles bound for one mole of albumin.

For the concentrations used (10 to 100 mcg/ml) tibric acid protein binding capacity was greater than that of the other drugs but tibric acid was not able to modify the protein binding capacity of chlorpropamide and sulpha (fixed 30 mcg/ml concentrations of chlorpropamide and sulpha with 1:1 to 1:10 varying drugs/tibric acid ratios) In another series of experiments the inhibition of dicumarol protein binding by various drugs including tibric acid and clofibrate was studied.

The results showed that the degree of inhibition of dicumarol protein binding is lower with tibric acid (11-16%) than with clofibrate (30-38%).

INTERACTIONS OF THE CLOFIBRATE WITH ESTROGENS AND THE RESULTS IN FERTILITY

G. C. Pantaleoni and P. Valeri

Il Cattedra dell'Istituto di Farmacologia Medica di Roma, Citta Universitaria Piazzale delle Scienze, Rome, Italy

The ethyl p-chlorophenoxy-isobutyrate (Clofibrate) has been particularly studied as regards biochemical processes metabolizing cholesterol and fatty acids. Clofibrate interactions with the processes of synthesis and the hormonal secretion and generally with the functions connected with the production of gonadotrophic hormones have been studied less closely. We studied the effects of Clofibrate short-term administration on the fertility in the rat and in the rabbit and on the secretion of 17-ketosteroids and estrogens. These observations were performed in Sprague-Dawley and Long Evans rats treated for 10 days with 200-500 mg/kg/die of Clofibrate. During the treatment the observation of vaginal smears was continued daily recording the number of animals showing interruptions of the cycle.

The 10th day the animals were put in metabolic cages for the fluorimetric determination of total urinary estrogens and the spectrophotometric determination of urinary 17-ketosteroids. The radiommunology of estradiol 17β was carried out on the plasma. The decrease of urinary estrogens and, at the same time, of estradiol 17β on the plasma were found to be statistically significant and apparently essential for the alteration of the oestrus cycle with the dose of 500 mg while the dose of 200 mg/kg no significant variations were observed on the studied parameters.

EFFECT OF HYPERCHOLESTEROLAEMIC DIET AND A SINGLE INJECTION OF POLY-UNSATURATED PHOSPHATIDYL CHOLINE ON THE ACTIVITIES OF LIPOLYTIC ENZYMES, ACYL-CoA SYNTHETASE AND CHOLESTEROL ACYLTRANSFERASE IN RABBIT TISSUES

J. Patelski, Z. Waligora and A. N Howard

Department of Biochemistry, Medical Academy, 60-781 Poznan, Poland, and Department of Investigative Medicine, University of Cambridge, Addenbrooke's Hospital, Cambridge CB2 2QQ, England

In rabbits fed a 1% cholesterol diet for 12 weeks the following were found: in serum, a decrease in lipase and no changes in phospholipase A and cholesterol esterase activities; in the aortic wall, decreased cholesterol esterase and cholesterol acyltransferase activities and no changes in phospholipase A, lipase and acyl-CoA synthetase activities; in the liver, increased phospholipase A, cholesterol esterase and cholesterol acyltransferase activities, and decreased lipase and acyl-CoA synthetase activities.

A single intravenous injection of polyunsaturated phosphatidyl choline (100 mg/kg) in 4% sodium deoxycholate solution (1 ml/kg) in control and hypercholesterolaemic rabbits resulted in different effects on the enzyme activities. The diet-independent and heparin-like effect of the drug on lipase consisted in increased activities of the enzyme in serum and liver and decreased activity in the aorta. Diet-dependent effects on the enzyme activities were as follows: in serum, decreased phospholipiase A activity in control and increased phospholipiase A and cholesterol esterase activities in hypercholesterolaemic rabbits; in the aortic wall, decreased cholesterol esterase and elevated cholesterol ester synthesis/hydrolysis ratio in control, and increased phospholipase A activity and lowered cholesterol ester synthesis/hydrolysis ratio in hypercholesterolaemic rabbits; in the liver, increased phospholipase A and cholesterol acyltransferase activities and decreased acyl-CoA synthetase activity with the ratio of cholesterol ester synthesis/hydrolysis elevated in control and unchanged in hypercholesterolaemic rabbits.

ON THE ACTIVITY OF GLYCURONYLGLUCOSAMINOGLYCAN SULPHATE ON DISLIPAEMIC PATIENTS: MIDDLE-TERM STUDY

F. Pedrazzi, L. Bonazzi and F. Peterlin

Department of Geriatrics and Gerontology, Verona, Italy

Forty-nine geriatric outpatients underwent a checking of the blood parameters involved in the atherosclerotic disease at various time intervals, during a 60 day period of treatment with an acid sulphomucopolysaccharide, extracted from the pig duodenum (Glycuronylglucosaminoglycan Sulphate, 3 GS).

The parameters initially altered resulted modified at a statistically significant degree; this results was still evident also at a subsequent control, carried out on a group of 6 patients, two months after the drug's suspension.

LONGITUDINAL EFFECT OF POLYUNSATURATED PHOSPHOLIPIDS ON HYPERLIPO-PROTEINAEMIA

H. Peeters and V. Blaton

Simon Stevin Instituut voor Wetenschappelijk Onderzoek, B-8000 - Brugge, Belgium

Intravenous injection of polyunsaturated phosphatidylcholine (PUPC) lowers significantly plasma cholesterol (20%) in hyperbetalipoproteinaemia and modifies the enzymatic activity of the arterial wall. In plasma cholesterol esters it decreases the oleic (3%) and palmitic acid (2%) content and increases the linoleic acid (4.5%). Thus the drug can be related to the faster removal of cholesterol.

The longitudinal effect of peroral PU-PC) was followed on 47 selected patients with hyperlipoproteinaemia. Before initiating the therapy starting lipids levels were controlled at an interval of 14 days. Intravenous therapy with 20 ml PU-PC/day was given during 14 days and the patients further treated with 3 x 2 capsules of PU-PC. Blood samples were analyzed after 14, 46 and 120 days. Changes in plasma lipoproteins, in lipid profiles and in plasma fatty acid compositions were investigated. Phospholipids were separated in their main components and phosphatidylcholine was quantitatively determined   Fatty acids of plasma, of plasma cholesterol esters and of plasma phosphatidylcholine were examined by gas liquid chromatography.

In this longitudinal study a significant decrease of cholesterol was observed while phospholipids increased over the starting value and the C/PL ratio was normalized together with a percentual increase of phosphatidylcholine of 3.5%. Triglycerides remain rather unchanged over the whole period. The significant decrease of the oleic to linoleic acid ratio observed after intravenous therapy was not only maintained but further decreased. The obtained results are discussed in function of the type of hyperlipoproteinaemia. Type II hyperbetalipoproteinaemia is more influenced than other types of lipoprotein disorders.

TIBRIC ACID: A NEW, STRUCTURALLY DISTINCT HYPOLIPIDEMIC AGENT

J. N. Pereira and G. F. Holland

Central Research, Pfizer, Inc. Groton, Connecticut, USA

Tibric acid, 2-chloro-5-(cis-3,5-dimethylpiperidinosulfonyl) benzoic acid, is a new hypolipidemic drug structurally distinct from existing agents which reduce plasma lipid levels in rats at oral doses as low as 5 mg/kg/day. In two day rat experiments with the drugs administered in the diet, tibric acid was approximately 10 times as potent as clofibrate. Administration of either tibric acid or clofibrate results in marked increases in the activity of the hepatic mitochondrial enzyme, α-glycerophosphate dehydrogenase More prolonged feeding of either drug causes an increased liver size which is accompanied by an increased number of microbodies. No increase in liver lipids is observed. In rats tibric acid and clofibrate produce hypolipidemic effects which are related primarily to lipid reductions in the VLDL-fraction although limited effects are also observed in the LDL fraction. Sucrose-induced hyperlipidemia in rats was completely blocked by tibric acid and clofibrate. In dogs, oral doses of tibric acid in the range of 1-20 mg/kg/day lower fasting plasma cholesterol and triglyceride levels.

EFFECT OF ATHEROGENIC DIET AND POLYUNSATURATED PHOSPHOLIPIDS (PPL)
ON MOTOR AND EXPLORATIVE ACTIVITY OF RATS AND THE LEVEL OF CATE-
CHOLAMINES IN THEIR BRAIN

R. Pilecki, L. Samochowiec and K. Szyszka

Department of Pharmacology, Pomeranian Medical Academy, 70-111 Szczecin, Poland

The influence of atherogenic diet and polyunsaturated phospholipids (PPL) upon the
motor and explorative activity of white rats, and the level of catecholamines in their
brain has been examined. Sixty-eight white male Wistar rats were used for the investigation The animals were given: Group I - an atherogenic diet, Group II - received the
same diet, and the rats were simultaneously administered prophylactically PPL in doses
of 280 mg/kg, - 900 mg/kg; and 2,800 mg/kg in the appropriate subgroups; Group IV
received a basic diet. After 80 days the motor and explorative activity was examined, by
an open field performance of rats (ambulation and rearing were scored), and after the
animals had been killed, the lipids in the blood serum, as well as levels of noradrenaline
(NA) and dopamine were estimated by the Chang method. The influence of the therapeutic
application of PPL has also been investigated in the Group III. Rats had been given in a
period of 80 days an atherogenic diet, after which they were administered a basic + PPL
diet in doses of 280 mg/kg, 900 mg/kg, and 2,800 mg/kg in appropriate subgroups, and
finally the above mentioned examinations were performed. On hand of the obtained results it has been stated, that the 80 days atherogenic diet caused a decrease of motor
and explorative activity, as well as a diminution of catecholamines, whereas these
changes correlated with each other. A prophylactic PPL application prevents these
changes. A theraputic administration of PPL increases the level of behavioural activity,
and catecholamines in relation to the atherogenic group, being subsequently not treated.
The obtained results have been statistically significant.

EFFECT OF CLOFIBRATE ON INSULIN AND GROWTH HORMONE SECRETION IN
NORMAL SUBJECTS AND IN PATIENTS WITH CHEMICAL DIABETES

G. Pozza, G. C. Viberti, A. E. Pontiroli and A. Tognetti

Istituto di Clinica Medica 1[a] e Ospedale S. Raffaele, Universita degli Studi di Milano,
20122 Milano, Italy

Seven subjects of normal body weight and with a normal glucose tolerance test, and
eight patients with chemical diabetes have been treated with clofibrate, 3 gm per day for
ten consecutive days. The effect of arginine on insulin (IRI) and growth hormone (GH)
secretion has been evaluated in basal conditions and the day following discontinuation of
therapy. IRI secretion was significantly decreased after clofibrate treatment both in
normal subjects (45. 5 + 26. 21 vs 77. 4 + 13. 77 μU/ml at 30 min, p < 0. 05) and in patients
with chemical diabetes (35. 1 ± 6. 41 vs 53. 1 ± 7. 76 μU/ml at 30 min, p < 0. 02). GH
secretion was significantly increased in normal subjects after clofibrate treatment
(13. 6 ± 3 35 vs 7. 0 ± 1. 99 mg/ml at 60 min, p < 0. 02), while it was slightly but not
significantly decreased in patients with chemical diabetes. Triglycerides were signifi-

cantly decreased after clofibrate treatment in normal subjects (p < 0. 05) but not in patients with chemical diabetes. Cholesterol was slightly but not significantly decreased in both groups. Blood glucose levels in response to arginine were unchanged after clofibrate treatment.

EFFECT OF DRUGS ON ETHANOL INDUCED HYPERTRIGLYCERIDEMIA IN RATS AND HUMANS

L. Puglisi*, V. Caruso*, F. Conti**, R. Fumagalli* and C. R. Sirtori*

* Institute of Pharmacology of the University of Milan, and ** Vergani Division, Ospedale Maggiore, Milano, Italy

Ethanol induces, both acutely and chronically, an increase of plasma triglycerides and very low density lipoproteins. The mechanism of ethanol induced hypertriglyceridemia (hyperTG) is still under debate (Belfrage, P. et al. Acta Med. Scand. : Suppl. 552, 1973).

We tested the effects of several agents active on lipid and carbohydrate metabolism on hyperTG's induced by ethanol in rats and human. Hyper-TG in rats was accomplished by a three day administration of ethanol both ad libitum and by intubation. Drugs were usually given b. i. d. orally. TG rise was on the average about 60%.

Of the various oral hypoglycemics tested, the most active were tolbutamide and glyclazide, while phenformin was practically inactive.

Clofibrate was also poorly effective, while Cl1, a hypolipidemic derivative of 3-methyl-4-phenyl-3-butenoic acid, showed a remarkable activity. In humans hyperTG was induced acutely by oral administration of 60 g ethanol in orange juice after an overnight fast. A 30-100% TG rise occurred usually 4 to 6 hours later.

Clofibrate and Cl1 were both active in this test, but Cl1 showed a slightly higher activity.

The relationship between TG rise and insulin levels after ethanol and the various agents tested witll be discussed.

THE HYPOLIPIDAEMIC ACTION OF ST22

M. T. Ramacci, L. Pacifici and L. Angelucci

Sigma-Tau Research Laboratories, Pomezia, and Institute of Pharmacology and Pharmacognosy, University of Rome, Rome, Italy

ST22, a sulphur derivative of substituted nicotinamide (rat LD50 mg/kg 2100 os), lowered the plasma levels of free fatty acids (FFA), triglycerides and cholesterol in 17 hr fasted rats. 25 mg/kg had a 240 min lasting effect (peak at 45 min), with a moderate rebound in the FFA plasma level. No tolerance was found after 100 mg/kg os x 12 days in rats. 50 mg/kg s.c. reduced the lipolytic activity (LA) of noradrenaline (NA) by 70% in rats. 50 mg/kg i.v. suppressed the LA of NA by i.v. infusion in cats. 50 mg/kg os x 15 days lowered lipidaemia in rats fed on an atherogenic diet. The anti-lipolytic activity on epididymal adipose tissue from rats was evident at 100 micrograms/ml. 100 mg/kg x 3 prevented plasma biochemical lesions following CCl_4 treatment and increased plasma clearance and biliary excretion of bromthalein.

TRANSFER OF LIPOPROTEINS FROM PLASMA TO PERIPHERAL LYMPH IN MAN

D. Reichi, J. J. Pflug, A. Postiglione, M. Press and N. B. Myant

Medical Research Council, Lipid Metabolism Unit, Hammersmith Hospital, London W12 OHS, England

In order to obtain information about the transport of plasma lipoproteins across the vascular walls, we have followed the appearance of radioactive apolipoproteins in peripheral lymph obtained from the foot in four human subjects after intravenous injection of native lipoproteins labelled in their protein components. Two of these subjects were given injections containing LDL labelled in the B peptide with ^{131}I and VLDL labelled in the A and C groups of peptides with [125]I. The lymph lipoproteins were separated by ultracentrifugation and the lipoprotein peptides were separated by polyacrylamide gel electrophoresis. Radioactivity was measured in the peptide bands obtained by electrophoresis.

Radioactivity appeared in lymph in all the labelled peptides within 1 hour of the injection. The relative amounts of radioactivity present in the different labelled peptides in lymph differed considerably from the relative amounts present in the plasma. This indicated that the peptide composition of plasma lipoproteins changes during their passage across the vascular walls and confirms our earlier suggestion based on the distribution of lipoprotein antigens in lymph fractions of different density (Reichl et al, Clin. Sci. Molec. Med., 45: 313, 1973).

A NEW HYPOLIPIDEMIC AGENT, [(DH-990); 2-(3,5-DI-t-BUTYL-4-HYDROXYPHENYL) THIO] HEXANOIC ACID

A. A. Renzi, D. J. Rytter, E. R. Wagner and H. K. Goersch

The Dow Chemical Company, Midland, Michigan, USA

DH-990, 2-[3,5-di-t-butyl-4-hydroxyphenyl) thio] hexanoic acid was found to significantly lower serum cholesterol levels in normal mice, rat and monkeys. The serum
cholesterol reduction among these species ranged from 21% to 40%. Serum triglycerides
were significantly reduced in rats. The drug was active over a wide concentration range
(0.03-0.25%) when added to the normal diet of rats. Liver weight was slightly increased
while liver lipids showed no significant change. Radiolabeled studies in rats showed
DH-990 to be active in preventing the uptake by the serum and liver of orally administered
cholesterol 4-^{14}C. Hyperlipidemia in rats induced by cholesterol feeding (5% cholesterol,
1% cholic acid) was significantly inhibited by the addition of 0.25% DH-990 to the diet.
Rabbits fed 0.50% DH-990 in a diet containing 1.0% cholesterol and 4% corn oil showed a
significant and dramatic reduction in serum and liver cholesterol and triglyceride levels
At this concentration the drug markedly decreased the incidence of atherosclerotic lesions
in the rabbit aorta. DH-990 was found to be non-estrogenic and animal studies indicate
a low order of toxicity. Clinical studies with this agent have been studied.

EFFECT OF PROSTAGLADIN-E$_1$ ON THE SEVERITY OF ACUTE MYOCARDIAL
ISCHAEMIC INJURY IN DOGS

R. A. Riemersma, M. F. Oliver and O. D. Mjos

Lipid Research Laboratory and Department of Cardiology, Royal Infirmary, Edinburgh,
Scotland

The effect of a naturally occurring antilipolytic agent, prostaglandin-E$_1$ (PGE$_1$) on
the severity of myocardial ischaemic injury following acute coronary artery occlusion
was studied in dogs. Ischaemic injury was measured as the sum of S-T segment
elevations (ΣST) in epicardial ECG recordings from 10-12 sites 10 mins after occlusion.
ΣST, arterial concentrations of free fatty acids (FFA$_a$), and heart rate (HR) were unchanged by i.v. PGE$_1$ (0.6 μg/kg/min), while mean aortic blood pressure (ap) was reduced (p < 0.001) from 128 ± 12 to 109 ± 13 min Hg (mean ± SEM).

Isoprenaline i.v. (0.2 μg/kg/min) increased occlusion-induced ST from 15 ± 6 to
46 ± 8 mV (p < 0.001). The augmentation of ΣST induced by isoprenaline was less
(p < 0.001) during i.v. infusion of PGE$_1$ (ΣST = 36 ± 7 mV). Effects of isoprenaline on ap,
HR and regional myocardial blood flow (using microspheres) were not significantly
latered by PGE$_1$. During isoprenaline infusion FFA$_a$ were reduced by PGE$_1$ from
2022 ± 181 to 1387 ± 270 μEq/l (p < 0.005).

It is concluded that the beneficial effect of PGE$_1$ on the severity of the ischaemic
injury was probably related to reduced myocardial oxygen demand through inhibition of
catecholamine-induced lipolysis.

SECHOLEX IN THE TREATMENT OF HYPERBETALIPOPROTEINAEMIA TYPE II

S. Ritland, A. Lanner, O. Fousa, J. P. Blomhoff and E. Gjone

Med. Dept. A, Rikshospitalet, Oslo, Norway

The effect of Secholex, a bile acid sequestrant, on cholesterol (CH) was studied as well as its influence on intestinal absorption, gastric acid output, liver and kidney function, insulin release, fecal fat and nitrogen excretion, and bile acid concentration and pattern in jejunal aspirate after test meal.

Nine patients were treated with Secholex 3 g t. i. d. for 3 months and 5 g t. i. d. for 9 months. CH decreased from 461 mg/100 ml by 15% ($p < 0.05$) triglycerides (TG) increased insignificantly from 73 to 105 mg/100 ml, whereas phospholipids remained unchanged. In 5 patients who continued on Secholex plus clofibrate during 6 months CH fell by another 13% and TG by 10%. Serum-Ca and SGOT were slightly reduced ($p < 0.05$), whilst other electrolytes, albumin, gammaglobulins, vit. K dependent clotting factors, serum-Fe, serum-vitamin B_{12}, serum and erythrocyte folic acid, serum-vitamin A (fasting) and liver and kidney function tests were unchanged. Absorption of glucose, iron and vitamin B_{12} were unchanged and so were also gastric acid output, insulin release after oral glucose loading and fecal fat excretion, whereas fecal nitrogen excretion and fating insulin were reduced ($p < 0.05$).

In jejunal aspirate after test meal bile acid concentration and glycine/taurine ratio increased significantly. This may be due to compensatory increased bile acid synthesis. The changed glycine/taurine ratio may be explained by greater capacity for glycine-conjugation than taurine-conjugation.

No side effects were seen on Secholex, but two patients had to interrupt clofibrate therapy due to side effects.

EXPERIMENTAL RESEARCH ON METABOLIC EFFECTS OF HEPARIN AND MYOCARDIAL ACTIVITY

F. Rognoni, A. Zuffetti and G. Garzia

Via Legnano, 20075 Lodi, Milano, Italy

What Oliver et al. have showed, i. e. that during the acute phase of myocardium infarct those who present a high concentration of fatty acids in the plasma are more likely to suffer from dangerous arrhythmias, has created doubts on the therapeutic use of Heparin.

The authors, in order to establish the close connection between the effect on the lipid metabolism caused by Heparin and the myocardium excitability, have carried out a series of researches using the test of arrhythmias caused by chloroform and adrenalin.

With this experimental model, they could study the connection between the influence of Heparin on the concentration of lipids in the blood and the characteristic alterations of the rhythm of the conductibility and of the cardiac ripolarization.

Experiments on rats demonstrated that Heparin, dosed so as to create a considerable alteration of the lipid concentration, does not influence the myocardium excitability. Instead, it has been noticed that Heparin interferes with the cardiac conductibility.

EFFECT OF A NICOTINIC ACID ANALOGUE ON PLASMA FREE FATTY ACIDS AND VENTRICULAR ARRHYTHMIAS AFTER ACUTE MYOCARDIAL INFARCTION IN MAN

M. J. Rowe and M. F. Oliver

Departments of Cardiology and Clinical Chemistry, Royal Infirmary, Edinburgh, Scotland

Elevation of plasma free fatty acids (FFA) occurs immediately after the onset of acute myocardial infarction (AMI), and concentrations above 1200 uEq/l are associated with an increased incidence of serious ventricular arrhythmias. Under experimental conditions, arrhythmias, increased MVO_2 and decreased myocardial contractility occur with elevation of plasma FFA.

A nicotinic acid analogue (NAA), 5-fluoro-3-hydroxymethylpyridine hydrochloride which is metabolized as 5-fluoro-nicotinic acid, has been shown to lower plasma FFA in healthy men, during a noradrenaline infusion and during AMI in man (1). It seldom causes flushing and produces no significant haemodynamic effects.

This NAA has been given in a double blind trial to 40 patients within 12 hours of the onset of symptoms of AMI: 41 patients with similar criteria of AMI received identical placebo capsules. The dose used was 200 two hourly during the first 24 hours after admission to hospital. Nausea was not uncommon and vomiting was more prevalent in the treated group.

Plasma FFA were reduced after the administration of the NAA from high levels into the normal range in the majority of patients. On withdrawal of the NAA a rebound occurred to the pre-treatment values.

There was no incident of ventricular tachycardia in the NAA treated group in patients commencing treatment during the first 5 hours after AMI, provided FFA were rapidly lowered and then maintained in the normal range. When the NAA failed to produce sustained reduction of elevated plasma FFA, the incidence of ventricular tachycardia was comparable with that in the control group. The effect of the NAA on ventricular premature beats, including the R/T phenomenon, will be reported.

(1) Rowe, M. J., Dolder, M. A., Kirby, B. J., Oliver, M. D., Lancet 2:814, 1973).

EFFECT OF NICOTINIC ACID (NA) ON FATTY ACID INCORPORATION INTO ADIPOSE TISSUE (FIAT)

R. Rubba and G. Walldius

Semeiotica Medica, II facolta di Medicina e Chirurgia, Universita di Napoli, and King Gustav V Research Institute, Karolinska Hospital, Stockholm, Sweden

Low removal of circulating triglycerides (TG) from blood by periferal tissues, namely, adipose tissue (AT) is a common cause of hypertriglyeridemia (HTG). In the removal process blood TG are first hydrolized by lipoprotein lipase (LLA) to fatty acids (FA) which are then incorporated into adipose tissue (FIAT).

Low FIAT has recently been found to be common in HTG. In the treatment of HTG, NA has been found to be effective in lowering TG. In this study we have investigated if the well known TG lowering effect of NA could be due to increased FIAT and/or simultaneously reduced lipolysis.

Subcutaneous AT was sampled from patients undergoing abdominal surgery for non-acute non-complicated disease.

50 mg pieces were incubated in Krebs-Ringer bicarbonate buffer containing 2% albumin and 5.55 mM glucose, with and without NA (1 microgram/ml).

^{3}H palmitic acid and ^{14}C-glucose were used as tracers for FA and glucose.

FIAT and glucose incorporation into adipose tissue (GLIAT) were determined. FIAT values were corrected for medium FA dilution by "cold" tissue derived FA, according to Dole formula.

The fraction of medium FA incorporated during the incubation time (fractional FIAT) was also determined. Glycerol release was used as a measure of lipolytic rate.

Addition of NA increased both FIAT and fractional FIAT ($p < .005$).

Lipolysis was decreased ($p < .05$). GLIAT was not significantly affected.

These results suggest that the TG lowering effect of NA might be due to both an increase of the FIAT process and a simultaneous decrease of lipolysis, with reduction of FA flow from AT to the liver.

OCCUPATIONAL STRESS AS A FACTOR OF CORONARY HAZARD

C. Rusconi and G. Orlando

Cardiology Institute, Spedali Civili di Brescia, 25100 Brescia, Italy

Among stressors of modern life car driving deserves a place of primary importance.

Therefore we deemed it interesting to examine subjects operating professional motor vehicles in order to evidence the possible atherogenic effect of the stress peculiar to such a work. Our series included 300 subjects working for a company providing suburban bus service aged 21 to 59; 200 were drivers and 100 conductors (control group). We took the following parameters into consideration: diabetic and atherosclerotic familiarity, alimentary and voluptuary habits (paying the best attention to amount of alcohol and cigarettes daily consumed), myocardial infarction ascertained or angina pectoris, obesity, arterial pressure, cholesterolemia, triglyceridemia, blood sugar curve following oral load, electrocardiogram, limbs oscilligram Examination of the prevalence of ischemic cardiopathy has evidenced a clear difference in favour of drivers compared with conductors, especially for those aged 40 to 59. Examination of company's registers showed that also incidence of ischemic cardiopathy in the previous 15 years has a behaviour clearly in favour of drivers (20 cases) compared with conductors (5 cases), although the number of employees practicing the two functions is the same. Though behaviour of parameters we considered (with particular regard to factors of coronary hazard and known causes of hyperlipidemia) shows some differences, is not such as to justify by itself the remarkable different prevalence and incidence of ischemic cardiopathy within the two groups of workers. Consequently it is concluded that occupational stress is surely an important factor of coronary hazard.

TREATMENT OF HYPERLIPIDEMIC PATIENTS WITH CINNARIZINE

P. Saba, F. Salvadorini, F. Galeone, M. Guarguaglini and J. L. Houben.

Psychiatric Hospital of Volterra, Department of Medicine, Pisa, Italy

Twenty-two hyperlipidemic patients were treated with cinnarizine for a 6 month period.

During the clinical trial, total serum lipids, cholesterol, triglycerides, pre-β-lipoprotein and β-lipoprotein were monthly evaluated. In patients with clinical symptoms of peripheral circulation disorders, changes in plethysmometry pattern were also studied.

It has been observed that cinnarizine is a potent hypolipidemic agent, which may be administered continuously for a period now extended up to 6 months, without any decrease in its effectiveness and without evidence of toxic effects. The lipid-lowering ability of cinnarizine was especially pronounced in patients with hypertriglyceridemia only.

In the patients with peripheral circulation disorders, a good improvement in clinical symptoms as well as in plethysmometry patterns, was also found.

Although the therapeutical activity of cinnarizine in hyperlipidemia is evident, its mode of action remains unclear.

PHARMACOKINETIC AND CLINICAL STUDY OF A NEW HYPOLIPEMIC AGENT

G. F. Salvioli, R. Lugli and M. V. Baldelli

Istituto di Clinica Medica, Universita di Modena, 41100 Modena, Italy

Blood levels obtained in man after the oral administration of 2-chloro-5-(3,5-di-methylpiperidinosulfonyl) benzoic acid (tibric acid), a new hypolipemic agent (250 to 750 mgs single dose; 250 mgs t.i.d. for seven days) were evaluated using a gas-chromatographic method (Packard gas-chromatographic apparatus with a flame ionization detector).

The non-metabolized drug was detected in the blood up to 5-6 hours after the oral administration; after 750 mgs single dose schedule the peak was observed in the blood 2-3 hours after the administration.

The hypolipemic activity of the drug was studied in 8 hyperlipoproteinemic type IV patients, in 4 type II (a or b) and in 1 type V other patients, using a dose of 500-1250 mgs/die for 23-28 weeks.

At the end of the treatment a significant reduction in the average levels of cholesterol and triglycerides in the blood was obtained in type IV patients; in type II (a or b) and type V patients the average reduction obtained was 18% for triglycerides and 11% for cholesterol blood levels. No significant change of phospholipids in the blood was observed. The clinical and laboratory tolerance was generally good.

INHIBITION OF "CARBOHYDRATE INDUCED" HYPERTRIGLYCERIDEMIA" BY NICOTINIC ACID

G. Schlierf and G. Hess

Department of Medicine, University of Heidelberg, Germany

Previous studies have shown, that inhibition of lipolysis by nicotinic acid administered during the night prevents carbohydrate induced rises of plasma triglyceride levels in normals and type IV hyperlipoproteinemic patients.

The present study compared the effects of equal amounts of nicotinic acid admini-stered either during the day or during the night on 24 hour triglyceride levels. In 14 type IV patients, 24-hour plasma triglyceride profiles were measured twice on high car-bohydrate diets while two grams of nicotinic acid were infused over eleven hours either from 8-19 or from 20-7 hours. The course of 24-hour triglycerides was significantly different with the two conditions. When nicotinic acid was administered during the day, triglycerides rose at night similarly to placebo studies while the nightly rise of trigly-cerides on high carbohydrate diets was abolished with nicotinic acid administered during this time. Our findings suggest that the effect of nicotinic acid on plasma triglycerides will be most marked when administered at the time (night) when lipolysis is most active.

CLOFIBRATE, NICOTINIC ACID AND HEXANICOTINIC ACID INOSITOL IN ONE DRUG (DUPLINAL) FOR TREATMENT OF HYPERLIPOPROTEINEMIAS

R. M. Schmuelling. B. Schoene and M. Eggstein

University of Tubingen, Germany

The effects of a new drug (Duplinal) containing 400 mg of clofibrate, 25 mg of nicotinic acid and 150 mg of hexanicotinic acid inositol each capsule on the lipid metabolism of 9 ambulatory patients suffering from hyperlipoproteinemia were studied in a cross-over study of 10 months (2 months placebo, 2 months Duplinal 3 capsules per day, 2 months placebo, 4 months Duplinal.

Cholesterol levels decreased from the initial mean of 356 mg/100 ml by 27% after a treatment of 4 months (significance) level 2 $p < 0.05$).

Mean triglyceride levels decreased from 531 mg/100 ml by 68% ($2p < 0.025$).

Systolic blood pressure diminished from the initial mean of 152 Torr to 129 Torr ($p < 0.02$).

Thirty-seven parameters controlling hepatic function, blood cells, serum proteins, blood glucose, serum electrolytes and renal function remained unchanged during the 10 months of supervision.

VLDL METABOLISM IN A PATIENT WITH PRIMARY TYPE I HYPERLIPOPROTEINEMIA

G. Sigurdsson, A. Nicoli and B. Lewis

Department of Chemical Pathology, Royal Postgraduate Medical School, Hammersmith Hospital, London, England

Patients with Type I hyperlipidemia have normal VLDL triglycerides while their chylomicron triglycerides are grossly elevated, although triglyceride in both lipoproteins are believed to be cleared by the same mechanism, the enzyme lipoprotein lipase. We have studied the turnover of apo-B peptide in very low density lipoprotein (VLDL) in a 24 year old lady with primary Type I hyperlipidemia.

After injection of her own VLDL, labelled with I^{131} a specific activity-time curve for apo-B was derived after fractionation of delipidated apo-VLDL on a Sephadex G. 150 column. I^{125} labelled apo-LDL was injected simultaneously. From the exponential slope of these curves the fractional catabolic rates were calculated. The intravascular mass of VLDL-B peptide was measured using the tetramethylurea method of Kane. VLDL-apo B turnover was 876 mg/24 hours which was not markedly different from normal and was very similar to her turnover of apo-LDL, 806 mg/24 hours.

It is suggested that adipose tissue lipoprotein lipase may not be necessary for normal

VLDL catabolism. If so, it would provide an explanation for the normal VLDL levels in type I hyperlipoproteinaemia. It would also suggest that a different lipase is responsible for the removal of triglyceride from VLDL during the conversion to LDL.

CLINICAL EVALUATION OF TIBRIC ACID, A NEW HYPOLIPIDEMIC AGENT

C. R Sirtori* and G. Noseda**

* Center "Enrica Grossi Paoletti" for the Study of Hyperlipidemia, University of Milan, Italy; and ** Medizinische Propadeutische Klinik, Universitat Bern, Switzerland

Tibric acid (T. A.) (CP 18,524: 2-chloro-5-(dimethylpiperidinosulfonyl benzoic acid) a new hypolipidemic agent, was tested in patients with hyperlipoproteinemia as part of a cooperative study between the Italian and Swiss Center. Thirty-one hyperlipoproteinemic patients, classified according to the WHO Memorandum, and one normal subject took part in the study. There were 4 patients of type IIa, 20 of type IV, 7 of type IIb.

Various treatment schedules were tested, giving the drug in one or more daily administrations. T. A. is supposed to be effective due to an increased activity of hepatic α-glycerophosphate dehydrogenase, and even single daily administrations of the drug should be adequate for this mechanism to become operative.

Patients were followed for periods ranging between two months and over a year. Four out of the 32 discontinued treatment: one because of severe itching after two months, one because of diarrhea, and another because of nausea after a few weeks of treatment; one patient underwent a myocardial infarction after about 4 months.

Analysis of plasma lipid data showed that type IV patients followed two patterns: those with triglycerides around or below 300 mg% responded favourably to single daily doses of 500-750 mg; in those with higher levels, the effect of single administrations, even up to 1250 or 1500 mg, was seldom adequate. In these cases fractionation of the dosage, into three-four daily administrations, obtained at times very favourable results. Cholesterol was lowered (10-20% at the most) in type IIb patients, where the effect on plasma triglycerides was similar to that in type IV. Type IIa patients, all with relatively mild forms, had a 15% decrease.

Clinical findings, such as the potentiation of hypoglycemia in a diabetic patient on insulin, and the clearing of an eruptive xanthomatosis in another patient, will be described.

SOME CHARACTERISTICS OF A NEW HYPOLIPIDEMIC AGENT - BM 15.075

H. Stork and P. D. Lang

Boehringer Manheim GmbH, Medical Research Department, 5800 Manheim-31, Germany

BM 15. 075 (2-4-(chloro-benzamido) ethyl-phenoxy-2-methylpropionic acid was found to be a potent lipid-lowering compound. In male rats, cholesterol and triglycerides were significantly reduced with doses of 6 mg/kg and 1 mg/kg, respectively. In comparative studies, BM 15. 075 was 20 times as potent as clofibric acid.

With 5 mg/kg, fructose-induced hypertriglyceridemia in rats could be significantly inhibited. Hypercholesterolemia in mice following Triton WR 1339 was significantly suppressed by 1 mg/kg. Higher doses were necessary in rats to interfere with the hypercholesteremic effect of dietary cholesterol + propylthiouracil. BM 15. 075 did not influence glucose and purine metabolism in animals.

Toxicity of BM 15. 075 was comparable to clofibrate. The half-life times in different animal species and man will be reported. Pilot studies in patients with hyperlipoprotein-emias were performed with daily doses of 300 to 600 mg. Results of these trials will be presented.

INCREASE OF FIBRINOLYTIC ACTIVITY AFTER ADMINISTRATION OF TIBRIC ACID

A. E. Tammaro and P. Giarola

Istituto di Gerontologia e Geriatria, Pavia, Italy

Ten aged patients with atherosclerotic hyperdyslipidemia were treated with tibric acid (1 g daily for 90 days). The following parameters were considered: cholesterol, triglycerides, lipoproteins, fibrinolysis, platelet aggregation, as well as routine laboratory tests, with particular respect to liver function tests. During and at the end of the treatment significant diminutions of some lipidic fractions, especially of trigly-cerides, as well as an increase of the fibrinolytic activity were observed.

EFFECTS OF FENFLURAMINE ON OBESITY AND HYPERLIPIDAEMIA IN PATIENTS WITH FUNCTIONING RENAL ALLOGRAFTS

S. A. Tomlinson and J. G Lines

Addenbrooke's Hospital, Cambridge, England

Obesity and hyperlipidaemia commonly occur in patients who have a satisfactory renal allograft[1]. Both of these complications are probably due to the continuous steroid therapy that is necessary to suppress graft rejection.

Fenfluramine has been shown to be an effective agent to reduce obesity[2,3] and there are some reports of its beneficial effect on abnormal plasma lipid patterns[4].

Double blind cross-over trials were conducted to compare the effects of fenfluramine vs placebo on the obesity and hyperlipidaemia of patients with functioning renal allografts.

Treatment with fenfluramine for 6 weeks caused a weight loss in 13 out of 25 patients. The maximum result was 12.5 kg. The average loss was 2 kg compared with small weight gains on placebo.

The usual abnormality of plasma lipoproteins in transplanted patients is a IIb pattern. With fenfluramine treatment some of these reverted towards normal.

Sixteen patients had hypercholesterolemia and in 11 the level fell with fenfluramine treatment. The average fall was 43 mg per 100 ml, i.e., 14% in 6 weeks, compared with a rise on placebo of 16 mg per 100 ml.

[1] Ghosh, P. et al., Transplantation 15: 521, 1973.
[2] Pawan, G. L. S., Lancet i: 498, 1969.
[3] Cameron, D. C. et al., Current Medical Research and Opinion 1: 153, 1972.
[4] Bliss, P P. et al., Postgrad. Med. J. 48: 311, 1972.

FATTY ACIDS IN SUBCELLULAR PARTICLES OF ISOLATED ENDOTHELIAL CELLS GAINED BY CELL-FRACTIONATION

B. L. Toth-Martinez and J Szegi

Normal and atherosclerotic rat endothelial cell preparations, containing individual cells, were subjected to cell-fractionation, and the following subcellular fractions were prepared and characterized by electron microscopy; cell membrane fractions, nuclei, mitochondria, desintegrated rough- and smooth endoplasmic reticular fractions, with polysomes and nucleoli, heavy- and light microsomes, lysosomes and liposomes.

Distribution of fatty acids in the cholesterol ester, tri-, di-, and monoglyceride fractions, and in the free fatty acid fraction was analyzed by gas-chromatography.

PROTECTIVE EFFECT OF SOME STEROIDS ON THE EXPERIMENTAL FATTY LIVER INDUCED BY AMANITA PHALLOIDES

R. Truhaut, J. R. Claude, J. M. Warnet and M. Thevenin

Groupe de Travail sur les Steatoses Hepatiques Toxiques, Faculte de Pharmacie de l'Universite R. Descartes de Paris, Laboratoire de la DGASS de la Prefecture de Paris, Paris, France

The accumulation in large amounts of fat in the liver is, in many cases, an early manifestation of an hepatic impairment. A number of ethiologic agents can produce it through different pathogenic mechanisms. The fatty liver induced by Amanita Phalloides seems to be due to an impairment of the hepatic beta-lipoproteins secretion, and is characterized by an increase of the level of liver triglycerides.

In previous studies, with Swiss strain mice and Wistar strain rats, we observed a sex difference in the response of animals intoxicated intraperitoneally by an extract of Amanita Phalloides: the females developed a marked steatosis and died with smaller doses, whereas the males presented a greater resistance.

The occurrence of a protective effect of adrogenic steroids towards the toxic effects of Amanita Phalloides, especially the fatty liver, has been investigated in this work. The data reported here show that Testosterone is able to prevent liver accumulation of triglycerides in Wistar strain female rats poisoned by the mushroom. In order to determine whether Testosterone is effective by its androgenic action or by its potency in protein sparing, we used an anabolic agent: the 19 nor Testosterone phenylpropionate. The effectiveness of these steroids were studied both on intact and ovariectomized female rats.

The results are discussed with regard to the biochemical interactions between these steroids and a toxin of Amanita Phalloides: alpha-Amanitin, on the hepatocellular protein metabolism in connection with an inhibition of RNA polymerase activities.

PRIMARY PREVENTION OF THE ISCHEMIC CEREBRAL AND CORONARY DISEASE BY USING A LIPID LOWERING DRUG: ETHYLNANDROL

M. Tsushima, E. Asano, Y. Hata and Y. Goto

Department of Medicine, Keio University Hospital, Shinjuku, Tokyo 160, Japan

A lipid lowering drug containing an anabolic steroid ethylnandrol (0. 75 mg) was administered three times daily to a group of 162 subjects screened from 568 persons over 40 years of age in three communities in the northern and middle parts of Japan. The plasma cholesterol and triglyceride concentrations, blood pressure, ocular fundi and ECG were examined once or twice a year from 1969 to 1974. The results of eight examinations so far performed, and the incidence of the ischemic cerebran and coronary diseases in the four years were compared with those of the control group in the same communities, possessing nearly equal distribution of age, sex, relative body weight and the other risk factors with those of the treated group. After one month of the drug administration, the mean cholesterol and triglyceride concentrations began to fall in the treated group by 2 to 39% and 3 to 36%, respectively. No significant changes were seen in the relative body weight, blood pressure, and the incidence of abnormal ocular fundi and ECG between the two groups. The ischemic cerebral and coronary disease occurred slightly less in the treated group; cerebral thrombosis 6 in the treated group vs. 6 in the control group, myocardial infarction 0 vs 2, while cerebral bleeding 3 vs 2, respectively However, the death due to these ischemic diseases had not occurred in the treated group in these last two years No side effects including liver disfunction and abnormal GTT were observed in the treated group.

EFFECT OF THE CHANGES IN MICROSOMAL PHOSPHOLIPIDS ON THE DRUG-BINDING CAPACITY OF CYTOCHROME P-450

I. B. Tsyrlov and V. V. Lyachovich

Novosibirsk 630049, USSR

The most essential step in the biotransformation of lipophilic drugs in microsomal "mixed-function oxidases" is the binding of drugs with cytochrome P-450 and consequentially the formation of a spectrophotometrically registered enzyme-substrate complex. It has been demonstrated that the Ks of this complex for several drugs does not correlate with their partition coefficient for distribution between the oil and water phases. On the other hand, it has been found that an increase in the microsomal lipid phase (after adding higher concentrations of microsomal membrane in vitro and after phenobarbital induction in vivo) leads to a 3-5-fold Ks increase. This decrease in the affinity for the type I substrate hexorbital is the result of a dilution effect for the substrate in the membrane. Only saturated concentrations of ANS (8-anilino-1-naphtaline sulfonate), which is possessed of a high affinity for microsomal phospholipids, are capable of displacing hexobarbital at the P-450 binding sites. It has been shown that this increase of the microsomal lipid phase is accompanied by a considerable growth in ANS concentration essential for the displacement of hexobarbital, even against a decrease in the affinity of P-450 for this substrate.

Spacially divided enzyme active centres for substrates I (hexobarbital, aminopyrine) and II (aniline, metyrapone) have also been observed to exist in relation with various phospholipid-dependent hydrophobic zones of the membrane. Incubation of the microsomes with increasing concentrations of DOC (sodium deoxycholate, 0.01 - 0.12%) converts P-450 into P-420 and increases the Ks only for type II substrates. The presence of CCCP (carbonyl cyanide m-chlorophenylhydrazone, 5.10^{-6} - 6.10^{-5}M) is, on the contrary, accompanied only by a rise in Ks for type I substrates. Both agents effectively inhibit the quantum output of ANS fluorescence, which evidences the decrease of hydrophobic interactions in the membrane. Their inhibition has a non-competitive character and they do not change the Ks of ANS for the phospholipids (Ks = 5.10^{-6} M). Thus, the heme group of P-450, which includes the binding sites for type II substrates, is located in the hydrophobic zone, sensitive to DOC. Type I substrates interact with the so-called "drug-binding protein" situated in other "CCCP-affecting" hydrophobic zone.

To sum up, we may say that the binding of drugs with P-450 is, to a great extent, a function of the lipophilic microsome membrane rather than a property of the substrate itself.

CLINICAL TRIAL ON A NEW ANTI-ATHEROSCLEROTIC EXTRACTIVE SUBSTANCE, GLUCURONIL-GLYCOSAMINE-GLYCANE

R Turpini

Medical Clinic, University of Pavia, 27100 Pavia, Italy

A clinical trial on the anti-atherosclerotic and anti-thrombitic activity of an extractive heparin-like substance with high clearing and anti-dislipemic action, glucuronil-glyco-samine-glycaen sulphate, was carried out.

In order to analyze the results of the treatment, 42 parameters were investigated, divided in the following 4 groups:

    a) investigation of fat metabolism: 9 parameters
    b) investigation of blood coagulation: 12 parameters
    c) investigation of cardiovascular system: 5 parameters

The patients, aging from 55 to 95 years, were maintained for 10 days under control, to investigate their basal conditions and the possible spontaneous changes; subsequently, were treated for 50 days with 18 mg/day of the active substance.

All the parameters were pointed out before and after 10 and 60 days of treatment.

The results show a sharp improvement, which is summarized as follows:

    a) favorable modification of cholesterol, α- and β-lipoproteins
    b) reduction of platelet adhesiveness and increase of antithrombin III and of plasmino-
gen
    c) improvement of oscillometry, photoplethismometry and EGG layout
    d) improvement of cerebrovascular demage's symptoms, with regression of weari-
ness, headach and troubles of bodily movements.

The statistical evaluation of the results, by means of a variance test for randomized blocks and of the X^2 Pearson's test, shows a statistically significant global improvement of the clinical picture and of the parameters separately evaluated.

DYNAMICS OF LIPID METABOLISM DURING INFUSION OF A BETA-MIMETIC DRUG (PARTUSISTEN) OR PROSTAGLANDIN $F_{2}\alpha$

V. Unbehaun, A. Conradt and C. M. Schlotter

Universitats-Frauenklinik, D-74 Tubingen, Germany

When 3 μg/min of the β-adrenergic drug Partusisten were infused for 4 hours to healthy pregnant subjects at term, as well as when Prostaglandin F_2 α was intravenously administered for therapeutic abortion in the second trimester of pregnancy, serum concentrations of free fatty acids, free and esterified glycerol, acetoacetate, 3-hydroxy-butyrate, triglycerides, insulin and total bilirubin were continously measured.

During infusion of 50-100 g Prostaglandin F_2 α/min concentrations of lipid-metabo-lites remained rather unchanged, ketone bodies and total bilirubin, however, rose signi-ficantly. Immediately after starting the infusion of the β-mimetic agent, acute lipolytic mobilization of fat reserves occurs. After 30 min free glycerol and free fatty acid levels have doubled High free fatty acid concentrations block the metabolism of acetyl CoA thus leading to excessive high levels of acetoacetate and 3-hydroxy-butyrate. Subsequently increased insulin concentrations enhance resynthesis of triglycerides, beginning from the second hour of infusion the ketone body concentrations decrease. After the end of the infusion initial normal levels are nearly reached within 1 hour.

EFFECTS OF NICOTINIC ACID ON THE INTRAVENOUS FAT TOLERANCE TEST (IVFTT) AND FATTY ACID INCORPORATION INTO ADIPOSE TISSUE (FIAT) IN HYPERTRIGLYCERIDEMIA (HTG)

G. Walldius and S. Rossner

King Gustaf V Research Institute and Department of Medicine, S-104 01 Stockhlom 60, Sweden

Decreased removal of triglycerides (TG) from blood to peripheral tissues is commonly found in hypertriglyceridemia (HTG). In the removal process, a) lipoprotein lipase hydrolyzes circulating TG to fatty acids (FA) which are then, b) incorporated into adipose tissue by the FIAT process. Low FIAT function has recently been suggested to be one possible defect causing low removal of TG and subsequent HTG. These present studies have been undertaken to find out how different methods designed to test the removal mechanisms in HTG were correlated and how nicotinic acid treatment affected these parameters. The removal of exogenous fat was determined by the intravenous fat tolerance test (IVFTT) with Intralipid (IL) and expressed as k_2 (%/min). A three hours continuous fat infusion was given and the content of exogenous fat (IL) left in blood after the infusion was taken to reflect the in vivo removal rate of IL. FIAT was determined as uptake of radioactive FA into subcutaneous adipose tissue biopsy specimens incubated in vitro. This process measures b) exclusively.

The k_2 value for IVFTT or the removal rate determined by the prolonged test as well as the FIAT values were significantly lower in subjects with HTG than in controls. Values for the removal rate as determined by the ordinary IVFTT or the prolonged fat tolerance test were positively correlated with FIAT values. Some subjects with type IV and type V HTG were treated with nicotinic acid for several months. The k_2 value as well as the FIAT values increased and plasma TG values were normalized. These findings suggest that the FIAT mechanism might influence and determine the in vivo removal of infused IL in HTG or that increased removal rate as determined by IL infusions increase the FIAT process resulting in uptake of FA in AT. Furthermore, the removal mechanism was stimulated by nicotinic acid treatment probably explaining the normalization of previously elevated TG values.

LIPID LOWERING EFFECT OF AMBERLITE XAD - 2 RESIN IN VITRO

A. Weizel and H. Rizk

Medezin. Univ. Klinik, Heidelberg, Germany

In vivo studies have shown a reduction of total cholesterol and triglyceride levels during hemoperfusion with Amberlite XAD - 2 resin.

In vitro studies were undertaken with isolated lipoprotein fractions. The VLDL triglyceride (YG) concentration decreased between 35-70%, the LDL TG concentration showed a fall of 20-40%, and the HDL TG were lowered between 30-60%. Total cholesterol reduction was 10-30% (VLDL), 20-50% (LDL), and 10-20% (HDL). There was no change in the total plasma protein concentration.

CLOFIBRATE RELATED HYPOLIPEMIC DRUGS: PROBES FOR ELUCIDATING MECHANISM OF ACTION AND STUDYING STRUCTURE-ACTIVITY RELATIONSHIPS

D. T. Witiak, W. P. Heilman, G. K. Poochikian, D. R. Feller and H. A. I. Newman

Division of Medicinal Chemistry, College of Pharmacy, The Ohio State University, Columbus, Ohio 43210, USA

For purposes of defining structural requirements for maximum antilipemic action of analogs related to clofibrate (Lipids 8: 378, 1973), probing into the nature of receptors which are either blocked or stimulated by clofibrate and classifying such sites according to their selective affinity and intrinsic activity towards various analogs (J. Med. Chem. 11: 1086, 1968; 12: 697, 1969; 12: 754, 1969; 14: 754, 1971; 14: 758, 1971; 16: 228, 1973), providing insight into the mechanism(s) of action of clofibrate (J. Pharm. Sci. 63: 199, 1974; 63: 203, 1974), studying the effect of structural changes on enzyme induction and drug-drug interactions (J. Med. Chem 17: 41, 1974; Proc. Soc. Exp. Biol. Med. 145: 281, 1974), and eveloping new leads for the design of hypolipemic agents we synthesized a series of acyclic and cyclic (2, 3-dihydrobenzofurans, chromans, and benzodioxanes) analogs. Recently, we have completed the synthesis for certain related biphenyl analogs, novel photodimers, and an enol-lactone which is considerably more resistant to hydrolysis by serum esterases than is clofibrate. The biological properties of twenty new compounds will be discussed in light of results obtained with older analogs synthesized in our laboratories. In vivo, all analogs have been assessed for their hypocholesterolemic and hypotriglyceridemic activity in the Triton WR-1339 hyperlipemic rat model. Selective effects on cholesterol levels on the one hand and triglyceride levels on the other have been observed for some of these compounds.

We are grateful to the National Heart and Lung Institute, U. S. Public Health Service, for support of this work through NIH grant no. HL-12740.

INFLUENCES OF POLYUNSATURATED PHOSPHOLIPIDS ON THE UPTAKE OF SERUM LOW DENSITY LIPOPROTEIN AND THE AORTIC WALL IN VIVO AND IN VITRO

T. Yasugi, T. Shimizu, M. Iijima, E. Sasa, T. Kinosita, M. Harada, M. Hatano and K. Oshima

The Second Department of Internal Medicine   Nihon University   , School of Medicine,
Itabashi , Tokyo, Japan

In vivo study, cholesterol fed rabbits were divided into three groups; first group as
a control, second administered EPL and the third administered essential fatty acid
for four weeks.   Three hours after the intravenous injection of cholesterol-^{14}C, the ra-
dioactivities of low density lipoprotein of aortic wall obtained from the three groups were
determined.   The radioactivity of EPL group was significantly lower than those of the
other two groups.

In vitro study, the uptake of cholesterol-^{14}C-labelled low density lipoprotein into
the aortic wall of rabbits grouped into two, one as a control and another in the EPL-
containing medium, was studied under the condition of low oxygen supply in the Warburg
apparatus.   Radioactivity of the EPL group was significantly higher than that of the
control.

Conclusion: In vivo study, the uptake of low density lipoproteins into the aortic wall
was significantly decreased by the EPL administration.   It may be speculated that EPL
may affect the solubility and esterification of cholesterol, and the outflux of cholesterol
from the aortic wall.

On the contrary, in vitro study, the uptake of low density lipoproteins into the aortic
wall was accelerated by the EPL administration and it may be suggested the possibility
that EPL repairs the injured tissue and increases the biological activity of the membranes
under the condition of low oxygen supply.

From these results, it may be concluded that EPL has an anti-atherogenic action.

EFFECT OF DB-3',5'-C, AMP ON BLOOD FFA, GLYCEROL, GLUCOSE AND IRI IN
NORMAL AND STREPTOZOTOCIN DIABETIC RATS

A. Zanoboni and W. Zanoboni-Muciaccia

2nd Department of Medical Phatology, University of Milan, 20122 Milan, Italy

Since there are only few reports about the metabolic actions of cAMP in intact rats,
our purpose was to investigate the lipolytic, glicogenolytic and insulin stimulating
activity of a cAMP analog, the N^6, 2'-0-dibutyryl derivative (DBA).

Three groups of male Sprague-Dawley, non fasting rats, weighing 250 ± 30 g, were
injected with DBA i. p. at the doses of 10-50 and 100 mg/kg, 30 minutes before killing.
Blood samples were taken for analysis of blood glucose, FFA, glycerol and plasma IRI.

Normal rats treated with DBA showed a significant increase of blood glucose concentrations and plasma IRI levels, more marked with the highest doses.   On the contrary,
plasma glycerol and FFA concentrations were markedly decreased by DBA.

The result of FFA and glycerol depression, i. e. antilipolysis, instead of lipolysis observed in vitro, prompted us to repeat the same experiment in streptozotocin diabetic rats, in order to clarify whether hyperinsulinemia was responsible for the aforementioned antilipolytic effect of DBA. Rats were given a single injection of 65 mg/Kg of streptozotocin i. v. , 6 days before the experiment; the rats had free access to food and water.

In streptozotocin diabetic rats, non-DBA treated there was hyperglycemia together with a normal range of plasma IRI levels; but, while DBA produced a further increase of blood glucose concentrations, it was not able to modify plasma IRI; moreover, plasma glycerol and FFA decreased after DBA treatment, showing at the highest doses the same pattern observed in normal rats.

Our observations show that DBA injected in vivo has an antilipolytic effect either in normal or in streptozotocin diabetic rats.

THE LECITHIN: CHOLESTEROL ACYLTRANSFER REACTION IN HUMAN BLOOD PLASMA FROM HYPERCHOLESTEROLEMIC SUBJECTS

A. Zucconi, F. Bellini, R. Chiostri, C. Bartoletti and A. D'Alessandro

Department of Gerontology, Florence University, Italy

The authors studied the LCAT activity in plasma from hypercholesterolemic subjects before and during treatment with clofibrate. The activity of the lecithin: cholesterol acyltransfer reaction is given either as percentage of labeled cholesterol acylated per hour or as μmoles CE formed per litre plasma per hour according to K. T. Stokke and K. R. Norum. No difference was found as far as the age of the subjects was concerned. In younger people the LCAT activity was 81 ± 19 μmoles and in the older ones it was 79 ± 21 umoles. An increase of LCAT activity was found in the hypercholesterolemic subjects (109 ± 26 μmoles), while the esterification percentage (3. 95%) was lower than that of the normal ones (5. 7%). In the hypercholesterolemic subjects treated with clofibrate no modification of LCAT activity was found if it was given in μmoles (86 ± 22), but the esterification percentage was still low (4. 19%). These modifications are not due to the different concentrations of the substrate, but they point to some alteration of the LCAT activity in the hypercholesterolemic subjects.

AUTHOR INDEX

(Underscored numbers indicate complete papers in this volume.)

SUBJECT INDEX

CPSIA information can be obtained at www.ICGtesting.com
Printed in the USA
LVOW021641140413

329061LV00005B/192/P